Text-Book of Homeopathic Materia Medica

Text-Book of Homeopathic Materia Medica

George Royal

Published by

FacsiMile Publisher
12 Pragati Market
Ashok Vihar, Ph-2
Delhi - 110052, India
Phone: 011-47034999
Email: www.facsimilepublishers.com
info@facsimilepublishers.com

Distribution Network
gyanbooks.com
India, USA, Canada, UK, Australia

ISBN: 978-93-5315-089-1 (HB)
First Published, 1920

2nd Impression 2025

Printed at: Gyan Press, Delhi.

TEXT-BOOK OF HOMEOPATHIC MATERIA MEDICA
Author: GEORGE ROYAL

Text-Book of Homeopathic Materia Medica

BY

GEORGE ROYAL, M.D.

PROFESSOR OF HOMEOPATHIC MATERIA MEDICA AND THERAPEUTICS OF THE STATE UNIVERSITY OF IOWA FOR 28 YEARS; SENIOR, EX-PRESIDENT, CHAIRMAN OF THE COUNCIL OF MEDICAL EDUCATION OF THE AMERICAN INSTITUTE OF HOMEOPATHY; MEMBER OF THE HAHNEMANN MEDICAL ASSOC. OF IOWA; MEMBER OF THE BRITISH HOMEO-PATHIC MEDICAL SOCIETY

PHILADELPHIA
BOERICKE & TAFEL
1920

TO

MY WIFE, ELLA J. ROYAL

AND

DAUGHTER A. JANETTE ROYAL, B.A.

IN ACKNOWLEDGEMENT OF

THE INSPIRATION AND ASSISTANCE GIVEN IN THE

PREPARATION, THIS BOOK IS AFFECTIONATELY

DEDICATED

PREFACE

This book is being published for the purpose of keeping a promise made the students of the College of Homeopathic Medicine of the State University of Iowa, viz., to put into book form the lectures delivered by the author. The method followed in these lectures is the result of experience. At the New York Homeopathic Medical College, the author had been taught that success in prescribing depended upon the ability of the prescriber to find in the symptoms which a drug produced upon the healthy the exact counterpart of the symptoms which diseases produced upon the healthy. After faithfully studying symptoms under Timothy Field Allen for two years and graduating in 1882, the author soon discovered that symptoms differed greatly in rank. Not only did one symptom differ in rank from another, *e. g.*, eructations from hemorrhages of the stomach; but that the same symptom differed greatly in rank under different conditions. Let me again illustrate by using the symptom "Blood in the stool". The amount of blood may be large or small, the color red or black, the form liquid or clotted, etc. These modifications helped somewhat in selecting the remedy but still the results were disappointing and we began to look for the cause of failure. Experience over a period of several years finally revealed the fact that two factors had been neglected in determining the rank of the remedy; first, the "elective affinity" of the drug; second, the effect which a drug can produce upon the part elected. Following this lead, study and experience soon demonstrated the fact that drugs do not have an "elective affinity" for the head, the chest or pelvis as a whole but for the tissues or organs which are found in these different parts of the body, *e. g.*, brains and nerves, skin and bones, uterus and blood vessels. Study and experience also taught that one drug may simply irritate a tissue or organ; a second may be able to irritate and inflame; a third may go one step further and produce functional changes, while a fourth may not only irritate, inflame; produce functional changes, but may also cause structural changes like ulcers, abscess, atrophy, etc. Let us now, with this knowledge in mind, return to the symptom "Blood in stool", and ascertain from what tissue or organ it came; further, what changes took place in the tissue or organ. It may have come from the mucous membrane, the submucosa, the hemorrhoidal veins. Fissures; ulcers or even congestion of the mucous membrane; ulcers or abscesses of the mucosa; rupture of a hemorrhoidal vein or some artery may have been the cause of "Blood in stool". Locating the cause will be of great help in determining the rank of our symptom, but let us not forget the modus operandi of our cause. Was the ulceration of the submucosa due to the action of the poison of typhoid on Peyer's patches or some slight traumatism in the rectum? From the above we see that a symptom may be the center of a group of symptoms, holding the highest rank in that group while the same symptom may rank the lowest in another group. About the time we had become accustomed to the above method of studying symptoms in groups, came our appointment to the chair of materia medica and therapeutics in the University of Iowa and that plan has been followed in our teaching. We use the word "Location" to represent the tissue or organ for which the drug has an "elective affinity", *e. g.*, mucous membrane, and then follow that tissue through the various parts of the body. Both grouping of symptoms and differentiation received a good deal of attention in our lectures. We have omitted differentiation in this work, reserving it for another book. The symptoms in quotation marks are of the two highest ranks, as found in Allen's Handbook and the leading repertories. In our private practice and clinics we use all potencies from ten drops of the tincture to the so-called 40 m. As to repetition of dose, we repeat. As to the frequency of repetition, we are guided by the following rule: the remedies which produce symptoms on the healthy in a short period of time, repeat at short intervals—minutes and hours; one which takes a long time to produce symptoms, repeat at longer intervals and continue for a longer period of time. As it is impossible to keep the time of all remedies in mind, we give the following: put in class 1 the gases, volatile salts, and those drugs which act directly upon the nerves; class 2, the earthy salts and those drugs which act upon the blood; class 3, compounds of the first and second classes to be repeated at medium intervals. For auxiliary treatment such as diet, exercise, rest, change of climate, we are guided by the modalities of the drug, *e. g.*, conditions which are worse from motion, advise rest, etc. As to diet, there is a sad need of reliable information. Anyone who would write a book on the dietetics of each remedy would bestow a great boon upon the human race. The remedies discussed are the polychrests and those of the others which have been most frequently and successfully used by the author. The latter include those which have been most recently proven and come into use. No claim is made for anything newer or better than is found in other text-books on materia medica. The method of presenting the old is not wholly original. We have gleaned from all our text-books on materia medica but more especially from Allen's Handbook, Clark's Dictionary and Boger's Synoptic Key. We hope that by following the method of grouping the symptoms in their study of remedies, undergraduates and busy practitioners may become more accurate and successful prescribers.

GEORGE ROYAL.

DES MOINES, IOWA,
May, 1920.

INTRODUCTORY LECTURE TO HOMEOPATHIC MATERIA MEDICA AND THERAPEUTICS

As Homeopaths prescribe remedies for their patients upon the "totality of the symptoms" presented by their patients, it is apparent that a thorough knowledge of symptoms is necessary in order to prescribe homeopathically. Not only is it true that you must have a thorough knowledge of a symptom to prescribe homeopathically, but it is also true that in proportion to your knowledge of symptoms will be the accuracy, the success of your prescription. Therefore, we will devote the first hour of our course to the study of symptoms.

Let us define a symptom as the manifestation of disease. It shows that the condition or function of some tissue or organ of the body is abnormal. You remember I told you when you were freshmen that a person was perfectly healthy when his tissues and organs were perfectly normal and functioning perfectly.

The essentials of a symptom are location, sensation and modalities. Of the three essentials of a symptom modality is the most important. By location we do not mean the head or leg or hand but some tissue or organ. As all organs are composed of more than one tissue we can only speak of them as locations when we think of them as a whole and functioning as such. Let me illustrate by taking the region under the left nipple. Beneath this we have such tissues as the skin, fascia, muscle, periosteum, bone, pleura and a portion of the heart which we consider as an organ composed of several tissues. All of these tissues are supplied by another tissue, *i. e.*, nerve tissue.

The sensations indicate the tissues involved, *e. g.*, a sharp, shooting, lightning-like pain indicates a nerve; a pulsating pain indicates an encapsulated organ; a sharp, splinter-like pain indicates an ulcerated mucous membrane or skin.

By modality we mean that which makes a condition or sensation worse or better. We speak of them as aggravations (agg.) or ameliorations (amel.). To illustrate, a pain is agg. or amel. by heat, cold, position, exercise, eating, time of day, etc. The brain is the most important location, because the homeopathic physician individualizes each case and the brain is the most important part of the human body.

Symptoms may be divided into many classes:

Objective and Subjective Symptoms.

An objective symptom is one which may be recognized by an observer who has the use of all his senses, *e. g.*, color, a murmur, an odor, a taste, heat, coldness, smoothness, roughness, etc. A subjective symptom is one which is perceived or imagined only by the patient himself, *e. g.*, a pain, an illusion or delusion in regard to sight, hearing or sensation.

Which of the two should rank the higher? That depends whether or not your patient is intelligent, reliable and rational. As I have stated above, we Homeopaths individualize and in this process the mental symptom should be given the highest rank. Therefore, if the patient be perfectly normal mentally, the subjective symptoms should be given the highest rank. A mental symptom is always a subjective symptom. But we find so many of our patients unreliable, irrational and wanting in the kind of intelligence necessary to accuracy and we have so good an opinion of ourselves that we prefer to believe our own senses rather than those of our patients.

Dynamic, Functional and Pathological Symptoms.

Our second class includes dynamic, functional and pathological symptoms. A dynamic symptom is difficult to define. Some consider it the purest kind of a subjective symptom; others understand by a dynamic symptom the manifestation of some condition which we are unable to detect by any of our senses, due to the fact that we have not as yet instruments of precision sufficiently developed.

Pathognomonic and Characteristic Symptoms.

A pathognomonic symptom is the distinguishing symptom of a disease or condition, *e. g.*, the peculiar rash and odor of measles, the primary and secondary fever of smallpox, etc. A characteristic symptom is the distinguishing symptom of a drug. It is to the drug what the pathognomonic symptom is to the disease, *e. g.*, agg. of all the symptoms by means of sleep under Lachesis. You ask if there are diseases and conditions which are agg. by sleep, *i. e.*, are there patient who really feel worse as the result of sleep? Any one of five years' experience will tell you that any conditions resulting from improper elimination are worse after sleep, especially is this true of uremic headaches or headaches resulting from constipation.

TOTALITY OF SYMPTOMS

Probably there is no expression in our homeopathic literature more confusing than "Totality of symptoms." In our text-books, in our journals, we find almost as many definitions of the phrase as there are writers. Let us as students and teacher reach some clear understanding on the subject at the beginning of our year's work. The first thing I want you to understand is that totality is not a numerical totality. Three symptoms out of fourteen may determine the totality. If this last statement be true symptoms must have different degrees or rank. There must be higher and lower degrees or rank of symptoms. And it is a fact that most writers on materia medica and repertories divide and arrange the symptoms into five groups or classes, according to the importance each writer gives a symptom.

How do we establish the rank of a symptom? There are many ways. When speaking of the essentials of a symptom, I told you that mental symptoms (those showing abnormal condition of the brain) should be given the highest rank and modalities the second rank. I have always put sensations in the third class. The pathological symptoms, I have been in the habit of putting in the fourth class. In the fifth class, I have put all the so-called "common" symptoms, such as lack of hunger, thirst, diarrhea and other functional symptoms which may be easily caused by errors of diet, exposure to cold or heat, etc. But the above only touches the surface of our subject, and one would be poorly equipped whose knowledge of symptoms was not clearer and deeper.

Going a little deeper into our subject we find that certain mental symptoms rank much higher than other mental symptoms, certain functional higher than other functional, and pathological higher than other pathological. How did Allen determine that a certain symptom should appear in large black type in his Hand Book, denoting the highest rank; or how did Boenninghausen decide what remedies should be in capital letters in his repertory or Knerr what ones should be marked with the heavy double lines in his repertory? The conclusion was reached from several view-points. If they found a *peculiar, unusual* or *striking* mental symptom they gave it the highest rank. Let me illustrate. A man came into our clinic who said he had something like a lizzard in his stomach. It had been there for thirteen years. This insect caused much distress in the man's stomach, his joints and the left side of the head, when the insect was active, and the insect was active when a storm was "coming up" but would quiet down as "soon as the storm broke." Here was not only a mental symptom but a peculiar symptom and a marked modality. Such a symptom would receive next to the highest rank.

Another illustration: Nearly all the provers of a certain drug had pains in the joints and other symptoms agg. just before a storm but the agg. ceased when the storm broke. A peculiar modality. Such a symptom would receive next to the highest rank.

A third illustration: Half of the provers of a certain drug had diarrheic stools, cutting, twisting, grinding pains in the abdomen (enteralgia and enteritis), the pain amel. by hard pressure on the abdomen also by hot drinks. Five drops of this remedy in a cup of hot water cured without a failure in five hundred cases to which it was given. The symptoms appear in black type in Allen, "caps" in Boenninghausen and doubled lined in Knerr. We call such a symptom a verified symptom.

Now for the application of that illustration. We take a case and find fourteen symptoms. Only three of these symptoms appear under Colocynth but they are all of the highest rank, the first one because it is peculiar, the second because it is a modality, and the third because it has been verified a thousand times. All of the fourteen symptoms are found under Nux, but all of them in the lowest rank. Expressing the highest rank by the numeral five and the lowest by one, we find that Colocynth represents fifteen and nux fourteen. And we say Colocynth has the "totality of symptoms".

Besides the peculiar symptoms, the verified and the symptoms reported by a large majority of provers, I have found another symptom to which I attach much importance. I call it a reasonable symptom. You will not find it under that name in your text-books so I will describe and define it by illustration. Several years ago while we were proving a certain remedy here in our college, there were certain head symptoms, subjective symptoms, reported by the majority of the provers. Then followed certain other symptoms, diarrheic stools, etc., but not until the provers presented yellow sclera and the laboratory tests demonstrated bile in the urine could I give the proper rank to the head and stool symptoms. The fact that certain causes will always produce the same results when operating under similar conditions should be recognized and remembered in our study of symptoms.

ACONITUM NAPELLUS.

Make-up: Robust, healthy, neurotic.

Loc.: Circulatory system, nerves.

Sen.: *Fear;* burning; sticking; tearing; shooting.

Mod.: Agg. in warm room; stimulants; motion; open air. Amel. in open air; lying on back; bending double. (You will note that open air both agg. and amel. This is true of both special and general conditions.)

Leaders: *FEAR; great restlessness; intense thirst;* rapid, wiry pulse; high temperature.

With exceptions enough to prove the rule, Aconite is always indicated at the beginning, the very outset of a disease. Even the exception is more apparent than real, *e. g.,* a condition which called for the remedy years before but which has not changed, will yield to the drug.

There is only one drug which will be found to present a greater number of symptoms when using the repertory and that is Sulphur. Aconite acts as a prophylactic, Sulphur as an energizer. Keep in mind the fact that Aconite is used as a prophylaxis in seven out of ten cases for which it is indicated and that the symptoms calling for it are premonitory of many conditions. This is especially true of diseases of the respiratory organs and mucous membranes. You should never give Aconite, however, with the hope of aborting such diseases as typhoid or smallpox.

Circulatory System.

Brain: *Aconite* will *prevent* and *lighten* convulsions due to disturbed circulation of the brain caused by fright, shock, exposure to the sun or cold air, the poison of pneumonia, scarlet fever, etc. The condition is always acute, never dependent upon a *chronic* constitutional taint or diathesis. The characteristic symptoms of the drug are especially helpful in this condition; the cause is the next most important guide. If there be delirium the patient raves about dying, of being afraid of a crowd, etc.

Head: "*Fullness in sinuses,* with heaviness and *feeling* as if *something would come out;* stitching in the muscles of the temples; *stitching, aching* in the vertex *better* from motion *in* the *open air;* scalp feels as if hair stood on end; stitching under the scalp; sensation as if the scalp were swollen and numb; scalp *sensitive to touch.*"

With the headaches you have the high temp. and the hot, flushed face; internally the head feels hot, pulsating, bursting.

Eyes: "Bloodshot; *sensitive to air;* enlarged feeling of the balls, as if coming out of the orbits and stretching the lids."

Useful for acute inflammations of the various tissues of the eye, first stage before exudation has taken place; also for acute agg. of chronic diseases.

Ears: "*Sensitive to every noise;* roaring; ringing."

Controls *inflammation* of the *external ear,* sometimes including tympanum. The *parts* are *hot,* the *pains excruciating;* the *cause cold air.*

Nose: "*Epistaxis;* blows out bright red blood in morning."

Will check flow of bright red, hot blood. The patient fears he will bleed to death.

Throat: "Redness; *dryness;* throat seemed to swell; swelling of tonsils; burning."

For acute inflammations, never for chronic or after induration, exudation or ulceration have taken place.

Stomach: "Pit sensitive to touch; anxious pulsation in pit with shooting pain; *Thirst for cold water;* vomits after each drink; vomiting of dark grumous liquid; of mucus; of greenish-gray, watery substance; of green masses with diarrhea of the same."

Useful for the above condition at the *outset of eruptive dis-*

cases; following a severe *shock;* after *suppression* of *menses* or *perspiration.* The patient is always *thirsty,* restless and *anxious.*

Abdomen: "Swelling; *sensitiveness;* burning."

For the first stage of inflammation and engorgement of any abdominal or pelvic organ. High temperature, extreme sensitiveness are your leading symptoms.

Anus: "Bleeding hemorrhoids; burning and heat in hemorrhoidal vessels."

Will help in recent cases of protruding, bleeding hemorrhoids; also for the first stage of dysentery.

Urinary Organs: "Burning in neck of bladder when not urinating; *anxious desire;* anxiety on beginning to urinate; *urine dark* and *hot;* deposits blood."

We find it useful for three conditions, first, retention of urine in infants; second, acute agg. of chronic prostatitis the result of cold; third and most frequently, for acute inflammation of any part of the urinary tract.

Respiratory Organs: "*Sensitiveness to inspired air;* hoarseness; dry, hoarse, ringing cough; *cough* with *expectoration of bright blood; fear* of *suffocation.*"

Has rapidly aborted, in the *incipent stage, laryngitis, bronchitis, pneumonitis,* spasmodic and membranous *croup* and *pleurisy.* It is for aborting diseases of the respiratory organs that Aconite has won its brightest laurels. It is for disturbances of circulation that Aconite is most frequently used.

Brain and Nerves.

As Aconite is useful only for the first stage of diseases of the other tissues and organs, so it is for the brain and nerves. Its action never goes beyond the stages of irritation and inflammation. Three-fourths of the cases are simply irritation. The irritation is marked, the inflammation high. The duration of time for both is short. The pains are sharp, shooting, sometimes burning and cutting. The sensation is generally along the entire course of the nerve. Let me again state that *Aconite produces no structural changes.* Also remember that in most cases the *disturbance* of the *blood supply precedes* the *irritation* and *inflammation.*

I will give you only a few of the algia symptoms caused by the drug.

Head: "Sharp; jerking; stitching; shooting; drawing."

The neuralgias are usually of the scalp and skull. The pain follows the nerves and leaves a numb sensation.

Eyes: "Shooting in supraorbital ridge, branching across forehead to scalp, temple, cheek and into teeth, worse from pressure; vision dim, lost; photophobia."

The *causes* of these *eye symptoms* are: *overstrain, taking cold;* foreign bodies in the eyes. The orbital nerve is most frequently *affected,* the ciliary next in frequency. We sometimes get a transient paralysis from cold. Nearly *always acute* cases, the *exception* being *agg.* of *chronic catarrh* and glaucoma.

Face: "Tingling; twitching; sharp; shooting; numbness."

The condition is usually the result of cold but it has cured tetanus.

Extremities: "*Drawing;* tense; stitching; sharp; numb."

You will find nearly all cases have numbness following the other sensations. There is also a feeling as if circulation were interfered with in many cases. The chief cause is checked perspiration.

Dose: I presume there is no remedy about which there are so many opinions as to the potency, and repetition of dose as Aconite. For all inflammatory conditions I use from 3x to the 30th and repeat at intervals of from 15 to 45 minutes. Especially is this my rule when the skin is hot and dry. I always leave an order to discontinue the remedy when perspiration begins.

SULPHUR.

Make-up: Spare; dirty, unhealthy skin; weak reaction; light complexion; red hair.

Loc.: All tissues and organs, because Sulphur is an integral part of every form of protoplasm. We will, however, pay especial attention to the *skin*, venous circulation, and *nutritive organs*.

Sen.: *All*, for the reason that it may irritate, inflame, produce functional and structural changes of any and every tissue of the body.

Mod.: Agg. bathing; suppression; when *heated*, in *bed* and from *woolens;* 11 A.M.; climacteric.

Amel. from motion and dry, warm applications.

Leaders: Stooped; lank; dirty; *old look in babes; skin festers* but *won't heal;* empty, all-gone feeling.

Skin.

"*Itching* on any and every part of body which, when scratched, turns to *burning;* formication over the whole body; *heat rash* on neck; groups of black points like *comedones* on forehead, but they cannot be squeezed out; black comedones on nose; *pimples*, inflamed, itching, burning red, irregular in various parts of body; itching *vesicles* on back of hands; *eruption, itching, burning* after *scratching;* itching *worse between the fingers*, on arms and legs, worse at night also in morning on waking, from *woolen garments.*"

Sulphur will help relieve all sorts of eruptions of the skin, *e. g.*, eczemas, acne, intertrigo, herpes, etc. Intense itching is marked in all groups. The itching is temporarily relieved by scratching but soon changes to burning if scratched. Water agg. all skin symptoms. For this reason children dislike the bath.

One word about the relation of Sulphur to acarus itch. Some object to its use locally because it suppresses the eruption and makes the patient worse. I have never observed any bad effects from Sulphur used to kill acarus unless some other skin conditions were also present. I always give the remedy high when I use it locally. However, if the patient is suffering from eczema, herpes, etc., when he contracted scabies, I use other local application to kill the acarus.

As important as any skin symptom is the *odor* emanating from it. This odor cannot be described but "stinking" comes the nearest to it. A well-to-do-farmer came into my office one day and said, "Dr., you must help me out. I *stink* so that the folks say I must eat and sleep out in the barn unless something is done." He added that frequent bathing only aggravated the condition. He had not been well since an attack of typhoid about a year before. Sulphur 30th cured.

Mucous Membranes.

Redness of eyelids and conjunctiva, nostrils, lips, tongue, throat, anus and vagina.

Eyes: "*Redness*, during the day; *itching* in evening; sticking and burning as from sand beneath the lids; cutting pain as if rubbed against spiculæ of glass and drawn in towards the pupil; necessity to close the eye, then burning in eye and lachrymation; *burning* and easy fatigue when reading; *aching* in ball in evening with weight and loss of vision; *redness* and *burning of lids* externally; agglutination mornings; jerking; *smarting* as from dryness of margin; vision dim; flickering; intolerance of sunlight with *weakness* of eyes and confused dark spots floating before them."

Sulphur has been successful either in curing or assisting in curing *eczema* of the lids, *blepharitis, styes* and tarsal tumors, catarrhal and traumatic *conjunctivitis*, parenchymatous *keratitis*, syphilitic and rheumatic *iritis*.

Bear in mind that in all eye troubles of Sulphur the *lids* are *red;* the pains are sharp, sticking, cutting, splinter-like; the photophobia is marked and that the modality "worse from the touch of water" is usually present.

Nose: "*Inflammation* of wings with swellings; *itching* of nostrils with burning and soreness worse of margins with swollen feeling; dryness; sneezing morning and evening with sensation as if cold were coming on and *discharge of mucus* mixed with *blood; odor of old, offensive mucus* on blowing nose."

For ***nasal catarrh*** acute, *chronic* and *ulcerative,* with the above. The odor, and redness of the membrane are the two most prominent of the several groups.

Mouth: "Tongue coated yellowish-white; *dryness* of the palate, in morning, with insipidity and *stickiness; bloody,* salty *saliva* in morning, after eating; *taste* pasty, *bitter,* coppery, in the morning on waking; *between* bitter *taste,* when tasting, the food has a good taste; *sour, vinegary* taste all day; sour *eructations after* drinking *milk; offensive* breath."

You will notice that these symptoms do not represent any condition of the mouth itself, like stomatitis, but are very prominent in the gastric and other groups of the drug.

Stomach: "*Appetite increased,* ravenous (Calcarea carb., Lycopodium, Cina and Iodium) and *if he does not eat headache, lassitude* and *necessity* to *lie down* follow; App. *lost* as soon as he sees food; he feels full in abdomen and has aversion to food when he begins to eat (Lycopodium); sour, empty *eructations* during the day, worse after eating; eructations tasting of bad eggs; *nausea* every morning, also before meals; faint, empty, sinking feeling *before meals; vomiting* of *food in* the *evening* which was *eaten* at *noon;* full feeling after eating a little (Lycopodium); heaviness in pit; distress from *milk,* which is *vomited curdled.*"

Please note that there is but little inflammation and structural change but much irritation and great functional change in the above group of symptoms. Sulphur is most frequently used for *dyspepsia* presenting many of the above symptoms. To understand the importance of dyspepsia let us look for the causes of it. The most frequent *cause* is *suppressed eruptions.* In taking your case always look for the history of eruptive diseases and other eruptions. The *abuse of alcoholic beverages* is another cause. Here we may find an exception to "no structural changes" for gastric ulcers may be present. In this group also you will usually find "redness of the orifices" especially of the eyes and rectum, also the "*faint, empty, sinking* feeling."

Anemia and diseases of the blood which will vitiate the gastric and other secretions of the digestive tract are frequent causes. *Catarrh* is both a cause and an effect. A knowledge of diet which agrees and also disagrees is very helpful in the treatment of Sulphur patients. A farinaceous food may cause dyspepsia and it always agg. the symptoms. The Sulphur child will vomit milk soon after taking it.

Intestines: "*Trembling* day and night *with diarrhea; gurgling;* stitches; *emission* of *offensive flatus*, smelling like sulphureted hydrogen; *griping* before and during stool, the stool more frequent, liquid and horribly offensive; so sensitive that clothes pressed disagreeably.

Rectum: "*Sticking* (Æsculus) agg. in the evening, taking away the breath; *cutting* during normal stool; *crawling* in the evening when sitting, with *biting* as from worms; itching during the day; *straining* at stool, also, before and after; *fullness;* sensation after stool as if something remained; *tenesmus*, in morning after waking, then a copious fluid stool; *urging* at night, cannot lie or sit on account of sticking and sore pain in the anus, it seems as if it had been pressed out, worse when retracting the rectum; ineffectual urging."

Anus: "*Hemorrhoids* (Æsculus, Aloe, Pulsatilla) increased *congestion of hemorrhoidal vessels;* burning; sticking; bearing down, with tenesmus; itching around it, at border, with sore feeling."

Stools: "*Fluid;* semi-fluid and *frequent*, soft and frequent in morning; pappy, yellowish-green, *copious, fetid* in morning, then feeling of perfect health; tough, gluey, fetid, so *urgent* that some escaped prematurely; slimy; *hard* and difficult only every two, three or four days; *scanty* and unsatisfactory."

After hearing me give so many symptoms under the four sections of the location m.m. you may ask "What is the use?" My reply is that every symptom has a different meaning, often representing a different condition in patients whom Sulphur has cured. Let us take for illustration "tenesmus." That one word suggests *dysentery* and when you add "bloody," "slimy," "mucous" stools; temperature; thirst and restlessness you have the complete picture of dysentery, generally chronic. Take the word "urging." *Under what conditions* and in what groups *has urging high rank?* Irritation will cause marked urging. What causes irritation about the anus of the Sulphur patient? Seat worms. What symptoms other than urging do worms produce? "Itching around border of anus with sore feeling," "burning after scratching," "variable appetite," "nausea and vomiting," emaciation and restlessness. In the same manner we could take up the *various forms of diarrhea, peritonitis, colitis,* hemorrhoids, etc., and group the symptoms in each.

A careful study of the *symptoms* of the mucosa of the digestive tract will demonstrate that most of the *conditions* which Sulphur will relieve are the *result of mal-nutrition.*

Urinary Tract: "*Dragging,* pressing sensation in the *bladder* in morning after urinating; *frequent urging* at night; constant *urging* and desire, with scanty urine; frequent urging; *urine* copious, scanty; turbid, *offensive,* covered with fatty pellicles; sticking, *burning,* itching, in the *urethra* (Cantharis, Mercurius cor.) when urinating."

Useful for *urethritis* specific and non-specific; *catarrh* of the *bladder;* nocturnal enuresis; and sometimes *chronic nephritis.*

Sexual Organs: "*Redness* and burning of the meatus; itching, burning of vagina so that she could not sit; papules and vesicles of vulva; a *corrosive,* yellow *leucorrhea.*"

Here, as under stomach, close study is required to correctly interpret the symptoms. What causes the "*redness?*" I have found the symptoms the result of "seat worms." The worms would crawl up into the vagina, cause the *itching*, the patient would rub the parts and cause redness and *burning* so intense that the little victim "could scarcely sit." These two symptoms should be added to the group I gave you under anus to complete the picture caused by seat worms in little girls. Leucorrhea and pruritus are the other two conditions most frequently found.

Respiratory Organs.

Larynx: "Drawing at times, with dryness; hoarseness in morning; *cough* from rawness in larynx with shooting pains in chest, *with heat in head* and eyes and *cold* hands; *dry* cough in evening before sleep, worse than during the day, waking him at night; dyspnea at night; sticking pains in sternum worse walking quickly and ascending stairs; sticking pains in sternum extending into the back, from the right side into the scapula; *pressure* and oppression of *chest; anxiety* and heaviness (Phosphorus); sensation of mucus after raising of which respiration was easier; *weakness* at night; weakness *when talking*."

Useful for *asthma*, for the various forms of *bronchial* and *laryngeal catarrh* with the cough mentioned above; for *pertussis* with the attacks of suffocation. It has some reputation for aborting pertussis in the early stages. For this purpose it is given internally and *burned in* the *room* of the patient. Many cases of *chronic asthma* with the dry cough agg. at night, the burning in chest, and fits of suffocation have been relieved by sulphur. Very often used in *pneumonia* with the following group of symptoms: The stage of solidification is prolonged, the temperature climbs a little higher, the cough becomes a little drier, hectic flush appears on the cheek, the pulse a little more rapid and weak, the head and extremities become hot, the restlessness is increased. All this in spite of the use of the *apparently* indicated remedy. Unless some change takes place soon an abscess will form in the lung.

Give a few doses of Sulphur 30th at intervals of two hours and after a few doses resolution will take place, thereby avoiding suppuration.

For *hydrothorax,* chronic, following such remedies as Bryonia. And finally for *incipient tuberculosis* especially *of girls at* the age of *puberty* (Calcarea, Pulsatilla, Phosphorus). The symptoms are: *Menses do not appear* (though all the other symptoms of maturity are present), the appetite is variable; *digestion slow* with *sour eructations;* dry hard stools; air hunger; hands, feet and head hot; feet burn at night and a *dry, hacking cough.*

This like the pneumonic conditions is a dangerous one and only the use of Sulphur, proper diet and exercise will prevent the development of *pulmonary t. b. c.* The appearance of the menses is the best evidence that the Sulphur is succeeding, and when they appear discontinue its use.

Blood and Thermic Centers: The *changes* found in the *blood simulate* those found in *malarial* and *eruptive fevers.* With the former you usually find the torpid liver, constipation and agg. at night. It seems to do the most good in those forms of eruptive fever where the eruption is slow in appearing or where there has been a recession of it. Only occasionally have I found it useful during the active stage of an uncomplicated case of malarial fever but I have seen results of the mal-treatment of such cases cleared up by Sulphur. The same is true of the eruptive diseases such as scarlet fever and smallpox. Sulphur is never indicated if they run the regular uncomplicated course; but for complications and sequellæ, often called for.

That the *local* application of Sulphur to the throat has cured diphtheria is vouched for by many physicians and laymen. I have seen good results from the combined use of the local and internal exhibition of it as an intercurrent, but have never seen Sulphur complete a cure.

The THERMIC CENTERS are much disturbed by Sulphur. Hot and cold, chills and fever are symptoms which occur frequently and are of high rank.

Let me recapitulate some of the chief points: Chronicity of most of the conditions; *offensive odors;* dread of and aggregation from water; *redness of the orifices;* periodic weakness; *marked affinity for the skin.*

CAPSICUM ANNUUM.

This member of the Belladonna family is the diseased, degenerate one. In one way and another he has lowered all his vital forces, especially those of the M.M. The result is congestion, ulceration, etc.

Make-up: Plethoric; flabby; lazy one who has abused himself.

Loc.: M.M. blood; *ears.*

Sen.: *Chilliness;* burning; biting.

Mod.: Agg. Drafts of cold air.
Amel. Continued motion.

Leaders: *Red purplish* color of M.M. and *nose* which is *cold.*

Ears: "Swelling on bone behind the ear, painful to touch (Tellurium); tearing behind ear, in concha; pain deeply seated with itching beneath the left ear with every cough as if an ulcer would open."

I am sure I have *aborted otorrhea* and *mastoid disease* in many cases by the internal and external use of Capsicum, and that I have given prompt relief in many more cases of *otalgia.*

Take a fleshy, flabby dark haired child with the above symptoms who wants to lie on a hot water bottle but howls with pain if anything cold touches his ear and Capsicum will relieve in a few moments. How do I use it? Internally in the 3rd., externally I have a good strong tea made from the pepper pods or ground red pepper. Make a poultice of corn meal and hot water, then pour your hot pepper tea over it and apply it over the ear and go home and sleep. (These cases usually come about midnight.) I have *used* it with *success* in mastoid *disease,* early stages, when the tenderness was extreme, and it seemed as if the meninges of the brain must become affected. *If suppuratiin has taken place, however, do not fail to operate.*

Mucous Membrane.

Throat: "Spasmodic contraction; pain on swallowing if inflamed but when not swallowing, drawing pain as from a swelling; pain during a paroxysm of cough, as if an ulcer would break."

Has *often* been *used for laryngitis* of *drinkers* and *smokers.* As you examine the *throat* it is of a deep red, *purplish,* color; dry, except in spots which are *ulcerated.* Use a good strong pepper tea for a gargle and give the 6th. I used it with success in one case of *diphtheria* in a fat, unhealthy child whose brother had been cured of diphtheria by Apis. When this child came down, just as the brother was recovering, I at first used the Apis, but when the uvula and adjoining parts began to slough and the child had regular paroxysms of chills I changed to Capsicum and an improvement soon set in. The child was too young to gargle so we used the tea as a spray.

Rectum and Stools: "*Tenesmus; Urging* to stool after *drinking,* but *only a little mucus passed;* feeling as if he would have stool as soon as he drank anything but only a little passed, hemorrhoids with burning and biting in the anus."

"Small, frequent; stools of mucus; at times mixed with blood and causing *tenesmus,* preceded by flatulent colic in the epigastrium."

Capsicum has served me in a few cases of *dysentery* with the above symptoms of which the *urging after drinking* was of the highest rank and *chilliness after stool* was the next most important. The tenesmus is marked; often you also have with the tenesmus of the rectum tenesmus of the bladder. In a few cases pain in the back was present.

Hemorrhoids with burning and tenesmus of rectum and

the pain in the small of the back. *Chilliness* is the 2d ranking symptom of this group.

Sexual and Urinary Organs: "Tenesmus; strangury; frequent almost ineffectual efforts to urinate (Mercurius cor., Cantharis); sticking in fore part of urethra when not urinating; *burning in orifice* before, during and after urinating; burning, biting after urinating."

Sometimes useful for *impotency* in old sinners, when the *testicles are atrophied,* the scrotum sore, and *the history of gonorrhea* in the record. It may also help during the acute stage of gonorrhea if there is excessive burning in the prostate and there is chilliness during the act of micturition.

I never have met that odor from the lungs which indicated a threatening abscess but I have used it for what I call a whisky cough, viz., a violent shattering cough which shakes the whole body. The odor with it is somewhat putrid.

Blood.

For conditions simulating pyemia, diphtheria, scarlet and intermittent fever. With the first the *temp.* is *high,* sweat profuse but *chilliness predominates.* In the two fevers, *chilliness* is the *ranking* symptom and *offensive discharges* the *second.*

BELLADONNA.

Make-up: Plethoric, full-blooded, active.

Loc.: *Brain; nerve centers;* M.M.

Sen.: Throbbing; cutting; dryness; hot; twitching.

Mod.: Agg. *Heat; P.M.;* motion; checked sweat; light; noise.

Amel. rest in bed, *equalizing circulation.*

Leaders: *Active congestion; wild, furious, delirium; prominent, sparkling eyes;* red, *dry,* hot *mouth* and *throat not relieved* by *water;* the suddenness and rapidity of all symptoms; *convulsions.*

Brain and Nerves.

Mind: "*Delirium* with heat, *springing out* of *bed, laughing,* constant *talking* with livid face, *injected* and protruding *eyes, dilated pupils, throbbing carotids,* full, hard, rapid pulse and inability to swallow. Furious; bites, strikes, tears everything to pieces; continually spitting at those around her, anxiety with desire to flee."

The delirium which Belladonna has often helped is a furious one, as the above symptoms from cases of poisoning show. Some of them need explanation, *e. g.*, the women tear off the clothing not for the purpose of exposing the person as do the Hyoscyamus patients but for the purpose of escaping from some imaginary enemy. For the same reason the Belladonna patient screams, bites, strikes, always at someone who is opposing them.

There is always the hot head, great excitement, protruding eyes, with the delirium which occurs in such diseases as scarlet fever, occasionally the first stage of typhoid, bronchitis, pneumonia, puerperal sepsis and erysipelas. I have met this form of delirium in a few cases of suppressed menses or lochia.

Head: Aching with intolerance of light, noise and odors; ruch of blood with pulsations in the cerebral arteries and throbbing in head (Glonoine, Ferrum phos., Ferrum); confusion; *pressive* pains agg. coughing, stepping (Bryonia); pain as if the brain rose and fell with every step; amel. strong pressure; shooting, stabbing pains from one temple to the other; sensitiveness so that even pressure of hair causes pain (China, Sulphur)."

The most frequent condition Belladonna relieves is a *violent hyperemic headache* with the above symptoms and especially the modalities. I have found it the *result* of *concussion*; and *reflex* from *uterus* or *ovary*, rarely from *kidneys*.

Belladonna is also frequently indicated for *apoplexy*, the very early stage. I have on several occasions found it useful for *meningitis* sometimes *cerebro-spinal* but more often accompanying *erysipelas* when it *extends* from the face to hair. The last case of the kind I used it fòr was a man of 40 who had had an operation on the septum of the nose. About 24 hours after, bright red, erysipelatous swelling spread up between the eyes over the forehead and in less than 12 hours into the hair. The temperature went up to 105.5, pulse to 140, hard and full, and the man began "fighting the devil" as he called his brother-in-law and the specialist. He was given Belladonna 6th, five drops every 30 minutes and poultices of scraped raw potatoes were applied, over the head. The hair was cut short. The symptoms subsided as quickly as they had arisen.

With children especially, the symptoms are amel. by putting cold to the head and something to the feet to draw the blood from the head. I use mustard water, horse radish leaves, or simply a hot water bottle. This amel., by *equalizing the blood* as I call it is the ranking modality of Belladonna.

Eye: The use made of atropine in eye work will be taught you in that department. We use it according to our law for *exophthalmus* when your *ranking* symptom is *dryness* of the eye so marked that the lid will not move over the protruding eye balls. You also have the rapid (Ferrum phos.) bounding pulse. Let me warn you against the use of Belladonna for the *pains of glaucoma* which greatly resemble those of Belladonna. Never give it low for that condition and watch closely if you give it in the 30th or 200th.

I have used it for spasms of the lids (Agaricus) when there was twitching of other muscles of the body which twitching was worse just as the child was going to sleep or perhaps had fallen asleep and was wakened by the twitching.

Face: "Tetanic closure of the jaws on attempting to pour down liquid; twitchings; *tearing pains on inner surface of corners* of jaws, agg. during deglutition."

For *"lockjaw"* (Stramonium); often for *facial neuralgia* with the twitching of muscles, flushed face and dilated pupils.

Spine: "Dartings, as if from knives, in the bones of the spine; gnawing in the dorsal spine."

There are three conditions we use Belladonna for in this section; *lumbago* when the pains are severe, acute, have come on suddenly, and shoot down over the hips into the thighs and legs. The pains are often cramp-like.

Irritability of spine with pressure upon the dorsal spine so severe as to cause screams. Cough which sometimes accompanies this condition, causes marked agg. *Hyperemia* of the spine with all sorts of difficulty in walking, due in most part—to loss of co-ordination. Do not think of locomotor ataxia for the loss of co-ordination for which Belladonna is indicated is temporary and yields to treatment in a short time.

Extrem.: "Sense of *stretching and twisting;* shooting pressure on top of shoulder; *paralytic drawing pressure,* upper arm and fore arm with weakness, cutting, shooting, pains in muscles above the knee only when sitting; pain in thigh and legs as if bruised, as if brittle, with shooting and gnawing towards shaft of the bone; tearing in joints obliging him while sitting to keep the feet in motion amel. when walking, tearing pressure in the middle of inside of leg."

Useful for *neuralgia* and *neuritis* especially of the *sciatic* with marked *sensitiveness agg.* from *pressure.*

Sleep: "*Sleep restless; the child tosses about, kicks and quarrels in sleep* (Hyoscyamus); *irrational talking and difficulty in keeping them in bed; starting and waking when falling asleep* waked constantly by fearful dreams and twitching."

I have put the sleep symptoms of Belladonna in this location because they are the result of hyperemia of the brain. The hyperemia is often reflex but occasionally due to cerebritis. *Anything which* will *draw* the *blood from* the *brain* will *help* the sleep condition. You will find that such *patients have hot heads* and *cold feet.* Belladonna children usually sleep with the eyes half open.

Mucous Membranes.

Eyes: "*Staring; projecting; sparkling;* glassy; inflammation; and a wild expression; dryness; stiffness; heat."

Belladonna has been a disappointment to me in purely inflammatory condition of the conjunctiva. I rarely use it for other than the conditions mentioned under the nerves.

Ear: "*Tearing downward in the middle and external ear;* thrusts in middle with pinching; ringing; roaring; sensitive to loud tones."

Although some of the above symptoms may belong under the heading "nerve," *i. e.,* otalgia, still I have never found a case of "Earache" calling for Belladonna without there was inflammation.

I place it only a little below Capsicum for earache. The *modality amel. from cold* is the *ranking symptom* of the ear group.

Nose: "Dryness of the Schneiderian membrane; blowing out of mucus mixed with blood; smell *sensitive,* the smell of tobacco is intolerable."

Belladonna is *useful* only for *acute inflammation,* acute *coryza* or cough. With either you have the inflammation of the eyes and lids with the dryness and heat. The nose is swollen and red.

Mouth: "*Drawing in* upper *teeth* all night; deep *redness* of *papillæ* of *tongue* with swelling; tongue dry interfering with speech, dry and retracted, dry and swollen, hanging from child's mouth; dry *crimson color* of *tongue,* of lining of the cheeks; lips, also of roof of mouth and pharynx which looked burned."

For the early stages of *glossitis, stomatitis* and *pharyngitis* with intense inflammation. There is a glazed condition and dryness but water will not relieve. The tongue is usually coated white and the red papillæ protruding is what gives us the "Strawberry tongue" which is one of the pathognomonic symptoms of scarlet fever.

Throat: "*Feeling as if too narrow when swallowing; dryness with difficult swallowing; regurgitation* of liquids, sometimes solids when attempting to swallow."

For the *first stage* of many *throat conditions* with the *intense congestion and great dryness.* Not useful after the acute becomes chronic, with moisture and catarrhal discharges. It has *aborted* many cases of *simple tonsilitis* by its prompt action.

Stomach: "Unquenchable thirst for cold water; incomplete eructations; hiccough; nausea and vomiting after eating; shooting, cutting in pit of stomach forcing him to bend backward and hold his breath; *hard pressure* agg. after eating; burning and sensitiveness to touch in region."

For *gastritis with* the *violent vomiting.* I wish you would bear in mind that in cases of measles calling for Belladonna we have vomiting.

Abdomen: "*Tumefaction with tenderness to touch; pain as if sore and raw; tenderness on pressure; cutting, now here, now there;* pain in a spot as if seized with nails, a griping, clutching, clawing, pain; heat (*with anxiety*) in abdomen, chest and face."

Belladonna is used successfully for *peritonitis, metroperitonitis,* hepatitis, *enteritis* and other abdominal troubles.

Always for acute troubles with intolerance of pressure (Lachesis) with heat and tenderness.

Rectum and Stools: "Squeezing, constrictive pain in rectum, alternating with shooting jerking pain into perineum; *tenesmus,* a constant pressing and urging towards anus and genitals, alternating with painful contraction of anus; urging to stool which is thin, frequent, but ineffectual or scanty and hard."

The only use I have ever made of Belladonna in this section was for *dysentery,* the first stage with *marked* inflammation, the mucous membrane of the anus swollen and everted. The *stools* were *green mucus* and *blood.*

Urinary Organs: "Pressure in vesical region at night, tenesmus, *urine retained; passed in drops;* urine deep red."

The only one of the above symptoms in first rank is "*urine retained.*" Many times have I relieved *retention* of urine by a few doses of Belladonna 6th. Remember that Belladonna is for *retention*, Stramonium for *suppression* and Hyoscyamus for *involuntary voiding* of urine. With the Belladonna *dysuria* of women and children you have marked excitability. Belladonna has something of a reputation for *acute nephritis*, with the severe pains in the region of the kidneys. Belladonna at first *flushes* the *kidney*, giving us increased amount of urine followed by decreased.

Sexual Organs.

Fem. Sexual Organs: "*Metrorrhagia, the blood having a bad smell; menses too soon;* urging as if everything would fall out; amel. lying and sitting erect, agg. sitting bent and walking."

I have found it the best remedy for *extremely offensive menses.* A case in point was a large, full-blooded, bright student aged 24, who came to the clinic with the following statement "Doctor, I want something for an offensive flow at the sick time." In answer to questions she added, "I menstruate every three weeks, I flow seven or eight days, but the bad odor is only the first three days, when it is so bad, I keep my room. Pain and clots first three days then bright red." Belladonna 30th, 5 drops night and morning for two months relieved all the symptoms.

The only other condition for which I have found Belladonna helpful in "hemorrhage with a bad smell" was in *puerperal metritis.* In this group, I have also found the feeling "urging as if everything would fall out" (Sepia, Lillium tig.), and often retention of the urine.

For *dysmenorrhea* when the pain comes during the first three days of the period, the flow being *dark,* clotted, *offensive.* For *suppressed menses* when the head and mental symptoms are of equal rank with the uterine which are: prolapsus, ovaritis and sensitiveness of the mammary glands.

Respiratory Organs.

Respiratory Organs: "Constriction of larynx; *painful dryness of larynx* with aversion to all drinks; dryness of larynx making voice husky and often inducing dry cough; *hoarseness* especially after crying; aphonia; respiration, short, rapid, oppressed, difficult."

For the first stage, when there is a high grade of inflammation and congestion, of *laryngitis;* both *spasmodic* and *catarrhal croup; whooping cough* and *spasms* of the *glottis.* With all of these conditions you have a good deal of hoarseness due to hyperemia, hot face, hot head, and soreness, except in chronic laryngitis.

Skin: "*Redness as in scarlatina* suddenly spreading over the body with heat and exaltation of all faculties; scarlet eruption like scarlitina on face, arms, and trunk; red scaly eruption on lower parts of body as far as abdomen: *pustules* on *cheek and nose, rapidly filling* with pus, *becoming covered with a crust;* sensitiveness to touch."

The best remedy for the early stage of what is *called "cat boils"* with marked *inflammation* around them also very *sensitive* to touch. For *erysipelas* when the skin is shiny and red, high temp., often delirium of the violent form. The *disease comes suddenly* and *spreads rapidly.*

No remedy has helped me so much for *scarlatina* as Belladonna, both as a *prophylactic* and to *reduce* the *temperature,* relieve the *delirium* and to *prevent* post-scarlatinal *nephritis. But now take note.* It is as useless for an irregular eruption as the same amount of sac. lac. You should use Pulsatilla, Bryonia or any indicated remedy for that form of Scarlet Fever. Belladonna is not indicated except in the smooth variety with the "*Strawberry tongue,*" the nausea and vomiting and scanty urine.

Belladonna has given results in all potencies from the 3rd to the 1m. I also use a 1 to 2000 solution of the tincture for local application.

HYOSCYAMUS.

Make-up: Neurotic.

Loc.: Brain nerves; muscles; blood.

Sen.: Jerking; twitching; restless; fear.

Mod.: Agg. *Mental effects;* fright; touch; noise; sitting up.

Leaders: *Nymphomania,* carphologia.

Brain and Nerve.

Mind: "*Raving,* delirious; restless; would not stay in bed; with ludicrous actions, like monkeys; ridiculous action like a dancing clown; violent and beats people; bit, scratched and nipped at every one who interfered with her violent efforts to get out of bed; carphologia, muttering to himself; lively delirium; sings love songs; talk is more animated than usual, also absurd, irrational as if a man were present who was not; hands in constant motion; now clutching the air, now pulling off bedclothes; jealous; dread of drinks; foolish; unconsciousness."

The most frequent use I have made of this long list of mental symptoms is *nymphomania* of the most furious character. The *patients* were "wild" with excitement, *uncovered for* the *purpose* of *exposing* themselves. Get into a man's lap, embrace him, etc. The eyes were bright and sparkling; the pupils dilated. The *cause* in most cases is *menstrual irregularities,* usually *suppressed.* In *one case* the *cause* was *cystic ovaries* and it was after the ovaries had been removed that she was given the remedy though the attacks came at the time of the menses before the operation.

Delirium comes next in frequency. Often delirium tremens when objects seem very large. His friends, or imaginary objects, are going to injure him or take him from home, the patients are very suspicious, refusing to eat or drink, wanting to get off by themselves. *Fear* sometimes leads them to strike and bite in supposed self-defense (Belladonna).

Mania, most frequently *puerperal,* of the *excitable form. Obscenity* is a symptom of this group and the *nymphomania* may be mixed with it. Here also we have the *suspiciousness* which may result in forced feeding because the *patient fears* there is *poison* in her food. With this condition, as with the delirium tremens, *objects* and persons *are abnormally large.*

There remains another form of *delirium* for which Hyoscyamus is occasionally useful. Here we find *carphologia.* The patient will lie quietly in bed, his *eyes fixed,* the *fingers* constantly *moving,* picking at, tearing, or tying knots in imaginary objects, every now and then *laughing* out loud or uttering a *cry of delight or pain.* The evacuations are involuntary, the *tongue dry,* so that speech is indistinct.

Eyes: "Distorted; staring; squinting; red; wild; brilliant and rolling about; *pupils dilated* and insensible, *small objects seem very large;* conjunctiva injected; vision dim and short."

These symptoms belong for the most part in the mental groups, though not of high rank. Aside from that they may be found in two groups, one being *spasms* of the *ocular muscles,* causing rolling and distortion; sometimes *strabismus.*

Urinary: "Paralysis of the bladder; urine retained."

I have never found a case for which Hyoscyamus did any good where the urine was retained. I have met a few cases of *suppressed urine with* the *manias.* The *paralysis* of the *bladder* I have always met in the *low* type of *fevers.* It is a functional condition expressed by "involuntary micturition." As stated above involuntary defecation usually accompanies it.

Resp. Organs: "*Hoarseness; cough at night;* frequent; dry cough, hacking tickling spasmodic cough, worse at night, on lying down, from cold air, eating and drinking, talking or swimming."

One of our best remedies for *acute aphonia caused* by *emotion,* especially *fright.* The other symptoms are also of nervous origin, in fact purely nervous. The *cough* is *dry* in that group with one *exception,* viz., *pertussis* in which I have seen a little *mucus,* making the *cough* a little *loose* and the *voice rough.*

Extrem.: "*Trembling;* twitching of hands and feet; convulsions now in the upper, now in lower; toes cramped, flexed, when walking or lifting the foot."

Now if we *take* our *location* "muscles" in connection with the above we will have the following picture called *chorea.* The symptoms are: *clutching motions* of the hands; *twitching* of *lips* and *cheeks;* all sorts of *grimaces, indistinct speech;* distorted eyes; *difficult deglutition* all agg. by excitement.

Blood: Conditions *simulating typhoid* and *scarlet fever* of low type. With this condition you find the brain and sphincters symptoms mentioned above.

Sleep: "*Sleeplessness, caused by long continued exhilaration;* all night he tried lying on one side and the other but could not lie quiet, only toward daybreak, with general sweat more about the neck; *restless* sleep; laughing expression during sleep; *starting out of sleep.*"

One of the best remedies for sleeplessness caused by excitement (Coffea); also for nervous children who cry in sleep, twitch, tremble and wake in fright.

STRAMONIUM.

Stramonium helps her other two illustrious sisters, Belladonna and Hyoscyamus, in supporting a reputation for producing cerebral excitement with all its dire results. It is more useful for suppression of excretions and secretions than the other two. There are so many symptoms in black types that I must omit most of them except in the grouping.

Make-up: Neurotic.

Loc.: Brain; nerves; muscles of the throat; skin.

Sen.: Jerking; twitching; cramping; dryness.

Mod.: Agg. after sleep (Lachesis), bright objects, suppression; fright; light; company.

Brain: *Delirium; noisy, frightened by strange objects; under impression of danger, clinging to the persons; sees horrifying things more at his side than in front of him; either chasing or fleeing from imaginary objects; usually black bugs, dogs and beasts which seem to spring out of the floor or dropping from the ceiling; rage on attempt to administer liquids, spasms of the pharynx so that any thing taken choked him or regurgitated; AVERSION TO FLUIDS; apprehension, starting up in fright; shuddering as from fright,* etc., etc. (if you care to, look up the other four-fifths in Allen)."

Before explaining the above symptoms I want to add those in black type under throat. "*Spasms on attempting to swallow; constriction, spasmodic,* with paralysis, dryness of fauces with redness and *difficult swallowing,* especially of *water.*"

I consider it the best remedy for *threatened hydrophobia.* And even after the symptoms have developed I would push Stramonium tincture in five-drop doses till I obtained some kind of result. For in addition to all the above, which belong to the *hydrophobia* group, we have "*expressions of terror*" under face and *dribbling* of *glossy saliva* " under mouth."

Stramonium has cured *delirium caused* by excitement also by the poison of various *fevers.* The delirium is *always wild, full* of frightful hallucinations and delusions. The patient screams from fright, clings to the mother; will not be left alone. The *objects* of Stramonium are *black,* of Belladonna *red.* Like Hyoscyamus the *objects are very large.* This last symptom is most frequent in the *delirium tremens* group." In this connection Stramonium patients may also imagine that they themselves or some parts of themselves are abnormally large.

I had a patient, a young man of 20, who had never been ill till he contracted measles. The eruption was slow in coming out and had receded twice, at which time the temp. went up and the delirium appeared. He was lying in bed when I first saw him, with his eyes fixed on the ceiling, then he would jump. For a few minutes he was quiet, with eyes shut, then he would open them, turn to the corner of the room, follow up the wall to the ceiling and there seemed to fix his eyes for a few minutes and then jump. After he had repeated the above actions three times I made an effort to rouse him and succeeded enough so that he told me that he knew it was not so but that it seemed that big spiders, big as turtles, crawled up the wall, over the ceiling and then would drop with the intention of putting out his eyes, but as he shut his eyes too quick the spider crawled off the bed over the floor, up the wall and tried again. *There was another high ranked symptom* in this group, viz., *no urine had been voided for 30 hours* and the bladder was empty. Stramonium 30 restored the function of the kidneys in four hours and the mental symptoms ceased.

How much and how often did I give it? Five drops in water every 15 minutes, till he voided. I have demonstrated many times that Belladonna *causes* and cures *retention* of urine; Hyoscyamus *involuntary* micturition and Stramonium *suppression* of urine and the many conditions arising from two of the abnormal functions of the urinary organs.

Head: "*Rush of blood to; vertigo* as if he would *fall forward* and to the *left;* throbbing in vertex and occiput; bores head into pillow, bends head backwards."

There are only two conditions for which you will find Stramonium useful, viz., *hydrocephalus, cerebro-spinal meningitis.* I never knew Stramonium to completely cure this condition. But it palliated while Apis and Calcarea phosph. cured.

The *cerebro-spinal meningitis* is *accompanied* by a severe *congestive headache,* the pains being so severe that the patients are besides themselves, you have the throbbing pains in the vertex and occiput.

TABACUM.

Make-up: Neurotic; spare; relaxed.

Loc.: Nerves; *stomach;* sphincters; *heart.*

Sen.: Vertigo; weakness, as if struck by a hammer; as if stomach were relaxed; as if seasick.

Mod.: Agg. motion; pressure; warm room; stimulants; evening.

Amel. *Vinegar;* cold to head; weeping; vomiting; open air.

Leaders: The *terrible* sinking at the stomach, the cold sweat, the relaxation of sphincter.

Brain and Nerves.

Mind: "Blunts all the senses."

Head: "Aching relieved in the open air; heaviness; *vertigo;* shocks; sensation of rush of blood."

For neuralgic headache accompanying the gastralgias. Amel. by cold. The pains come suddenly (Belladonna) as from a blow, going from one temple to the other.

Stomach: "*Nausea* with *relaxed* sensation in stomach; *paroxysmal, as in seasickness* with vertigo and cold sweat; nausea almost faintness; amel. open air; violent vomiting; sinking at pit."

For *gastralgia* when the *pain begins* at *cardiac end* of *stomach* and *extends* over shoulder into the *left arm.*

Abdomen: "*Painful distention* of abdomen; pressing pains in lower abdomen."

To these two symptoms add *vomiting* violent, sometimes of *fecal matter; cold sweat;* pinched face and you will have the picture of *incarcerated hernia* which Tabacum will help. The cause of the incarceration is a relaxed ring and contraction of the abdominal muscles. (Cocculus.)

Stools: "Resembling those of cholera; urgent, painless, frequent, profuse, gushing."

Occasionally useful for *cholera infantum* with the above stools plus the feeble, irregular pulse, the icy coldness of the extremities; the deathly pallor of the face; the nausea and *vomiting,* the latter of which is *amel. by uncovering the abdomen.*

Heart: "*Precordial oppression* in paroxysms worse at night with *palpitations* between the shoulders; *violent palpitation* (Thea, Spigelia); action weak; purring tremor."

The most frequent use I have made of the drug is for *acute dilatation caused* by *shock or* violent *physical exertion.* You will find in this group in addition to the above the pain running over the shoulder into the arm and the *cold sweat.* As you know, a great majority of the men rejected by the army because of heart trouble suffered from *dilatation* and *mitral regurgitation.* The sphere of action of Tabacum is the most restricted of the solanum family. Allen calls attention to the fact that it causes degeneration of nerve tissue as witnessed by atrophy of the optic nerve (Strychnia). That it soothes the excited, irritable nerves is claimed by most users. I don't know.

THE ALKALIS.

Today, as we take up the study of the Alkalis, we may with profit divide them into two general groups, viz., the alkaline salts and the alkaline earths. Among the former are the salts of sodium, potassium and ammonium. The latter are the salts and earth of calcium, magnesium and lithium. The potash group includes *Causticum.* The *alkalis affect all tissues* of the body *hence* their *location is general.* For the same reason they produce every known sensation, and every modality also applies to them. As the group has an "affinity" for any and every tissue or organ in the body so some of them have the *power to* produce all of *the four conditions* on any or all tissues, *i. e.*, irritation, inflammation, functional and structural changes.

The groups also furnish *remedies for* nearly all the *diatheses,* Calcarea for the rachitic, Kali carb. for the rheumatic, Natrum sulph. for the hydrogenoid, etc.

The *conditions*, for which we look for help to the alkalis, are usually *chronic*. They are deep acting remedies.

Auxiliary treatment is not only useful but often necessary with this group. Especially is this true of diet and climate.

The alkali family is a large one and possesses many strikingly different traits. But there are, on the other hand, many family resemblances which when grouped together make up what we, teachers of materia medica, call the "alkali cachexia."

Because the alkalis act deeply the misuse or abuse of them may cause irreparable harm and for this reason you should be familiar with their action, also familiar with their antidotes.

My old teacher of materia medica, T. F. Allen, speaking of the alkalis, said: "As a rule they are devilish in their effects, insidious and disorganizing, profound tissue changes resulting often, quite out of proportion to the amount taken. I am of the opinion that more chronic disease predisposing to pernicious and incurable maladies, is produced by the almost universal habit of drinking alkaline waters than by any other of the numerous habits of the civilized world. They lay the foundations for tuberculosis, cancer, gout, with their numerous progeny, etc."

External Action: Let us look a little more carefully into the action of the alkalis. Take the skin. A weak solution dissolves the superficial epidermis, making the skin soft and soapy. But increase the strength and your concentrated solution destroys the skin, also the tissue beneath and leaves an ulcer.

Internal Action: They act the same on the mucous membranes. The secretions are dissolved, the surfaces are reddened and softened by the weaker solutions, while the *stronger solutions produce ulceration*. In the stomach, they lessen and neutralize the formation of the acid by combining with the acid of the stomach and forming salts. In addition to dissolving the mucus, etc., of the intestine, the alkalis draw from the blood, and other tissue, fluid and in this manner cause diarrhea.

These alkaline salts, formed in the stomach and otherwise, are readily absorbed into the blood, increasing the alkalinity of the blood. It will give you a better understanding of their action if you bear in mind that the alkalis and their salts are eliminated by the kidneys at the same time increasing the amount of the urine, increasing the solids, increasing the alkalinity but decreasing the acidity.

Let us now examine Prof. T. F. Allen's statement as to what the alkalis will do in the light of this statement of the action of the alkalis. Here is a patient whose ancestors for four or five generations have suffered from cancer. As a result of some error of diet he contracts gastritis with overacidity. That patient is given some alkali in large doses till the mucous membrane of the stomach reddens, softens and sloughs, leaving an ulcer. Are not the prospects good for that ulcer developing into a cancer? We may draw the same conclusion for the tubercular and other diatheses.

I use this illustration knowing full well that many of our younger pathologists claim that there is no cancer diathesis—that there is nothing in the idea of heredity.

So much for what the alkalis as a group will do if given in large doses or medium-sized doses continued over a long period of time. Let us now inquire into the action of a few of the individuals of the group and learn for what conditions they are used, and in what doses they produce the pernicious results we have intimated.

When I began the practice of medicine, one of the alkalis which was almost universally prescribed by the majority of physicians was the chlorate of potash. It was prescribed for sore throat. The druggists, noting the demand for it in filling prescriptions, advised it for sore throat to every customer. The result was that most every one carried tablets of Kali chloratum in their pockets, taking them themselves and giving them to their friends. About five years later, the intelligent, observing physician noted that chronic interstitial nephritis followed the use of the drug, and then through our journals and from our medical meetings the cry of alarm and protest against its abuse arose, but not till thousands of lives had been sacrificed.

Passing over many others of the group which have had their day from that time to this, let us take bicarbonate of soda. The stomach specialists use it almost as freely as borax is used for cleansing purposes. Today, the stomach specialist prescribes it for "acidosis" and the layman takes it and gives it for "sour stomach." The specialist's dose is from 5 to 20 grs., the layman's dose usually four times as large, *i. e.*, "a heaping teaspoon in half a glass of water." The physician, to neutralize acids, gives it just after meals as little diluted as possible; if he wants to change the reaction of the blood he gives it between meals in very large quantities of water; if for diabetic coma he administers it intravenously or as a rectoclysis.

I feel it is unnecessary for me to say more about the pernicious action of the alkalis not only when used as "Alkaline Waters" but also when prescribed by physicians or taken by the laity without a prescription. I feel sure you will agree with Dr. Allen's saying that the results are "devilish." Knowing these facts, what are our duties? First—to educate our patients and the public, Second—to know and administer the antidote. How shall we educate the public? By talking to our patients, by discussing the subject in our medical meetings and having our discussions published in the papers; and finally by writing the facts for the health columns of the large dailies. We should state freely what we mean by "Alkaline Waters", namely, Vischy, Pluto, Abiline and the many other preparations found in all drug stores of the country. I have stated what we mean by the alkaline salts and earths, mainly the sodium, potassium, ammonium, calcium, magnesium and lithium groups and their combinations and compounds.

Antidotes.

For this task the physician trained in homeopathic principles has a decided advantage. I mean that the homeopathic physician who "takes the case" as he should, inquires further into the habits of his patients as to their food, *drink*, sleep, and so forth, will ascertain whether the symptoms the patient presents are due to the use of alkalis or to other causes. Having found such to be the fact, that fact becomes a part of the "Totality of Symptoms" which will lead to the antidote. It would take altogether too much time to give an antitode for each of the many alkalis. More than that, an antidote to Kali chloratum or Natrum bicarbonate for a patient suffering from the chronic effect of either drug may differ from an antidote required for the acute effect of either and still more might it differ from the antidote required for the individual patient suffering from either. I believe, however, there is a rule we may take for our guide if we do not care to rely upon the law of similia, and yet wish to take into account the action of the drug we are attempting to antidote. That rule is to give another remedy of the same group or family, the one most resembling the one we wish to antidote, for example Kali carb. for Kali nitricum; Lithium carb. for Natrum muriaticum. My experience has led me to believe the chemical or other antidote given in our books is in a great majority of cases the one which we find indicated when we select it upon the "Totality of Symptoms." For that reason I nearly always select my antidote as I select any other remedy, that is, upon the "Totality of Symptoms."

I want to add, at this point, that there are no cases for which what I call adjuvant treatment, namely, proper diet, exercises, etc., are so helpful, yes, so essential to a cure, as these we have been considering. Of course you will discontinue the drug which has caused the condition, and often when that is done and the diet and exercise corrected, your patient will be cured without any other remedy.

Let us now take up the potash family. We find twenty kalis in Clark's Dictionary. Let us remember that the potashes have an "Elective Affinity" for the motor centers of the heart, *i. e., motor centers of the heart muscles.* Paralysis of the heart is the result of large doses. The other locations are *mucous membranes, kidneys, blood and glandular organs.*

The general sensations therefore are: sharp, sticking, aching, weak, chilly, etc., corresponding to the tissue or organ involved and the stage of disease.

The modalities are: Agg. morning; after sleep; cold; exertion. Amel. warmth, rest, and by a diet which is nourishing and rich in blood making properties. I will only mention the groups of symptoms under each compound after giving the "make-up," "location," "sensations" and "modalities".

Kali Aceticum.

Make-up: Weak, dropsical patients.

Loc.: Kidneys and lower intestines.

Sen.: Weakness, trembling, griping and gnawing.

Mod.: Agg. morning, except the headache which is 4 P.M. The Urinary group is as follows: Amount greatly increased; urea greatly increased; reaction strongly alkaline; color yellow; odor either sweet or ammoniacal; specific gravity high.

Conditions: Diabetes and Polyuria.

The Intestinal Group: Gnawing in the stomach; distension of abdomen. Agg. after eating; free watery stools; bleeding hemorrhoids; weakness following stools; musty offensive perspiration.

Kali Arsenicosum.

This is the much used and abused "Fowler's Solution," also called "Liquor Arsenicosum." The symptoms resemble Arsenicum more than kali.

Make-up: The restless, nervous, anemic.

Loc.: Nearly every tissue in the body, but especially the skin, blood and kidneys.

Sen.: Itching, jerking, twitching, burning, nausea and constriction.

Besides these we have the following: "Sensation of a ball rising from the pit of the stomach to throat causing suffocation; "As a red hot iron in rectum." "Head feels large;" "burning and numbness of tongue; tongue feels too large." These four symptoms should be given highest rank whenever found in the potash group.

Mod.: Agg. at night on undressing; warmth.
Amel.: Belching.

Kali ars. has three prominent skin groups, viz., Herpes, Eczema, and Psoriasis. Besides it is used in the exanthemata and miliary rash. The herpetic patients needing the remedy present the following: Eruption on any or all parts of the body except scalp. We first have papules, then vesicles, then pustules which dry and form scabs and then fall off, leaving sores varying in size from a line to a third of an inch.

There is intense itching, greatly agg. by warmth, while undressing and at night. The cicatrices remain dark colored for some time, in fact the entire skin loses its freshness and becomes dry, inelastic and muddy. The sclerotics become yellow; the appetite poor.

I also want to mention a case of epithelioma of the lower lip which had been treated by arsenic paste but which returned after several years. The patient did not wish to have the paste used again so I gave him Kali.ars. 3x three grs. morning and evening for eight weeks. The result was a complete success.

The Kali ars. eczemas have dry, scaly eruptions, the scales are larger than those of Ars. alb. and with them a little moisture (just enough to diagnose eczema), scratching that increases the amount of moisture which sometimes forms cakes or scabs. The psoriasis begins on the arms and legs, spreading over the body. The itching is intense and there are the same modalities as under herpes. The skin after the eczema is redder than after the herpes.

KALI BICHROMICUM.

Make-up: Light complexion, flabby; lazy.

Sen.: Sharp; stinging; sticky.

Loc.: *M.M.;* skin; ligament; joints.

Mod.: Agg. *Cold open air,* undressing; *beer; 2–4 A.M.;* suppressed catarrh.

Amel. heat.

Leaders: *Thick, tough,* stringy, adhesive secretions; absence of fever.

Mucous Membranes.

Eyes: "Inflammation, in the morning with yellow discharge and agglutination of lids; sensitiveness; margins of the lids red; a yellow purulent discharge in inner canth. in morning; itching with lachrymation and photophobia, agg. evening and night, with pain as from sand in them; *white, granular elevations, surrounded by redness* of the conjunctiva; pustules on the cornea with surrounding indolent inflammation; red, raw, rough feeling, of the margin of the lids so that winking causes rubbing against the balls, "burning in margin."

Kali bich. is very useful for many *sub-acute conditions* of the eye all of a *sluggish* nature with very little photophobia.

Some of the conditions are: *granular lids* with *burning* sensation, with scanty exudation; *ulceration* of the *cornea* the ulcers being small, punched, deep; *catarrhal conjunctivitis* with *morning agglutination;* the latter stages of iritis *generally syphilitic.*

Ears: Nothing marked from the provers but clinically we find it useful for otorrhea after rupture of drum when the discharge is yellow, very *tough* and *stringy.* We had a clinical patient with the mucus so tough it could be drawn out four inches from the drum before it loosened.

Nose: *"Septum ulcerated away, in the upper part, as far* *as its articulation with the vomar and ethnoid, and purulent inflammation of the whole nasal mucous membrane;* septum dotted with minute ulceration; sticking in side on blowing nose with discharge of greenish, offensive masses (Pulsatilla); discharge through posterior nares had a disagreeble taste; ulcers in external border of nostrils; nose swollen at root and hot; nose seemed thick and full; *dryness with pain in root* at the beginning of stopped catarrh extending to the temples, burning, sore feeling at root extending into the frontal sinuses; *plugs;* clinkers which if torn away too soon cause bleeding and soreness."

This last symptom is the ranking symptom of this section. Just a word of explanation as to how such large clinkers can form on the ulcers which I have described as deep, and smooth as if punched. It is that several ulcers are so close together that the mucus from all of them, as that oozes from their mouths, runs together and forms a scab which then adheres to the ulcerated surface.

For *chronic inflammation* of the *frontal sinuses* with the sore, *stopped up sensation.* The stringy *mucus* may stay in the sinus for some time before it is discharged. When this is true the discharge becomes of the consistency of oil.

Your sensations are nearly always those of *obstruction;* the exception being the *sharp sticking pains* of *ulcerations.* Occasionally Kali bich. is useful for *nasal polypi* (Phosphorus, Sanguinaria nit.).

Tongue: "*Smooth, red* and *cracked;* red and dry; yellowish-white; aphthous patches on; dryness."

You will find the first symptom during a *low chronic form of dysentery.* The other conditions for which the drug is useful are *aphthous stomatitis and syphilitic ulceration* of the tongue.

Throat: "*On the side of the root of uvula, an excavated sore, with reddish areola, containing yellow tenacious matter; hawking* of *much gelatinous, tenacious mucus* in the morning; feeling of adherent mucus in morning; sensation of a hair in fauces."

First, for *diphtheria;* many cases have been cured when there were profound prostration, *lack* of any *acute, painful sensation,* profuse perspiration, weak, soft, pulse, some infiltration of cellular tissue and the tough tenacious exudation.

In addition to the diphtheritic ulceration we have *ulceration* of the *posterior wall* of the *pharynx* with the well defined punched edges, and the *cheesy exudate* forming clinkers. For *follicular ulceration* of the *fauces* and finally and most frequently for *chronic* catarrhal inflammation of the entire throat.

Stomach: "Thirst; longing for beer; nausea with hot eructations and sweetish, flat saliva; *vomiting* of a pinkish glairy fluid; digestion disordered by meat (Pulsatilla); *burning pains* in pit after dinner with salivation *extending* to *mouth* (Sanguinaria nit.)."

For the *dyspepsia of drunkards* or others using malt liquors, with the nausea and vomiting after eating, and flatulency. For *ulceration* of the *stomach* with soreness in small spots here and there and the nausea and vomiting. For *chronic gastric catarrh* with the above symptoms plus a thickly coated tongue.

Abdomen: "*Distention;* rumbling after stool, after eating, with griping, then a retraction of the anus; nausea; sticking pains and soreness to pressure."

For ulceration and catarrh of the duodenum, Kali bich. stands second to no other remedy, with jaundice, light stools, and dark urine.

For gastro-enteritis with the discharge of stringy mucus, and the bilious vomiting.

Stools: "Diarrhea profuse, constant, involuntary, of mucus and blood; of brown frothy water; dysenteric stools with gnawing at navel and ineffectual straining."

We have two conditions; *dysentery,* second *diarrhea.* The diarrhea is like that of Rheum, *i. e.,* frothy, brown, watery stools with some pain about the navel and slight tendency to strain after stools. It has been used for a periodic dysentery coming on in the spring. The stools are painful, a little tenesmus; the tongue is dry, red, cracked. The stools most frequent in the morning. Occasionally for dysentery following diphtheria (Mercurius) with mucous stools occasionally streaked with blood, and patches on the tongue (Taraxacum, Natrum mur.).

Urinary Organs: "Burning in bulbus urethra and glands of the urethra when urinating and after; sometimes when passing urine; urine scanty and red."

For *sub-acute urethritis* with the sensation that a drop of urine could not be expelled without much straining. There is usually burning pain in the fossa navicularis and bulbus urethra.

Sexual Organs: "Pain in penis; constriction in morning after waking; erections."

Clinically we find Kali bich. useful for *chancre*. The make-up of the patient, *i. e.*, fat and fair, plus the peculiar tenacious cheesy discharge from the ulcers are the leading symptoms. Kali bich. has helped many cases of very tenacious leucorrhea, yellow in color. Also for *pruritus* of the vulva with marked burning and excitement agg. during hot weather.

Respiratory Organs: "Mucus in bronchi and nose in the morning without catarrh; burning in bronchi when coughing; mucus obliging hawking; intermitting scraping with soreness in morning; pressure agg. talking; *hoarseness* in morning agg. till noon, amel. eating; dry cough agg. expectorating thick, yellowish-white mucus; voice rough; cough after meals; cough with expectoration as tough as pitch and which can be drawn out in strings; marked dyspnea in the morning as if the mucous membrane of the bronchi were thickened."

The best remedy we have for *catarrh* of the *pharynx, larynx, bronchi,* and *nose.* Note the chronic nature of the condition also the *tough tenacious mucus,* the ulcerations, the *agg. morning* and *eating, amel. lying down* and warmth.

The condition in this section which most often calls for this remedy is *membranous croup,* in the last stages. The symptoms are: *hoarseness, loose cough;* barking cough; *gagging* because there is much tenacious mucus, *pulse soft* and *weak, marked* prostration, profuse sweat, the sawing respiration; *gasping for breath,* cool skin.

Also for *spasmodic* and chronic *bronchitis,* with the wheezing in lung, the tough tenacious mucus which is difficult to expectorate and sometimes causes choking.

Skin.

"Dry eruptions like measles, cover the whole body; small pustules over the body similar to smallpox (Tartar emet.); hot, dry and red skin all over the body; ulcers full of serum; *ulcers* dry with overhanging edges, a bright red inflamed areola, hard *dark spot* in *center;* under skin is found a hard, movable knot, like a corn with a small ulcerated spot in the middle; the hard, knotty spot remaining after the ulcer healed; skin rough in ridges."

First, for *simple ulcers* with the peculiar *smooth edges* and the sticky exudation. All the more indicated if the *cause* of the *ulcers* is syphilis. *Lupus,* of the sluggish variety, painless, indolent (Graph., Ars., Mez.). Occasionally for *measles* with low temperature; conjunctivitis; with the stringy, tough discharge from nose and throat; the hoarse, croupy cough (Elephantiasis).

Joints.

Back and Extrem.: "Periodical wandering pains along the bones; cracking in joints agg. motion; stiffness of shoulder joint; violent aching pain, like a gathering in small spots in sacrum, a steady throbbing pain agg. night hindering sleep amel. in day, when up, and walking about."

Now and then for *neuralgia* of *sacrum* and *coccyx.* For *syphilitic periostitis* with the wandering pains along the bones. For sciatica of the left side amel. walking and bending the leg, agg. lying, standing, sitting and from pressure. For *rheumatism* which usually comes in the *spring*.

The make-up is your ranking symptom in this group, *viz.*, *fat, fair, sluggish.*

I never derived any benefit from the medium potencies. Use the 2d or 3d or the 1m.

KALI BROMATUM.

Make-up—Loc.: *Brain* and *Nerves* of *spine;* skin.

Sen.: Aching; restlessness; nervousness.

Mod.: Agg. *Sexual excesses;* mental exertions; emotions. Amel. When occupied.

Leaders: Depressive delusions; hebetude.

Brain and Nerves.

Mind: "Inability to express oneself; weak, so that in talking substituted one word ending in 'tion' for another; memory lost, with amnesic aphasia (Cannabis ind.) for single word or one syllable is constantly dropped, or two words are always interchanged; delirium."

For *various forms* of mania, 1st, *Acute mania* when the *patient* is *sleepless,* easily *excited,* afraid of being poisoned (Hyoscyamus); is being pursued (Belladonna); 2d, *Suicidal* mania with mental degeneration; the trembling of the muscles and weakness (Argentum nit.).

Profound melancholia with marked excitability, full of all sorts of *delusions* especially *religious; night terrors* of children after being *frightened,* when the child *wakes* up *shrieking* and *trembling* (Stramonium).

Cerebral anemia with coldness, at first excitability, but soon changing to drowsiness and even coma, with twitching of the muscles (Belladonna for hyperemia).

As you all know the other school uses it in massive doses to suppress epileptic convulsions. They do not expect to cure except in a few cases. They admit that it is a choice of two evils, viz., the continued attacks or cerebral degeneration.

There is only one sadder sight than that of a patient gradually sinking into idiocy under the influence of Kali brom. and epilepsy and that is of a patient rotting under Mercurius and syphilis.

But some cases of epilepsy are cured by massive doses of the Bromide of Potash; and some cases are also cured by the potentized drug. When the convulsions are severe and the *effects* on the mind as stated above, *come early,* especially for women when the attacks come at time of the menses, when there is increased sexual appetite, often ovaralgia and marked acne, Kali brom. will cure in massive doses and also in the 30th. Next to Lachesis, it has done more for me in what I call "menstrual epilepsy" than any other drug.

Throat: "*Anesthesia* of the mouth and throat; *dysphasia* of liquids (infants), can swallow only solids."

Many cases of anesthesia of the mouth and throat, the result of excesses in alcoholic beverages, have been helped by the drug in the 3rd. In this same line persistent hiccough has been cured when due to the excessive use of tobacco.

Sexual Organs: "Excitement during partial slumber agg. in bed usually with erections and emissions which awake him; appetite diminished, then lost; debility; impotency."

As you know it is our best remedy for controling the sexual appetite of our soldiers, especially our young married men, when away from home; Clark says, "I have often known a few grains of the salt given at bedtime to permanently relieve youths who were troubled with erections and sexual excitement on going to bed. It might have acted as well in the attenuations but it could not have done better."

It will control exaggerated sexual desire in women who suffer from pruritus. I have frequently used it in the 3rd for extreme nervousness of the extremities, the weakening memory, and insomnia the result of sexual excesses.

Respiratory Organs: "Dry, hacking, paroxysmal, fatiguing cough like whooping cough, agg. night, with difficult respiration."

For *spasmodic croup* recurring *every night;* also for the same cough of drinkers and smokers.

Skin.

"Acne on forehead and cheeks; acne pimples with yellow tips."

Kali brom. is one of our best remedies for *acne which comes* with every *monthly period.* There is but little sensation accompanying it. Also, for the same condition when masturbation is the cause (Caulophylum).

KALI CARB.

Make-up: The t. b. c. diathesis; fair; large.

Loc.: *Muscles* of *heart, uterus* and of lumbar region; *BLOOD;* serous and M.M.

Sen.: *Weak;* sharp; sticking; pulsating.

Mod.: Agg. *COLD; lying on painful side;* 2 to 3 A.M. after labor; during rest.

Amel. Warmth.

Leaders: *The agg. from cold;* little sacks over the eyelids and beneath the eyebrows; pains in the lumbar region.

Kali carb. is the most prominent member of the Kali family in *weakening* the *heart* and *causing* profound *anemia;* also in *promoting* tissue *waste, increasing* the amount of uric acid and *urea.* The patient takes cold easily (Hepar, Hydrastis) hence he dreads a draft of cold air. There is a marked lack of reaction. Owing to the anemia the excreting and secreting glands fail to functionate properly and we have some disturbance in every tissue and organ. Next to Sulphur it is the best general energizer we have. The Kali carb. patient, especially the child, has a lifeless expression, a sickly look, marked pallor, pale lips, haggard and exhausted countenance.

Mucous and Serous Membranes.

Eyes: "White of eye red; capillaries injected; swelling of eyes and lids with pain on reading by candle light; excoriation and suppuration in corners of the eyes."

Useful for many *chronic conditions of* the eye when you have the characteristic *bag-like puffing* of the upper lid. Also for *asthenopia* after these chronic conditions.

Ears: "Tickling, cracking, singing, roaring noises; inflammation and swelling within the ears, with pain about them."

The *chronic otitis* of the drug is usually associated with the same condition of the nose. The pains are sticking and stinging, are from within outward, with much soreness and tenderness about and around the ear (Silica, Tellurium).

Nose: "Thick; red; burning; ulcerative pains in nose; stoppage of; blowing offensive matter from nostrils."

Dry catarrh is the name we give to the above symptoms. In addition, some *hoarseness* and *cough;* also frequent *epistaxis,* the blood being pale, are *accompanying symptoms.*

Throat: "*Mucus agg. in morning* in back of throat only *loosened by much hawking, tenacious* so that it *can* be *neither* completely *swallowed nor hawked up;* sticking in pharynx as from a fish bone (Hepar) if he becomes cold; swallowing difficult, food descends esophagus very slowly."

For *pharyngeal catarrh,* and catarrhal stricture of the esophagus with a feeling of a lump which cannot be swallowed and sticking pains extending to the stomach (Ign.).

Stomach: "Eructations of water after midnight and in the morning; sour eructations; *nausea on* every inward *emotion* but *when fasting* there is only *retching;* nausea as if to faintness, amel. lying down; feeling as if cut to pieces in the morning with *external sensitiveness of the epigastric region; feeling as if full of water;* heavy swollen feeling in epigastric region after eating; uneasiness starting from pit, then eructations of acid food."

Indigestion most frequently calls for Kali carb. The symptoms are ***bloating,*** weak feeling, ***sour eructations;*** sensation of a lump in stomach, pulsations, also soreness (Lycopodium, Calcarea carb.). *Dyspepsia* of *old, weak people.* Ice water or anything cold will agg. the stomach symptoms.

Abdomen: "*Distention of ab.* (Carbo veg.) *after eating* even a little (Lycopodium); incarcerated flatus; *sticking* in the hepatic and inguinal region; in a spot in hepatic region sore to touch; pinching in hepatic region like pleurodynia; pain in liver when walking; heat in liver."

Hahn. tells us that many of the conditions of the drug are accompanied by or caused by *chronic hepatitis.* In addition to the above ab. symptoms the patient has constipation with stools like sheep dung but light in color, the yellow, itching skin, marked agg. from cold air, not much temperature, much flatulency. The sharp sticking pains usually mean *hepatic calculi* or the *after effects* of the same.

Rectum: "Burning and griping in rectum after stools; ineffectual urging with feeling as if the rectum were too weak to expel stool (Hepar); hemorrhoids, swollen, bleeding during natural stool and protruding with a hard stool."

Stools: "Like sheep dung, painful and difficult (Natrum mur.); constipation during menses; stools soft and insufficient."

As stated above the *stools* are *large, hard, light,* and *painful, with chronic* hepatitis also with *chronic dyspepsia,* but occasionally we find a soft, light-colored stool after the two conditions have existed for a long time, either condition indicating a sluggish liver and lack of elimination of bile.

Respiratory Organs: "Easy choking when eating; raw pain in larynx on coughing; cough as early as 3 A.M., repeated every half hour; tickling, suffocative cough that affects the chest, from tickling in the throat (Phosphorus) at 5 A.M. as from dryness of larynx; cough with cramp in the chest so that she could not speak without redness of the face and general sweat; expectoration of small round lumps of mucus

(Stannum); feeling as if there were no air in chest; arrest of breath wakens him at night."

Kali carb. has a very wide field in this section. It has cured many patients, suffering from *subacute or chronic catarrh* of the air passages; *pertussis; asthma; pneumonia; pleurisy;* and *tuberculosis.*

As we have not the time to go into all the symptoms of the six groups let us fix in our minds a few general symptoms, *e. g., the 3 A.M. agg.*, the agg. *from cold* of any kind, viz., air, food, drink, bathing, etc., especially changes of weather; the *scanty difficult expectoration,* viz., little, round balls of mucus sometimes with a little blood in the center; the *sharp, sticking, cutting, pains;* the swelling under the eye-brows. How do I explain the expectorations? The mucus comes from ulcerated surfaces or from small cavities. It is tenacious and torn loose after much coughing and hacking and as it is detached it rolls into balls leaving the part next to the ulcer or raw surface of the cavity (the bloody) in the center. Remember the diathesis also the make-up of the drug. If you bear in mind the modalities, you will never send a Kali carb. patient to the cold North pine woods.

Back and Joints: You will find many symptoms coming from the membranes and coverings of the joints, in fact too many to enumerate. You will note however that they are the sticking, bruised, throbbing, jerking, drawing, etc., which indicate all conditions from a simple irritation to suppuration and sinuses.

Here again your *modalities* are the *ranking symptoms,* but do not forget that the t. b. c. patients often suffer from joint affections.

Heart and Pulse.

"Sticking in the precordial region; anxiety preventing sleep after 2 A.M.; palpitation on least exertion."

You should bear in mind the fact that all potashes have weak hearts so as to advise your patients against undue exertion.

Rarely, you will find a patient will come to you for cardiac inflammation with all the other symptoms of the drug so prominent that it will cure.

Sexual Organs.

Male: "Emissions followed by weakness, desire lost."

These two symptoms appear in the group which indicates that your diathesis has become a dyscrasia.

Female: "Soreness before, during and after the menses; menses too early, too profuse and too long lasting (China, Calcarea carb.); menses acrid causing soreness and eruption of the thighs."

For *menorrhagia* with the above symptoms; *suppression* of the *menses* with nose bleed (Bryonia), sharp pains in the abdomen, the sour eructations and distended abdomen, sensitiveness to cold and weakness; puerperal metritis with suppression of lochia, distended abdomen (Terebinthina) *not much temperature* and the diarrhea; *threatening abortion* due to the weakness of the uterine muscles. For the last condition the patient should be kept warm in bed for several weeks and given Kali carb. 30th.

Blood.

Anemia, due to the effects of t. b. c., in general and then reaction agg. all the conditions we have enumerated. Sometimes the anemia is associated with or simulates the changes which take place in rheumatism.

KALI CHLORICUM.

Make-up: The typical Kali.

Loc.: *M.M.;* skin; blood.

Sen.: Sticking; burning; aching; smarting.

Mod.: Agg. Jar, cold.
Amel. Nose-bleed.

Leaders: *Gangrenous ulcerations of the mouth*, disorganization of the blood and glandular organs. The chlorate is the most poisonous of all the potashes. It depresses all the vital forces very rapidly, disorganizes the blood, and produces pathological changes in most tissues. You remember I cited its pernicious use as a wash or tablet for sore throat. Let me cite you another case in which it was used, for fibroid tumor, dissolved in water: "Felt dull and stupid; dizzy on stooping and rising; headache over the eyes; objects appeared double beside each other; *face so swollen she could hardly see on rising in the morning;* smarting of tongue; appetite diminished; flatulency of abdomen; urine increased; terrible dreams; great coolness, shivering on cold days; general bloated feeling." Post-mortem of patient who died from taking the drug and who died in convulsions were: "blood disorganized; liver, spleen, and kidneys found softened and filled with the disorganized blood."

I am relating the above facts in order that you may refrain from using the drug in large doses, also that, knowing its ill effects, you may warn your patients and friends against the indiscriminate use of this poison. You ask: "Does it have a place in homeopathic therapeutics?" Yes, very useful in a narrow field, which we will now consider.

Mucous Membrane.

Mouth: "Symmetrical ulcers on the side of the tongue; mucous surface of tongue, mouth and lips covered with follicles and gray based ulcers with the mucous surface red and tumid; salivation acid."

Our most frequent and successful use of the drug is for *stomatitis, aphthous* and *GANGRENOUS*. It was used for the latter form in a large children's home saving over 90 per cent. of the inmates who had it. The symptoms were as follows: "ulceration and sloughing of the mouth and throat; extreme fetor of breath; albumin and blood in the urine; cough; dyspnea; throat red and edematous; submaxillary blands swollen and sore; stools diarrheic sometimes bloody; nose-bleed."

Stools: "Liquid; thin; mucous; blood and mucus mixed."

For dysentery when the stools are almost clear blood (Mercurius cor.); frequent; with great prostration and the severe cutting pains as from knives.

For the stomatitis, use weak solution for a gargle if the child is old enough and a swab if he is not, and the 3rd or 6th internally.

KALI IODATUM.

Make-up: Low vitality; rheumatic.

Loc.: *Glands;* lungs; blood; membranes.

Sen.: Tearing; burning; stitching; constrictive.

Mod.: Agg. *Heat* of room or clothes (Mercury); lying on the affected side.

Amel. Cool air.

Leaders: Allen says: "The use of the drug in massive doses for symptoms of secondary syphilis . . . should not be included under the proper homeopathic application of the drug."

On the other hand, Clark says: "In active secondary syphilis, in ulcers of the constitutional type, and in cases of subacute rheumatism, iodide of potash will generally do what is expected of it. That its action is specific is generally admitted; and *specific* is the same thing as *homeopathic*." Clark then adds, "I rarely find occasion to use it in lower attenuations than the 30th."

I have used it as I use all remedies in various strength according to the temperament of the patients. It has undoubtedly been proven that those patients who are saturated with syphilis or with mercury, or both, will not only need but can stand massive doses which are sometimes given. Harm is frequently done when the salt is given for diagnostic purposes in large doses when the case proves to be non-specific. But as you can get all the pros and cons on the question from the other side, let us take up the study of the drug in our usual way from the homeopathic standpoint.

Glands and Glandular Organs.

It is because of its power to absorb extraneous tissue from glands and glandular organs that has given the drug the title of "The liquid knife." There is no doubt that Kali iod. does absorb gummatous *tumors* of these organs, which includes the brain, presenting certain symptoms. Let us take this location up by sections.

Head: "Stitching on stooping, tearing or jerking sensation in sinuses in the evening, transiently amel. by pressure; *aching* in the sinuses and ethmoid bones; pains in vertex as if it would be forced asunder with external heat in vertex."

You will find that the *drug will absorb* the tumors and *relieve pains* like the above, also frontal headaches due to catarrh when the frontal sinuses and root of the nose are involved. The *pains* are *pulsating, violent,* lancinating, *amel.* in *open air* (Pulsatilla, Kali bich.) *and pressure* (Gelsemium Silica).

Salivary Gland: Bloody saliva with disgusting taste; salivation (Mercurius); flow of mucus and saliva with offensive odor.

This condition has been most frequently found in the *salivation of pregnant women.*

Liver: For gummata of the liver when there is enlargement, dull or *throbbing,* sticking pain; marked tenderness of liver; hard, lumpy, difficult stools.

Testicles: Compressive pains in the testicles as if being drawn back into pelvis; atrophy of the testicles (Codium, Staphisagria); "Swelling of the thyroid gland with sensitiveness to touch and pressure; swelling and suppurating of the submaxillary glands."

Thyroid and Submaxillary: In all glandular troubles which are non-syphilitic, the action is much less violent than Iodium but not so slow as Baryta or Calcarea carb.

Lungs.

Trachea and Larynx: "Voice lost; dry cough morning and evening with soreness of larynx; short hacking cough from rawness in throat; dyspnea on ascending stairs, with pain in region of the heart; short breath."

Three conditions in this section: *catarrh* of the *larynx* where there is *rawness* and *soreness* as if the parts were *granulated*. For *asthma* and a *catarrhal cough*. With the asthma and catarrhal cough you also have rawness and the sense of granulation but an *expectoration like soap-suds,* which is the *ranking symptom* of the group.

Chest: "*Sticking* deep in middle of chest; in right costal region behind the sternum agg. evening; *sore* pain in upper part of chest when sitting bent over, amel. becoming erect; amel. moving about; soreness in middle of sternum, extending to shoulders; pain as if cut to pieces; oppression."

The condition in this section for which I have received the most help is that of *pleuritic exudation* following a severe attack of acute pleurisy when there was marked dyspnea, a constant hacking, distressing cough, agg. lying on painful side and the agg. of the already short breath on suddenly lying down. It has obviated the necessity of aspirating or other method of evacuating the exudate in many cases and assisted in absorbing what remained after operating, in a few cases.

It has also been used for *hydrothorax; chronic pneumonia* with the general catarrhal symptoms of the nose and throat, also *pneumonia* associated with the pleuritic effusion as stated above if you have the profuse exhausting night sweat (China) and salivation, with dyspnea. You note that the conditions are very similar to those of Iodatum but there is far less temperature and emaciation.

Blood.

A *condition* which *simulates gonorrheal* or *syphilitic rheumatism.* We find the *subacute* variety both *articular* and *neu-*

ralgic; the pains are always agg. at night (Mercurius); very little temperature; a good deal of swelling especially of the joints; the pains are boring, worse at night, driving the patient out of bed and causing him to walk about.

KALI MURIATICUM.

Make-up: The potash, *i. e.,* all complexion and build.

Loc.: Connective tissue; epithelium, glands.

Sen.: Snapping; lightning like; swollen.

Mod.: Agg. rich, fat food or pastry (Pulsatilla); motion; warmth of bed; in morning.

Leaders: *Light-color* of tissues, of eruptions, of exudations, of secretions; toughness, of exudate, blood clots too quickly, hence embolism, hard swelling, etc.

We are indebted to Schuessler for introducing this drug to the profession and for many of its symptoms. Kali mur. has not been proven to any extent. Schuessler says of it: "It is contained in nearly all the cells and is chemically related to fibrin. It will dissolve white or grayish-white secretions of the mucous membrane and plastic exudations." Again: "When the cells of the epidermis lose molecules of Kali mur. in consequence of a morbid irritation, then the fibrin comes to the surface as a white or whitish-gray mass; when dried this forms a mealy covering. If the irritation has seized upon the tissues under the epidermis, then fibrin and serum are exuded, causing the affected spots on the epidermis to rise in blisters. Similar processes take place in and below the epithelial cells."

All that I can give you is based upon the indications given by Schuessler and records of cases reported in our journals.

Ears: "Snapping and noises in the ears; deafness; swelling of the external ear; cracking noises on blowing the nose."

It is for curing *chronic, obstinate ear troubles* that the drug has won its reputation. My teacher, Professor Houghton, gives the following group: "*Proliferous inflammation of the middle ear,* with obstruction of the Eustachian tube; retraction of the drum which is lighter in color than normal; exfoliation of the epithelial layer of the tympanum; dull pain in the ear; deafness; sore throat and swelling of the glands about the ear." Dr. H. advised the use of the 3rd and 6th.

Eyes: "Discharges from the eyes of white mucus; yellow or greenish matter; sacks of matter on lids; feeling of sand in the eyes."

Our eye specialist praises it as a remedy for *inflammation* of the eyes of *scrofulous persons;* for *Kerato-iritis* with *pus* in the *anterior chamber;* for *choroi-retinitis* with hazy, vitreous, and parenchymatous keratitis. With most of these conditions you have the catarrhal conditions of nose and throat.

Nose: "Stuffy cold in head with thick white phlegm in nostrils."

For nasal catarrh.

Throat: "Tonsils excessively swollen; swallowing very painful, even water; tough stringy whitish mucus; hawks up offensive, cheesy mucus in small lumps."

We have found that with the above we usually have sneezing and sometimes profuse secretions of mucus.

Skin: "Dry flour-like scales on skin; eruptions on skin, white contents."

For *eczema,* albuminoid and other eruptions *resulting* from *vaccination* with bad lymph (Thuja); also from *suppressed menses* or other deranged uterine function. With these conditions you always get enlargement and sometimes suppuration of the glands which drain the affected area.

Schuessler gives *abscesses, boils, carbuncles,* erysipelas, *herpes, ulcerations* and *warts,* but the drug has not been well enough proven to verify such claims. There is one condition, however, in which Schuessler claims it to be a specific, for which I feel he is justified in doing if he will specify the symptoms. I refer to *epilepsy* of *extremely nervous children who suffer from dyspepsia, with urticaria* as the *ranking symptoms,* or when such children have had the peculiar eruption of the drug suppressed by mercurial or other ointments or washes, then he will be perfectly justified in the claim. Use any preparation from the 3rd to 30th.

KALI PHOSPHORICUM.

Make-up: *Neurotic.*

Loc.: According to Schuessler, *cells* of *brain*, nerves, muscles, blood, and *intercellular fluids.*

Sen.: Morose; irritable; tearful; burning; soreness.

Mod.: Agg. after eating; before menses; by cold; noise; when tired.

Amel. Out of doors; pressing temples; when the menstrual flow begins.

Leaders: *Kali phos.* is the *great American remedy* for the brain and nerves. You remember I told you that Nux was the great American remedy for diseases of the digestive tract because of what and how the American people eat and drink. In the same manner no people abuse their brains and nerves as do the Americans. Everything, our education, our business, our pleasure, we rush at a killing pace under the highest excitement. As a food to nourish our brain and nerves under such conditions or as a remedy to restore them after the collapse Kali phos. has no equal. This statement is proven by symptoms produced and by confirmation of the work of the provers.

Because I know he will help you understand its action, I will again quote Schuessler: "Disturbance in the motions of its molecules produces: (1) In thought cells: Despondency, anxiety, fearfulness, tearfulness, home-sickness, agraphobia, weak memory. (2) In vaso-motor nerves: First small and frequent pulse; later retarded. (3) In sensory nerves: Pains with sensation of paralysis. (4) In trophic fibers of Sympathetic Nerve: Retarded nutrition; even total arrest in a limited area of cells and then softening."

Taking the above as a basis and guide Schuessler outlines

the numerous conditions for which Kali phos. is indicated and will relieve.

I will give you from this long list the conditions I have relieved and then we will group the symptoms for each. They are: *Hypochondriasis; brain-fag;* nervous insomnia; hysteria and that other undefinable condition *neurasthenia;* syncope: adynamic typhoid fever; nervous dyspepsia, etc.

Brain and Nerves.

Mind: "Morose; irritable; tearful (Pulsatilla); aversion to being talked to (Ignatia); flies into a passion and can hardly articulate (Platinum); easily startled; cruel to husband, to baby; apprehensive; completely exhausted after moderate mental effort (Picric acid)."

For *hypochondriasis* when the patient *wants* to *be by himself,* objects to being advised, *insists he is all right,* has light-colored offensive stools, *emissions without erections;* urine scanty and loaded with phosphates; is chilly; has a cold moist skin, with *offensive sweat.*

Brain fag of business men with *insomnia,* cannot get to sleep till toward morning and then they soon become covered with a light but cold, clammy sweat; awake unrefreshed with a foul breath, brown-coated tongue, no appetite; trembling of hands; profuse, painless, urgent stool on waking; spine sensitive to touch. You get the same group from women, mothers who have worried through a long sickness of a babe (Cocculus), or society women who have gone through the season of excitement, etc. These women in addition to the symptoms mentioned for men will have irregularities of menses, usually amenorrhea, and the occipital headache (Picric ac.) and vertigo (Cocculus). For insomnia *with* an *active mind.* The patients take their sorrows, their pleasures or their business to bed with them (Scutellaria, Coffea). When they do sleep, they dream lascivious dreams, talk in their dreams, are sometimes hard to waken, but when wakened are cross, peevish, or angry because they were awakened. Sometimes they awake startled and are surprised that burglars are not in the house.

Hysteria when the patient laughs and cries, shuts herself up in a room and moans and sobs, covers herself with bed clothes and screams, trembles and shakes so she wants to be held, voids urine in small amount every few minutes, has globus hystericus; feeling as if tongue cleaved to the roof of the mouth. The patient is readily startled into any or all of the above by a noise or touch.

Head: "Woke with pain in occiput and loins, amel. lying on back, passed off after rising; violent tearing pain in forehead and sense of fatigue before the menses, amel. lying down and on menses appearing."

Kali phos. will help those intense *headaches* which *result* from deep *emotions* and physical efforts. In addition to the local symptoms given above you have the *insomnia* of the drug and the menstrual irregularities. The *pains* are *amel.* by a *good sleep,* by being out in the fresh, open air, by nourishing, easily digested food and by gentle motion or massage. The agg. are from bright sun or light, noise, pressure, violent motion and at night. The menstrual headache is the most frequent (Actea, Sanguinaria, Natrum mur. and Sepia).

Eyes: "Eyes twitch; tire with reading; eyes blurred; black spots moving before eyes; a throbbing pain in eyes agg. sunlight; eye balls ache and are tender." We have *weakness* and in some cases *paralysis* when due to sexual excesses which yield to the remedy. *"Water secretions"* is the ranking symptom of these groups. You will find the tired feeling and weakness of the legs second in importance. I have found it useful for newly married people who come to me for the weakness of the eyes.

Ears: "Fulness; singing; surging; cannot endure noises; yellow discharge from ruptured drum."

The *otalgia* and *otitis* are frequently found in Kali phos. patients. The fulness is the *symptom* which is marked in the otitis preceding otorrhea.

Extrem.: "Back lame as from a fall, with pains extending down into the legs; fidgety feet (Zinc. val.); twitching in muscles of arms and legs; *weak, tired feeling,* amel. by gentle motion."

The above you will find distributed in the other groups, simply signifying the low tone of the nervous system.

Sexual Organs: "Sexual instinct depressed; impotence; emissions without erections; utter *prostration and weak vision* after coition; stitching all through the pelvis and uterus; pain in the left side and ovary, shooting across the sacrum to right ovary; sharp bearing down pains during menses; sense of fatigue after menses (Picric ac.)."

Occasionally useful for *ovaralgia* and *ovaritis* but most useful for irregular menses and the prostration which follows.

In men, we find complete loss of power in most cases. As this is usually caused by excess, the history will show that there was at the beginning increased passion, sometimes priapism. Under the term *excess* I include masturbation as well as coition.

Mucous Membranes.

There is but little under this heading but you will find that what *catarrhal discharges* there are have a *yellow* color. In fact Kali phos. is a *picture* in *yellow* as Kali mur. was a *picture* in gray or white. I use Kali phos. in the 3rd in most cases. The 30th for extremely nervous people.

CAUSTICUM.

Causticum belongs to the potash group, being a solution of potassium hydrate.

Make-up: Weak; low vitality; anemic; no ambition.

Loc.: Brain and nerves; muscles of bladder and respiration, M. M.

Sen.: Weakness; suffocation, trembling; sharp.

Mod.: Agg. *cold,* dry *winds;* drafts; 3 to 4 A.M.

Amel.: A cup of cold water.

Leaders: Warmth of bed; paralysis of various parts; spurting of the urine when coughing (Pulsatilla, Drosera).

Brain and Nerves.

Mind: "Morose, apprehensive whenever anything happens; inattention and distraction; absent-minded."

The Causticum patients are slow in learning to walk and talk. The older patients are weak and anemic, having no desire and but little ability to undertake anything either mental or physical.

Eyes: "*Lids involuntarily close* (Rhus tox., Sepia), *heaviness* of the *upper lids* as if they were agglutinated to the lower and could not be easily loosened; *photophobia* with necessity to wink."

One of our best remedies for *weakness* and even *paralysis* of the upper lids, caused from *taking cold* or after *scarlet fever*. It may cause *asthenopia*. There is much inflammation of the lids and *a sensation* of *sand under* the *lids*. *Causticum* has *often arrested cataract*. *Diplopia due* to the *paralysis* of ocular muscles. Vision dim, agg. turning eyes to the right.

Ears: "*Re-echoing* of her *own words* and steps, also of sounds with difficult hearing; roaring in ears."

Causticum has checked the progress of *Meniere's disease* when the ranking symptom was the re-echoing of one's own voice, the second symptom in importance being *vertigo*. Amel. getting up from the reclining position in P.M.

Face: "Tension and pain in the jaws so that they were difficult to open; difficulty in eating; *rheumatism of* lower jaw."

Very often useful for *neuralgia* of the face of rheumatic patients. The cause being exposure to cold air, agg. damp cold.

Throat: "Tension in throat; sensation of tightness and suffocation, obliging him to open the neck band (Lachesis)."

Paralysis of the muscles of the throat after scarlet fever and from taking cold.

Stools: "Frequent ineffectual urging; stool passed better when partially standing."

Paralysis.

Urinary Organs: "Micturition so easy he is not sensible of the stream, and can hardly believe in the dark that he is micturating; involuntary mic. while coughing and blowing the nose (Pulsatilla, Phosphorus, Zinc.); involuntary at night in sleep."

There are two conditions I have frequently verified: 1st, *nocturnal enuresis,* where the child wets the bed as soon as he falls asleep (Ignatia) and the spurting of urine every time the patient moves the abdominal muscles of the abdomen; 2d, for retention of urine after labor.

Respiratory Organs: "Muscles of larynx do not perform their function and inability to speak a loud word; hoarseness agg. morning and evening, arrest of breath while speaking or walking rapidly; irritation to cough agg. in the morning, with every inspiration."

This is one of the most important sections of this location. We often cure *aphonia caused* by *taking cold.* The *aphonia may be complete or* we may *have partial paralysis* of the cords, so that he strikes an octave above or below what he tried for. It is a grand remedy for difficulty of voice of singers, and public speakers (Phosphorus, Alumina, Nux vom.).

For a nervous cough, with spurting of the urine agg. by warmth of bed, *amel.* by *sips of cold water.*

Back and Extrem.: "Drawing, bruised pain in region of coccyx; tearing now in one joint now in another, at one time severe, at another slight; uneasiness in the morning in bed; weakness and trembling."

The trouble is more that of paralysis though there may be some rheumatism. The leading symptoms of the group are *drawing* or sense of shortness of the tendons and muscles and the trembling indicating partial paralysis. The agg. are motion; cold, damp; storms (Rhus tox., Rhododendron).

Mucous Membrane.

Eyes: "Pain, agg. touch; *sensation as from sand* (Natrum mur.); *rubbing* and *burning with dryness* and *photophobia;* itching agg. open air."

With the ptosis and disturbances of vision we frequently have *blepharitis,* agg. in open air and *granular lids.*

Nose: *We have a* dry, catarrhal *condition* of the nose usually with the coryza, frequent sneezing, and stopped up feeling. It usually follows an acute laryngitis and pharyngitis. You will find ulcers in which the discharge has dried into crusts.

Throat: "Hawking of clots of *mucus which* he *cannot* loosen enough to *get up* but *must swallow,* with pain in the throat pit."

Catarrhal *laryngitis* and *pharyngitis* with the *inability* to *get under* it and expectorate it (Kali carb.).

Rectum and Anus: "Frequent sudden pressing-piercing pain in rectum; frequent and ineffectual urging (Nux vom., Silica); hemorrhoids with sore pain on walking; H. with itching, sticking pain and moisture about anus, agg. walking, at stool (Æsculus, Silica)."

The only use you will make of Causticum here is for *hemorrhoids* with fissures, sometimes fistulas which interfere with passage of stool (Silica).

Female Genital Organs: "Biting in pudenda as from salt during and after micturition; leucorrhea flowing like menses and of same color."

For leucorrhea with the above symptoms in weak debilitated patients, *great weakness* and *agg. night.*

CALCAREA.

The **calcarea group** is without question the *most important* of any group of our materia medica. I am speaking of groups not of single remedies. Calcarea carb., Sulphur and Lycopodium form the great trio of antipsorics. The *calcarea com-*

pounds have an elective affinity for and *affect* most profoundly *every tissue* in the body, the blood and through it every secreting gland, the skin, the bones, muscular tissue, etc. etc. All secretions are vitiated, *i. e.,* altered in quantity and quality. The same may be said of all the tissues. The *Calcarea group meets* the wants of persons suffering from any and *all diathesis,* the rachitic, the scrofular, the tubercular, the rheumatic, the neurotic, etc., etc. The dyscrasias the group produces are most profound, *e. g.*, cavities in the lungs, caries of the bones, especially the vertebræ, caseating and suppurating glands, leucocytosis, profound anemia, etc. The group comprises all the modalities. Calcarea carb. is the most important of the group and its preparation is the best proof of the genius of Hahnemann as a chemist.

CALCAREA CARBONICA.

Make-up: "*Fat, fair, flabby* and *forty; bone tissue* too soft and *not properly distributed;* muscles soft and flabby; glands prominent."

Loc.: Glands; bone; muscles; female generative organs; and mucous membranes.

Sen.: "Cold; clammy; pulsating; weak; faint."

Mod.: Agg. from *cold; damp, cold;* working in water; at full moon; after eating; exertion, both physical and mental.

Amel. by inspiring fresh, dry air; after breakfast; in open air.

Characteristics: Big head; large; abdomen with stomach like an inverted saucer; *profuse, sour sweat about head and shoulders;* enlarged glands; cold, clammy feet; mind sluggish.

Glands.

Throat: "*Swelling of submaxillary glands* as large as hen's eggs, hard, with painful tension when chewing and sticking pains in when touched; swelling of tonsils, with elongation of uvula and feeling when swallowing as if throat were too narrow."

Abdomen: "*Swelling of inguinal glands* with pains; sensation as if inguinal glands were swollen; induration of the *hepatic region;* swelling and induration of the mesenteric glands."

Neck and Trunk: "*Hard* and *painful swelling* of *glands* of neck; pain in glands on turning head as if a tumor or boil would protrude; hard and strumous swelling of the *thyroid* gland; tumor between the shoulder blades; *suppuration* of the *axillary glands.*"

The *lymphatic glands* are those *most affected.* All glandular inflammations develop slowly. The glands are hard and the surface without discoloration till suppuration takes place. *After* pus forms and is evacuated the *hardness* and *swelling disappear slowly.* Often *fistulas remain.* You should not expect rapid results from the exhibition of Calcarea carb. and especially is this true of the glandular Calcarea carb. patients. I have given Calcarea carb. five to eight weeks to patients before either suppuration or absorption of the enlarged glands began. *Heat has* but *little effect* towards hastening suppuration but I am sure that the application of Iodine does hasten absorption. The Calcarea carb. glands are the only ones for which an early incision is not indicated and beneficial. If you assist the eliminative organs while giving Calcarea carb., the ill effects of absorption seem less than the effects from long draining through the fistulas which follow incisions of spontaneous evacuation. For this reason, unless the amount of pus be large, I begin with the 30th or 200th and wait for absorption.

Bones.

Head: From the nature of the case the symptoms we have for this locality are for the most part clinical. They are found in new born babes and in the first few years of childhood. There is plenty of bone material in the skull of the new born babe but it is not properly distributed or of proper quality. As the result, the bones are too thick in spots and none of the fontanelles are properly closed. The outer surfaces of the bones are spongy. Pressure, as from forceps, leaves a deformity.

Neck and Back: Because of the peculiar composition of the bone, the vertebræ being softer in some parts than others, there is pressure which causes irritation, inflammation, functional and structural changes which take place in all forms of curvature of the spine. Given early it will prevent many cases; given later it will check the disease and relieve the symptoms of pressure upon the spinal cord and nerves which cause so much suffering in these cases. Do not misunderstand me to mean by the above that Calcarea carb. will make indispensable plaster paris casts, braces, etc., used to correct curvatures of the spine, but it will in many cases assist them in securing the desired effects.

Extremities: The bones of the extremities are large, soft and, as in other parts, the material improperly distributed. The ends of the bones are not provided with the amount and quality of cartilage. The results are bow legs, large joints which easily suppurate.

Female Generative Organs.

"Menses too early and too profuse; menstruation delayed; menses suppressed; sterility; metrorrhagia; leucorrhea like milk during micturition; leucorrhoea with burning and itching."

The mental symptoms of Calcarea carb. are most pronounced just before the menses. They are "depression," "melancholia;" "*fear* of *going crazy* or that something dreadful is going to happen." The head symptoms which accompany the menses are "rush of blood to head with heat in it;" and "fulness." We also have the cold, clammy extremities.

I want to call your attention to the expression "delayed menstruation." I have found it in a group of symptoms exhibited by young women at the age of puberty, the diagnosis being incipient tuberculosis. If in addition to that symptom, you have the make-up of Calcarea carb., a variable and unnatural appetite, a night cough with expectoration of sweetish mucus, full feeling in and at times bleeding from the lungs, and marked anemia, you will get wonderful results. The breasts have developed and all other signs of maturing are present but the menses do not appear. Use the 30th for this condition. After the menses appear you may expect them to reappear too often and the flow to be too profuse. Attention to the patient's diet is a very essential auxiliary to the remedy in the treatment of these cases. I have cured two cases of *membranous dysmenorrhea* with the 30th. One was also a case of sterility and two children have been born since the cure.

Calcarea carb. is a good remedy *to modify* both the quantity and quality of *milk*. When the flow of milk is excessive, the child does not like it or does not thrive on it, the use of the 6th or 30th of Calcarea carb. will often secure the desired result. Give it three times daily for three or four weeks.

Mucous Membranes.

Eye: "Sensation as if sand or foreign body were under the lids; itching, swelling, redness and nightly agglutination of lids; during the day lids full of gummy matter with heat, smarting pains and tears."

For *scrofulous ophthalmia* and all sorts of *inflammation* resulting from *working in water*.

Ear: "Crushing; pulsating; cracking when chewing."

For chronic, scrofulous inflammation of the ear; deafness from working in water; for thickening of eardrum; mucopurulent inflammation, light colored discharge like paper wads. Sometimes polypi which are very sensitive and bleed profusely.

Nose: "Sore, ulcerated nostrils preceded by frequent sneezing; sneezing without coryza; fluent coryza; smell before nose as of bad eggs or gunpowder."

For chronic catarrh, nasal polypi and inclination to epistaxis in fat children who suffer from congestive headaches.

Stomach: "Loss of appetite, but when he begins to eat relishes food; empty eructations tasting of food; *nausea caused by milk;* nausea with flow of sour water from the mouth; *vomiting* of *sour water;* pressure in pit as if lump were in it."

For chronic, *acid dyspepsia* and *fermentation*, when everything turns sour. Calcarea carb. patients usually have enormous appetites and great thirst. They eat and drink to excess and *crave* all sorts of *undigestible things*. Everything taken ferments, causing distention, eructation and belching.

Abdomen: "Distention; hardness; pinching, griping, tensive pains in ab.; colic with cramp-like, gnawing, contractive pains in P.M. with vomiting of food which has soured."

For chronic entero-colitis with vomiting of sour matter, food, mucus, or both.

Anus and Stools: "Hemorrhoids protruding and swollen, causing pain even with a soft stool; burning during stool; stools at first hard then soft and pasty, sometimes perfectly white, always sour and terribly offensive."

For diarrhea stools large and as stated above; for ascarides with the enormous appetite and the diarrhea.

Bladder: "Frequent micturition at night; urine dark colored, without sediment; *urine sour smelling* at night."

For an inflamed, irritable bladder when the urine is abundant, fetid and *sour*.

Respiratory Organs: "*Painless hoarseness* so that she was unable to speak, worse in morning; cough at night; cough from a feeling as if a plug stuck in the throat and moved up and down; cough with the expectoration of sweetish mucus, worse at night; expectoration of blood and hawking with a rough and sore sensation in chest; respiration short on going up a slight ascent; urgent necessity to take a deep breath which caused sticking in chest."

For chronic *bronchitis* with hoarseness; tubercular diathesis when the upper part of the lungs is affected. With all conditions the symptom "Respiration short on going up slightest ascent" is the most prominent. You will also find that the expectoration is most free in the morning, while the cough is more troublesome during the night. The Calcarea carb. patients always perspire freely and lose weight rapidly in spite of the fact that they consume an enormous amount of food. Potency from high 1 m to 3rd.

Muscles.

Back: "Pressure between the shoulders which impedes respiration, worse from motion; pain in the lumbar region so that he can scarcely rise from a seat."

Extremities: "Cramp of entire arm; spasmodic tearing pain of forearm; swelling of the finger joints; swelling of knee; tearing and stitching in the patella on stepping when beginning to walk; weakness of legs and ankles as if they could not bear the body."

The muscles are always large but flabby. The patient is lazy, slow in his motion, which is often due to rheumatism of the muscles. The Calcarea carb. patient is some like the Rhus tox. patient in that he is stiff on beginning to walk but with Calcarea carb. the stiffness gives way to weariness.

CALCAREA PHOSPHORICA

Make-up: *Dirty white,* anemic, weak mentally, *poorly nourished.*

Loc.: *Brain* and nerve, bone.

Sen.: *Aching;* weak; colicky; sharp.

Mod.: Agg. from motion, thinking, wet, teething.
Amel. from rest.

As malnutrition is the key note of this calcarea, I would call your attention to its effect, especially on the bones and brain, as we study the drug.

Bones.

Head: The trouble here is not *improper distribution* of a sufficient supply but the *deficiency of supply.* The bones are not only too thin but too small. They feel like parchment paper and do not cover the brain so that the fontanelles are as wide open as in Calcarea carb.

Neck: The bones are so small that they do not support the head which is always abnormally large.

Extremities: The bones of the legs are so small and weak that the child cannot walk.

There is another use I have often made of the remedy, viz., to help unite fractured bones. I consider Calcarea phos. 3x or 6x second only to Symphytum to assist the union of bones. Calcarea phos. has absorbed nodular tumors of the bones which were very hard and painful.

Brain and Nerves.

The child's brain is proportionately too large for the rest of the body. The brain substance is also abnormal. The result is that the child is peevish, fretful and slow of comprehension. You may have cretinism.

Head: "Crawling as if ice were on upper part of occiput; head is hot, with smarting at the roots of hairs; aching worse after dinner, from exertion, on going into the open air."

The following constitute a group of symptoms which the remedy has helped. An anemic school girl, with dirty white skin, blue eyes, large head, at the age of puberty. She is backward in her studies but ambitious so that she studies hard to make her grades. The *result* is the *hot, aching head, icy cold feet, unusual hunger* for indigestible things, dyspepsia with an indescribable feeling in stomach, which is only temporarily relieved by eating; *green, undigested,* offensive *stools,* expelled with much flatus, and frequent, copious urination. If menstruation has been established the menses are too profuse and painful. For such a condition, known as "*school girl's headache,*" no remedy equals Calcarea phos. in the 3rd, 6th and 30th.

The next in frequency is a condition known as *hydrocephaloid, e. g.,* large head, thin bones, open fontanelles, peevish and irritable disposition, irritable stomach with abnormal desire and cravings, flatulency and the peculiar diarrhoea. These conditions are most frequently congenital but may follow exhausting diseases, like cholera infantum, typhoid fever and pertussis. For this condition I have found the 30th the best.

CALCAREA ARSENICOSA

Thermic Centers: This is what I call the kidney member of the family because it seems to act more intensely on this organ than any other. The next most important location is the thermic centers. The *Arsenicum* of the compound seems to have *eliminated* the *action* of *Calcarea on the bones.* It has also taken the cold producing properties out of the thermic center. I have in mind three marked cases of nephritis cured by the remedy. Two of the cases followed scarlitina, one measles. The symptom present in all three cases was "*SENSITIVENESS TO PRESSURE IN KIDNEY REGION.*" (So marked was this that the mother said she had wakened the child by putting her hand on the region unintentionally.) All three complained bitterly when even moderate pressure was made on the region. There was urging to urinate; *urine bloody, scanty,* and *highly albuminous;* temperature from 103 to 105.5; great restlessness and in one case delirium; great *thirst* and *vomiting;* dark, watery stools. All three were of the Calcarea carb. build. Two of them I saw in consultation after Arsenicum alb. in different potencies had utterly failed. Calcarea ars. 6th cured rapidly. The temperature fell, the restlessness ceased and finally the urinary symptoms disappeared.

CALCAREA IODATUM

This is the *dark complexioned* member of the family. It is also the *high temperature* member. The skin is not only dark but dry. It is also the *emaciated. skinny* member. The *glands* for which the Iodatum has a special affinity are the *mesenteric* and mammary. The *diathesis* is the *t. b. c.* Although the remedy has been used successfully for uterine fibroid, mollities ossium, tumors of the breasts and flatulent dyspepsia, the most frequent use I have made of it is for *enteritis* and *enterocolitis of tubercular patients.* The condition *usually follows* some *acute* attack like *cholera infantum.* The symptoms are: "Child dark, very emaciated; nothing but skin and bones; *abdomen enormously enlarged* (child looks like a young robin before its feathers have grown); hectic; a chronic cough, with expectoration, green and purulent if the child can raise it, rattling in chest if he cannot; with frequent green or varying colored, watery, mushy stools accompanied by much flatus; *skin* very *dry except* for the *night sweats.* Give Calcarea iod. 3x or 6x every few hours. Use pure cod liver oil by inunction. Use butter fats freely. Wash out the lower bowels every day or two with a normal salt solution of the temperature of the body. By the above treatment a good per cent. of apparently hopeless cases may be saved. Just one word in closing about the tumors of the breasts. They are nodular, freely movable, very tender to touch and excruciatingly painful when moving the arms; worse before menses.

CALCAREA FLUORICA

This is Schuessler's bone salt, found in the surface of bones and the periosteum. It has been used for bone tumors and other affections of the bones, *e. g.*, syphilitic swelling of the periosteum, want of or early decay of enamel or the teeth; also for induration of the glands which are of stony hardness until they break down and suppurate freely.

Better from warmth, worse from cold are marked modalities. I have used it frequently for the enamel of the teeth. For the bony tumors I prefer Calcarea phos. The most frequent as well as the most successful use I have made of the remedy is to cure patients of tendency to whitlow and to abate and relieve the pain of whitlow. For the first condition use the 30th once daily for two or three months; for the others use the 6th or 12th every few hours. I also use dilute fluoric acid locally while giving the remedy internally for the two latter conditions.

NATRUM CARBONICUM.

Make-up: Emaciated; anemic; light haired; leuco-phlegmatic constitution; lazy both mentally and physically.

Loc.: M. M.; digestive organs.

Sen.: Nausea, retching, distress, weak.

Mod.: Agg. from *heat* of sun and hot weather; errors of diet; *milk;* drafts.

Amel. Motion; mental exertion.

Mucous Membrane.

Eyes: "Burning in eyes agg. reading and writing, with dryness as if she had wept much; dryness and heat; ulcers about the corners, with stinging in eye so that she must shade it."

There are only two uses I have ever made of Natrum carb. for eye trouble, viz., dry *catarrh* and ulceration of the cornea. The indications for it in catarrh are the *burning* and *dryness* of the conjunctiva (Alumina). All such cases had the catarrhal nose group associated with the eye. For corneal ulceration in addition to the *burning* and dryness may be found photophobia with stinging, biting pains. I once took a case to Dd. Woodburn which he diagnosed "*ulcerative keratitis.*" He used Natrum carb. with his local treatment and cured the child.

Nose: "Ulcers high up in nostrils; stoppage with hard

offensive pieces from one nostril; *much nasal mucus passes through the mouth;* discharge of thin, yellow, offensive mucus; fluent, intermittent, stopped coryza; bleeding."

The Natrum carb. patient takes cold easily and has first a fluent coryza, then free during the day but stopped at night. Later the discharge becomes thicker, yellow, offensive. Much of it is post-nasal. The patients take cold from the slightest cause.

Throat: "*Violent hawking of thick mucus, that constantly collects again* (Calcarea carb., Pulsatilla); swelling of the submaxillary glands."

Stomach: "*Sour,* empty *eructations;* waterbrash; ineffectual retching in the morning; weak and easily disordered; scraping heartburn after fat food (Pulsatilla)."

I have found the above symptoms in *indigestion* when milk and fat would cause the *sour eructations* sometimes *vomiting, palpitation* and *distress about* the *heart.* The *stools* which were usually hard balls *became watery* at such times, preceded by cutting in abdomen and followed by burning in the rectum and sinking in the hypogastrium.

NATRUM MURIATICUM.

Make-up: Scorbutic diathesis; tired; dirty.

Loc.: Brain; *blood;* muscles; heart; glands.

Sen.: Tired; weak; chilly; throbbing.

Mod.: Agg. Heat of sun; hot weather; puberty; 9–11 A.M.
Amel. Open air; cool bathing.

Leaders: Craving salt; *herpes about lip,* dryness.

Brain and Nerves.

Mind: "**Excited**; *sad, weeping mood* the more he was consoled the worse he was affected (Ignatia); sad all day, apprehensive; disheartened, with palpitation; despair that deprived him of all power; easily startled; ill humor; anger at trifles; disinclined to mental work."

Very useful for *brain fag, hysteria* and *melancholia.* The *brain fag* group includes the ill humor, *disinclination* and inability to work, indifference; impaired memory and occasionally numbness of the extremities (Picric ac., Zinc.).

Only occasionally useful in *hysteria.* You have alternating *weeping* and laughter; menses delayed and painful; profuse, greenish acrid leucorrhea with smarting, itching; also constipation. Most frequently useful for school girls.

The *melancholia* is also more frequently found at *puberty* and the *menopause.* With the *sadness* and *weeping* you have the throbbing, heavy pain in the occiput (Picric ac.), chilliness, restlessness, constipation and palpitation. The patients are anemic (Chlorosis), have a poor appetite, a *patchy tongue,* with dry mouth. Such patients are always hopeless of the future. They want to be alone. Aside from the ages of puberty and the menopause this form of melancholia is sometimes found during pregnancy.

Head: "Aching all day; a. in the morning lasting till noon, agg. sneezing or coughing, amel. by compression; a. *as if it would burst* (Bryonia); *heavy* and *pressive pain above the eyes,* and in eyebals, so that opening lids was painful and difficult and he could read no longer, throbbing and *beating* pains *through head;* itching of scalp and falling out of hair; *sensitiveness* of scalp (China); vertigo."

Natrum has *cured several varieties* of *headache,* depending upon such causes as *intermittent fever,* when we have the *throbbing* ("beating like a thousand hammers") *during the chill and fever; headache* of *school children due to eye strain* especially to muscular orthenopia. This pain is mostly in the frontal region. For periodical headaches during the menses which are usually late, scanty and painful. The headaches come just before the menses and continue through. This melancholia is a prominent symptom of this group (Actea rac.). For the *nervous sick headache* (Nux vom., Sanguinaria, Spigelia) with the bursting, throbbing pains extending to neck and chest, with nausea, vomiting, heat of face, and constipation, exceptionally a profuse, watery stool. This headache is due to some error in diet (Nux vom., Graphites) and usualy there is sweating as it disappears. There remains the *anemic* headache. As a matter of fact the patients suffering from all the headaches we have mentioned are anemic which makes them susceptible. The anemic may be called the mother of all the others. In this group you must frequently find the vertigo, the patchy *tongue,* scorbutic bleeding gums, the great *weakness* and sinking *of* the *stomach,* the *sour eructations,* sometimes vomiting, fissure of the anus, general emaciation, irritable heart and greasy skin (Sulphur). The vertigo in all these conditions is amel. by lying down. While putting the above headaches under "Brain and Nerves" I realize that two of them at least could with equal propriety be given under "Blood."

Eyes: "*Eyes give out on writing or reading,* with pressure over the eyes extending into the head, amel. walking about the room; *letters and stitches run together;* objects become confused on looking at them; sudden darkness at 6 P.M. on looking long at anything, amel. by looking at another object."

Useful for a number of *conditions caused by* muscular *asthenopia,* especially when the *aggravation* is *any use of* the *eyes,* with burning and smarting as from salt, when the vision blurs after even a little use of the eyes or if the patient wakens in morning with blurring and headache (Iris) caused by reading the night before. For ciliary neuralgia, also paralysis of the internal recti muscles causing vertigo (Gelsemium) or strabismus.

Face: "*Sticking* in jaws followed by *burning* and numbness, agg. in evening."

I once cured a patient of *neuralgia* of the face for the above symptoms except that the attacks came at 9 A.M. instead of evening. The patient had had a severe attack of intermittent fever a few weeks before which had been *cured?* by quinine.

The intermittent had had all the symptoms of the Natrum mur. group. A few doses of the *200th cured* the *neuralgia*.

Back and Extremities: "Pain in back as if broken; pulsations in back; paralyzed weakness in the lumbar region nearly all day, amel. lying, agg. eating; trembling from weakness on rising from a seat, amel. continued walking; weakness in the morning especially in knees, amel. towards noon."

For the *backache caused* by *prolapsus uteri,* amel. by lying on something hard pressed up on small of back. Also for weak paralytic condition following fever and diphtheria.

Blood.

Heart: For *conditions simulating anemia,* diphtheria and *malarial fever.* Most of the symptoms we have enumerated under Brain and Nerves may be found in the anemic group. In addition may be found the following heart symptoms: "*Fluttering, palpitation,* on exertion especially ascending steps. Sometimes these symptoms are the result of anemia, again they may be the cause, more likely the latter when the patient has an hypertrophied heart and attacks of palpitation are agg. by lying on left side (Phosphorus). *Coldness about* the *heart* is a marked symptom of this group. Examination will show a marked diminution of the number of red blood cells and also that they are breaking down (Picric ac.). The blood changes in the *intermittent* are accompanied by "itching over the entire body," "chill from 8 A.M. till noon," "heat till evening," intense thirst with chill and heat but drinking does not relieve it. We find a *profuse sweat* which *relieves all* the *symptoms.* It is with this condition that we have the throbbing frontal headache, the heart symptoms just enumerated in the anemic group and prostration. In more than three fourths of the patients you will find the "sharp, sticking pains in region of the liver" during the apyrexia.

Skin: "*Itching eruption on margin of hair at nape,* temples and in brows; whitish hives on arms and hands becoming red after rubbing; red hives with itching over whole body; red tetter in hollow of knees; pimples on face; *painful vesicles below the septum of nose,* burning and filled with bloody serum; itching of the whole body."

Skin: The *skin* of the Natrum mur. patient *is greasy* (Sulphur). The conditions for which the drug is useful are: *eczema* especially of eyebrows; *warts* of the palms of the hands; *herpes circinatus; urticaria, hangnails* with dry cracked nails; and *purpura hemorrhagica.* Like Sulphur most of the symptoms are agg. by water. I have never found Natrum useful for the eruptive disease, or such conditions as furuncles, boils, etc.

Mucous Membrane: The symptoms of the mucous membrane have been given under the other locations.

Use it in the 30th, 200th and 1000th.

NATRUM PHOSPHORICUM.

Schuessler says "Natrum phos. is the remedy for those diseases which are caused by the excess of lactic acid." Hence for children who have been fed to excess with milk and sugar. The symptoms are: sour eructations, vomiting of sour, cheesy masses; yellowish green stools, colic with spasms, hot head, icy-cold feet, sour sweat (Calcarea carb.) and restless sleep. You will occasionally find such a group in bottle-fed babies. When you do give the 6th and change the baby's diet. I feel that I once saved a baby's life by giving Natrum phos. and liquid beef peptonoids. The child had been fed milk in all forms, also malted milk, barley water, etc. He was 9 months old. He had nothing except the peptonoids and plenty of water for three weeks.

NATRUM SULPHURICUM.

Make-up: Hydrogenoid constitution.

Loc.: Glands; liver; intestines; *nerve cells.*

Sen.: Fullness; stitching; rumbling.

Mod.: Agg. *Damp* weather, night air, cellars; late evening; lying on side.

Amel. *Dry* open or cool air.

Leaders: Sudden, spluttering, gushing, stools preceded by rumbling in the bowels.

Before taking up any location let us get Grauvogl's definition of "hydrogenoid constitution." He says: "It is the state in which there is extreme sensitiveness to damp, wetting, bathing, watery food, residing near water, especially standing water." Let me also quote what "Schuessler says when comparing Natrum sulph. and Natrum mur. "The action of the sodium sulphate is contrary to that of the sodium chloride. Both, indeed, have the faculty of attracting water, but the end is a contrary one; Natrum mur. attracts the water destined to be put to use in the organism. Natrum sulph. attracts the water formed during the retrogressive metamorphosis of the cells and secures its elimination from the organism. Natrum mur. causes the splitting up of the cells necessary for their multiplication; Natrum sulph. withdraws water from the superannuated leucocytes, and thus causes their destruction." The latter salt, therefore, is a remedy for leukemia.

From the above you see why we get results from our salt solutions which we inject into the body. Schuessler goes on to tell us that Natrum sulph. is a stimulant to the epithelial cells of the nerves and therefore stimulates the function of the kidneys, biliary apparatus, pancreas and intestines. Therefore if Natrum sulph. does not properly stimulate the sensory nerves of the bladder the child wets the bed. So also through the irregular action of Natrum sulph. on the nerves of the biliary apparatus we have too much or too little bile; too much or too little excretion from the intestines. So we explain the action of Glauber's Salts.

Liver and Intestines: "Painful sensitiveness of the hepatic region to touch, during a walk or to a sudden jar; stitches, throbbing, tension and lancinations in hepatic region; collection of flatus without evacuation of it, with pain in abdomen; flatus becomes incarcerated here and there; rolling, and grumbling with sudden pinching as after a purgative, then diarrhea; flatulent agg. difficult emission of flatus."

Fortunately we do not have conditions presenting such violent symptoms very often. The only case I have ever used it for was *hepatitis* caused by getting a good drenching in a boat on his way home from a shore dinner. The result was marked sensitiveness in hepatic region agg. lying on the left side, sallow skin, yellow sclera, dirty yellow tongue and spluttering stools, watery with some lumps. He came to me three weeks after the shore dinner saying he was getting worse instead of better. Natrum sulph. 6x three doses per day soon corrected the condition.

Stools: "Diarrhea, fluid, yellow in the morning, with full feeling in the abdomen and emission of flatus; knotty."

These are the only symptoms in the Handbook in italics, showing they come from the provers. From clinical reports however we find that these have been verified times enough to make them of the highest rank in any group. We also find from the clinical a great many similar symptoms caused by irritating the nerves of the tissues of the liver and intestines. The clinical symptoms also show that we have marked functional disturbances, *e. g.*, that the secreted bile is not excreted but absorbed by other tissues. We also have light red or bloody stools showing functional changes. You will find evidence of the lithic diathesis in many of the symptoms of the diarrheas that the drug will cure.

Mucous Membrane.

Eyes: "Pain in the evening when reading by candle light; with heaviness of the lids; agglutination in the morning with photophobia."

Useful for *granular conjunctivitis* with much redness of the lids (Sulphur). Unless you have the redness of the lids and evidence of the sycotic constitution as shown by excrescences and warts about the eye, nose, anus and other parts of the body, also, the rheumatic stiffness of the joints and the modality agg. *damp* you had better give Sulphur as an intercurrent and look up some other remedy.

Respiratory Organs: "Cough with expectoration, if he coughs while standing; stitches in the left chest with shortness of breath; cough with tickling in larynx agg. in morning after rising with soreness in the chest and rough feeling in the throat, *relief from sitting up and holding her chest with both hands.*"

Useful for a *bronchial catarrh* with the above symptoms plus a time *agg.* for the *cough,* viz., *3 to 4 A.M.* (Kali carb.). Also for asthma with the 3 to 4 A.M. agg. marked dyspnea. In both conditions you get your agg. from damp.

Urinary Organs.

"Stitching in meatus; burning during micturition; urine copious, urine scanty; urine with brick dust sediment, dark and passed more frequently than normal, so that she had to get up several times in the night. Pain in the small of the back with scanty urine."

When calculi are the *cause* you may *give it* with the utmost confidence in *cystitis, uretitis,* and *urethritis,* providing you have your diathesis and your modalities. Useful also *when gonorrhea causes* the *symptoms.* I had one case in an old man, in which an *enlarged prostate caused* retention of urine which in turn caused *all three conditions.* Use the 3rd and 6th.

NATRUM SALICYLICUM.

You are all familiar with the claim which is made for Natrum sal. in the treatment of rheumatism. Probably no remedy has been more used and abused during the past twenty years, than has Natrum sal. for this condition unless it be Colchicum. Yet no one can deny that both have done some good. The good or evil done by the drug seems to depend upon the amount given and the condition of the patient to whom it was given. Has Natrum sal. a place in our homeopathic materia medica and does it cure rheumatism homeopathically? Yes to both questions, but there are other conditions for which it is more frequently called for than rheumatism, viz., *Meniere's disease* and tinnitus aurium. The pathognomonic symptoms of Meniere's disease are vertigo, noises in the ears and deafness. The vertigo of Natrum sal. is agg. by raising the head from the pillow, amel. lying down; objects seem to move in a circle and to the right; the noises are almost constant, agg. lying down; the deafness is direct and perosseous. With the attacks of vertigo you sometimes have vomiting and unconsciousness.

Natrum sal. will cure *periostial rheumatism* when you have the parts hot, tender; swollen, red, a diffuse redness; when the pulse is irregular from 40 to 120, weak and soft; when the profuse sweat on exertion smells musty; when the temperature varies, increasing and decreasing with the rheumatic pains. Use the 3rd.

MAGNESIA CARBONICA.

Make-up: *Worn out;* exhausted; *sensitive.*

Loc.: Mucous membrane of the digestive tract; nerves of face and teeth.

Sen.: Lightning-like; throbbing; sharp; shooting; restlessness.

Mod.: Agg. *Night;* rest; noise; cold; touch; change of weather.

Amel. Walking about.

Leaders: *Green, frothy* stools.

Mucous Membrane of the Digestive Tract.

Stomach: "Craving for fruits and acid things in general; aversion to fresh food; *relish for meat;* acid risings; nausea and vertigo during a meal, followed by retching and vomiting of bitter or saltish serum; sharp pain in stomach with great sensitiveness to pressure."

A very useful remedy for *acid dyspepsia,* with the above aversion and desires. The most frequent cause is drinking milk. The other symptoms are *rumbling in abdomen* and distention, *followed* by frequent, green, liquid, frothy stools. For colic amel. by bending forward (Colocynth).

Stools: "Greenish; frothy; mucous (look like frog spawns), stools with cutting and griping pain; stools white, with shooting pains, white like tallow (Phosphorus); always preceded by griping worse on right side; diarrhea of sour smell; constipation with heart burn; frequent and ineffectual want to evacuate (Nux vom.) with scanty feces."

The diarrhea group belongs with the M.M.; the constipated with the nervous conditions. With the sour stools you always have the sour sweat. The child smells sour. Catarrh and improper diet are the causes.

Female Generative Organs: "Menses delayed, scanty and lasting but a short time; *menses more profuse by night than by day,* with dragging pains amel. pressure on the abdomen and stooping; no discharge of menses during the pains, only after them, and also at night when asleep; discharge glutinous, dark almost like pitch, difficult to wash off the napkin (Crocus)."

Magnesia carb. has helped me a few times to cure *leucorrhea* when the discharge was *whitish,* coming *after* the *menses.* The discharge was acrid and *preceded by colic;* amel. by bending forward (Alumina). I have cured one case of *vomiting of pregnancy* when the same leucorrheal discharge was present. The woman came *for relief* from *sour tasting,* sour *smelling vomit,* but stated that the *smarting* of the leucorrhea and *colic* before the discharge were as *annoying* as the morning sickness.

The discharge came when she relaxed, sitting, worse lying down. The 6th cured both conditions. Finally for *irregular menses* with the peculiarity of the discharge.

Respiratory Organs: "*Cough* excited by tickling in throat with a *serous and salty expectoration;* cough in the morning with expectoration of a yellow pus; expectoration of *tough mucus* and *blood tasting* of *salt* (Kali bich.); expectoration of tubercles as large as a pea, and very offensive."

I verified the "tough mucus and blood tasting of salt," also "expectoration of yellowish pus" in a child suffering from *bronchial catarrh.* Both symptoms were marked but no more so than the green, sour stools that accompanied them.

Nerves.

When we come to this location we find the sections are mostly in the head.

Face: "Tearing in left zygoma at night, better from sitting up in bed or driving her out of bed, both burning and boring as with a red-hot iron (Arsenicum) and with anxiety; pain, so that she must run from room to room all night, hold the painful side and wag the head; agg. remaining quiet."

Has cured many cases of *facial neuralgia* with the above symptoms plus the lightning-like shooting pains agg. by touch, or change in temperature. It also *cured* a case of *Tic* for me with these two symptoms differently expressed. The patient said: "The only way I can keep the thing still is to cover up so nothing can touch me." (Agaricus, Arsenic, Magnesia phos.)

Teeth: "Toothache beginning in the evening in bed and at night driving him out of bed; extending into the temple."

For *neuralgic toothache,* which is usually *accompanied by sour, bitter taste* of saliva. We have the same modalities as with the facial neuralgia and tic.

Abdomen: You remember we found one symptom here. "Colic amel. by bending forward." This means *enteralgia.*

I have never gone above the 6th but repeat often for the nervous conditions. I always give the magnesias in hot water—a tea cup full at a dose.

MAGNESIA MURIATICA.

Make-up: *Sluggish liver* and entire circulation.

Loc.: Nerves; liver; sexual organs.

Sen.: *Soreness;* cramping; burning.

Mod.: Agg. *Lying on right side; milk;* salt food; night; noise.

Amel. Hard pressure; cool, open air.

Leaders: *Stool dry, knotty* or of little balls; sharp drawings in hepatic region.

Liver.

"*Burning, tensive sticking* pains in the right hypochondria; sharp drawings in the hepatic region; aching in the liver when walking or pressing the part, agg. lying on right side; painful hardness of right side of the abdomen."

Stools: "*Hard, like sheep dung, difficult* (Opium), *hard, nodular, with pain in rectum;* hard and covered with streaks of blood; hard and knotty, then a soft one enveloped in mucus; *crumbly as if burnt.*"

Anus: "Hemorrhoids, pain during normal stool; smarting in after a hard stool; burning after usual stool with smarting."

I have put these three sections together before commenting on the liver symptoms because they are of the same origin and should be grouped together. The most frequently called for group we will call *congestion* and *enlargement* of the *liver.* In addition to the symptoms I have given under hypochondria, anus and stools you will find sour vomiting, offensive breath, yellow, sallow color of face and eyes, itching of whole body (jaundice); urine scanty, high-colored and sometimes albuminous; swelling of feet and legs. In a few cases I have found the stools to be gray in color instead of black. If your patient be a woman you will find the "*menses* delayed," "passed in black clots more when sitting than when walking."

Brain and Nerves.

"*Griping* in the temples in evening when lying down; *amel. pressing head with both hands* with feeling as if he would become dizzy and unconscious; aching amel. by wrapping up head; stitching in right side of head extending into the eye with necessity to press the eye together."

For *neuralgic headache* more especially around the eyes with *feeling as if the head would burst* (Bryonia); *agg. motion* and *fresh air*, but *amel. by pressure*. With the neuralgic headache may be found many of the hepatic symptoms. The symptom "amel. pressure" you should recognize when you see the head tightly bandaged. (Gelsemium, Silica.)

Stomach: "Violent hiccough during and after dinner; sensation as if a ball were ascending from abdomen into esophagus, amel. eructations; throbbing in pit of stomach."

Allen says that it has cured many cases of obstinate chronic gastralgia. The only use I have made of it was for nervous indigestion of children with the hard stools covered with blood.

Urinary Organs: "*Micturition only by exertion of abdominal muscles* (Causticum), micturition in drops and some always seemed to remain behind."

Helpful for *dysurea due* to *partial paralysis* of the muscles of the *bladder*.

Sexual Organs.

Female: "Leucorrhea agg. motion, amel, stool, with cramp in abdomen; menses delayed, sometimes scanty but more often profuse; menses thick and black."

Has proved useful for *fibroid induration* of uterus (Trillium, Black oxide of Lime), also for *scirrhus*. For the scirrhous induration of the uterus, the pains extend into the thighs.

With both conditions you have the abdominal symptoms and stools, also the black menstrual flow. Occasionally with the fibrous indurations you may have bright red blood alternating with the black. Finally for *irregular* conditions at time of menses, *e. g., hysteria with* marked *globus hystericus, diarrhea,* etc. A recent graduate sent to my clinic a young woman with a *profuse, black, liquid diarrhea* coming on with the menses and continuing for a week. During the other three weeks between the menses the stools were dark and constipated. Taking the case in the clinic brought out the fact that the menses were always accompanied by the neuralgic headache of Magnesia mur. and marked tenderness of the right abdomen. She had also had two attacks of "yellow jaundice" during the two years she had suffered from the "diarrhea during the menses." The doctor had overlooked Magnesia mur. because he did not have it in his list for diarrhea. In other words he was treating a condition and not his patient.

MAGNESIA PHOSPHORICA.

Make-up: Neurotic; thin, emaciated, dark.

Loc.: Brain and nerves.

Sen.: *Paroxysms; shooting;* lightning-like; *cramps;* paralysis.

Mod.: Agg. *Cold;* air or water; exhaustion; touch; at night. Amel. *Warmth;* pressure.

Leaders: The agg. drafts of cold wind; touch; at night; motion and the amel. warmth.

Schuessler did some excellent work when he gave us his study of Magnesia phos. in his tissue remedies. When it comes to location S. says: "It is contained in blood corpuscles, muscles, brain, spinal marrow, nerves and teeth" and "disturbance of its molecules results in pains, shooting, lightning-like or boring, cramps, paralysis." What causes disturb the molecules? The following are a few: Exposure to cold winds, cold drafts, cold water, *e. g.,* working in it, dentition, the use of the catheter

(Nux vom.). The above are only general statements which might apply to Calcarea carb. Dulcamara and others. To be able to differentiate between them we must study our locations by sections.

Brain and Nerves.

Mind: "Illusions of the senses; sobbing, crying, lamenting all the time about pain in the affected parts; depressed; drowsy, forgetful, inability to think clearly."

This remedy is often helpful for *melancholia with weak functioning of the brain.* Aside from the "drowsy, forgetful," etc., the most marked symptom is that the patient *wants to be* continuously *talking to* others about her pains. Isn't that true of all patients? No, the Ignatia patient won't say a word about hers but goes off and has it out by herself. It is recognizing and acting upon these facts that makes the difference between a good and a poor prescriber. The other condition for which our drug is useful is *brain fag.* Here again we get from school children: "I'm so tired, I can't study. It makes my head ache awfully."

Head: "*Excruciating, spasmodic, intermittent pains; shooting,* darting, stabbing, *shifting* from place to place, always amel. by external application of heat (Arsenicum, Silica); dull headache as if brain too heavy; severe pain beginning in the occiput, extending over their whole head; pressing pain in head down through middle of brain; severe pricking over the head and forehead as if rubbed with a fine brush."

Useful for what is so commonly *called nervous headache* with *diplopia,* sparks before the eyes, photophobia, increased lachrymation, *nausea,* flatulent colic, amel. by pressure (Colocynth). All these symptoms are agg. by cold and mental exertion and amel. by *hot* application.

For *congestive headache* with the flushed, red face, sensation of fulness agg. lying down, the pressive pain into the middle of the brain, nausea, chilliness and followed by marked prostration.

Eyes: "Double vision (horizontal); sparks, dark spots before the eyes on reading, rainbow colors; photophobia with increased lachrymation; twitching of lids; ptosis agg. right side; intermittent, darting pains in and above the orbit."

This group, for the most part indicates *orbital* and *supra-orbital neuralgia* from irritation, but you also note the effects of functional changes, *e. g.*, the ptosis and diplopia. Some might say the ptosis indicated structural change but I have never seen a case in which the ptosis did not clear up. Many cases are on record of *nystagmus* and a few cases of *strabismus* being helped by Magnesia phos, the latter being due to improper functioning of the nerves, never to pressure back of eye ball as in Apis and Hellebore. There is a marked tendency to the right side, and warmth, especially dry heat, greatly relieves.

Ear: "Sharp, intermittent pains behind the right ear greatly agg. by cold air or washing the face in cold water."

The above needs no comment. It simply means *nervous, spasmodic otalgia* amel. heat.

Face: "Neuralgia of right upper jaw and teeth, begins with great fierceness at 2 P.M. and lasts till it gets warm in bed; pains sharp, agg. cold, amel. heat, with face swollen as if stung by bees; boring, pinching, nipping pains driving him out of bed, soon spreading over entire right side of face; pains radiating all over right side of face from infra-orbital foramen; agg. touch, opening mouth, by walking or riding in cold air; convulsive twitchings of angle of mouth; sensation of painful contraction of jaw-point for several days, with a nervous backward jerking."

Too many symptoms, you say. Yes, but the *varieties* of *facial neuralgias are* also *many* when we consider the parts involved. We had already mentioned the *supra* and *infra-orbital.* Now we add *neuralgia* of the *jaw* and *angles of* the *mouth.*

You will note that the character of the pains and the modalities are neuralgic; also that there are no symptoms of degeneration of tissues, mostly irritation, very little inflammation.

Teeth: "*Toothache agg. after going to bed,* agg. by eating and drinking *cold things, amel. heat;* teeth sensitive to touch and cold air, could not brush the teeth with cold water for months; severe pain in filled teeth."

While typing these notes a dark, firm-fibered, nervous, married woman of forty came to me for relief from a most violent toothache and general prosopalgia. As bathing and swimming in the lake were new experiences for her she spent a good part of the day in the water. The sharp, jerking, twisting pains began about the antrum, spread over the face and terminated in a fearful twist in the teeth of the upper jaw. The agg. was marked from cold. Moist heat did no good but dry heat gave some relief. She went to a dentist who found the "teeth perfect" and turned her over to a throat specialist who insisted on draining the antrum but as she overheard the dentist say to the throat man that he was not sure he saw anything, the woman refused to submit. She came back to her cottage and after spending a sleepless night called me. She was given Magnesia phos. 3x grains 3 every half hour and heat through an electric bulb applied. She became easier that day, spent a better night, still easier the second day, a good sleep the second night and was out to a fish dinner the next evening.

Please note a new *cause. i. e., filling of teeth.* If you look up the records of the provers you will find that three of a group of seven had to give up the proving and go to a dentist for treatment. Also note that the filling *was silver.* I wish also to state that with the complaint of teething children, especially *during dentition, spasms without fever* are *frequent.* A few cases are on record of ulceration with the neuralgia, accompanied by swelling of the glands of the face, throat, and neck; also of the tongue.

Stomach: "*Spasmodic* pains in stomach, with clean tongue (Ignatia); intense, *cutting, shooting,* cramping pains in region of stomach and epigastrium, extending toward back and abdomen; flatulent distention of stomach, with constrictive pain amel. by warmth and bending double (Colocynth); a *cold drink of water starts* a *colicky pain in stomach* which radiates to bowels, very severe, *amel. by doubling up, rest* and *belching.*"

Hiccough is the condition which has been *most frequently cured* by Magnesia phos. There are several cases on record where the condition had been of long standing speedily cured. With one case the *hiccough* was *accompanied by sobbing.* This case had continued three days. Another case the hiccoughs at times occurred thirty times per minute. In this case the patient's life had been in danger for two months. A third case of hiccoughing with retching had continued for three days, night and day. The patient vomited coagulated milk, bile and mucus. I have found no drug in my 37 years experience that will cause and cure such severe hiccoughs as Magnesia phos. except Tabacum.

Gastralgia readily yields to the remedy. The symptoms are extreme soreness and tenderness to touch of the epigastrium; eructations, vomiting of food and bile, amel. by drinking hot water, sometimes by eating hot food.

Magnesia phos. will excel even *Arsenicum in relieving* the *burning pains, persistent vomiting* and *hiccough caused by cancer.* It seems to work best in those cases which "seemed to have worn out Morphine." It only palliates; it can never cure but I have had patients made comparatively comfortable for months by giving the 3x every two or three hours.

Urinary Organs: "Cutting pain in the bladder before urinating; restless sleep from urging; excess of phosphates; spasm of the bladder; spasmodic retention of urine."

I have used it for two conditions: *Spasmodic retention* of the urine, the result of the use of the catheter (Nux vom.) and *nocturnal enuresis caused* by *irritation* of phosphates (gravel). With the latter you find restless sleep and burning, rasping pains during micturition in the day time.

I will just mention in closing that in *dysmenia* (genuine menstrual colic) you find the same cutting, drawing, cramping pains as elsewhere, also the modalities plus amel. from the flow; but that the violent, dry, spasmodic cough with retching and choking is agg. in a warm room but amel. in open air.

Anything added to the above manifestations from the various sections of the nervous system would only mar the picture, so I will not mention any other location. I call it my homeopathic opiate. If homeopathists would study it more and the old school would try it occasionally much of the irreparable harm done by the almost universal use of aspirin would be avoided.

MAGNESIA SULPHURICA.

This remedy under the name of "Epsom Salts" has had a reputation as a "refrigerant cathartic" for centuries. Lately the old school has "discovered" that it is a good remedy for dysentery. The conditions which are better covered by it than by the other members of the magnesia family are those of the urinary organs? and skin. I say urinary organs because the cases of *diabetes* do not seem to be of hepatic origin. As you all know, when used as a cathartic Magnesia sulph. produces marked increase of the flow of urine, intense thirst, and dryness of the mouth. Taking these three as ranking symptoms and adding "loose evacuations," "repugnance for all food," "weakness," "emaciation," "sleepy in evening" and sugar in the urine, you have a good picture of diabetes.

The ***skin symptoms are*** in the line of *growths, i. e.*, warts and epithelioma. The warts of the soft, large variety, generally come on the face. I have succeeded in a few cases by substituting Magnesia sulph., after Thuja had failed. Many cases having all the ear marks of epithelioma have yielded to its use. One specialist reported eight cases. He used the crude salt three drams to the pint, and gave a teaspoonful three times daily.

LYCOPODIUM CLAVATUM.

Make-up: Lithic diathesis; lethargic.

Loc.: Digestive tract; urinary organs; liver; skin; mucous membrane.

Sen.: *Fullness;* dryness; sharp; sticking; of ball rising; distention; pressure of clothes.

Mod.: Agg. from eating *cabbage, beans* and *starchy food; warmth;* rest; before menses, 3 to 4 P.M.; from lamplight.

Amel. in open air; urinating; warm drinks.

Leaders: *Red sand in urine; a little food causes fullness;* much noisy flatulence; general acidity.

Before taking up our general groups I want to study with you a few of the general properties of the drug. It is one of the three great anti-psorics (Sulphur, Calcarea carb.). It once held a prominent position in old school medicine in the treatment of rheumatism, nephritis, flatulent colic of children and young girls, renal calculi, etc. It did and still holds a prominent place in the arts. About the only use made of it by the old school, today, is as an inert dusting powder. Our school not only considers it one of the three great anti-psorics but one of the leading polychrests. Why this difference? There are two reasons: first, by triturating (potentizing) we liberate the active principle of the drug; second, by our provings, our scientific investigations, we ascertain and classify the results of its action. The fact that it is an anti-psoric makes it an ally to a large number of remedies. Allen mentions sixteen. This means that it may be often called for as an intercurrent during the use of any of these sixteen remedies. It further means, as I have stated under Sulphur, that a thorough knowledge of Lycopodium is necessary to a good working knowledge of its allies.

Lycopodium is one of our leading *tissue remedies. Malnutrition* is the *keynote* of Lycopodium. As an energizer to awake from their lethargy and stimulate to action any or all the tissues of the body, Lycopodium ranks second only to Sulphur.

Digestive Tract.

Stomach: "*Appetite* after eating, though the stomach and abdomen are full and tense, *great; lost* and whatever she eats goes against her even to vomiting; *aversion* to food, especially to accustomed *coffee* and *tobacco;* sudden satiety with thirst and distention of stomach and abdomen; incomplete *eructations,* burning, rising into pharynx, where they cause burning; *sour E.,* the taste of which does not remain in the mouth, but the acid *gnaws* in the *stomach; waterbrash;* hiccough; distention and cramp; pain in pit in P.M. after eating a little; *pain* in the *epigastric* region *caused* by *cough; feels* as if *overdistended* in evening after eating only a little; digestion slow; discomfort after eating."

The above symptoms may be grouped to simulate *dyspepsia,* acid, atonic, *flatulent.* The satiety and fullness on beginning to eat is the most prominent. Solid food, especially that containing starch, causes more discomfort than liquids. It is one of the best remedies for bottle-fed babies. The babies are constipated and have freqnent eructations both empty and of food. Several cases of chronic indurations of the pylorus have been reported cured by it. With these cases I have always found induration with enlargement of liver. Constipation and hemorrhoids are often found in this group.

Here we find many of the same symptoms as under the location, stomach, but somewhat modified.

Abdomen: "Distention after eating, with tension, relieved by emission of flatus; sensitiveness of the skin, especially in epigastric region; bruised pain in region of liver worse to touch, on breathing; unpleasant and distended feeling in hepatic region if she eats to satiety; weight in left hypochondria when walking, sitting or lying, not affecting breathing."

For *chronic hepatitis with* heaviness; dull pain; *constipation;* itching, *yellow, dry skin;* brown spots; variable appetite: acid eructation and *flatulency. Gall-stones* with the urinary group. It palliates the suffering of *cirrhosis* of the liver.

With the latter condition and the chronic hepatitis you frequently have dropsy of the abdomen.

Urinary Organs.

Urine: "*Deposit* of *red,* yellow-red ***sand though*** the ***urine*** rather *clear;* urine dark, foamy, turbid, milky, with greasy pellicles on, and bloody; micturition painful, scanty, profuse, ceasing suddenly."

Bladder: "Dull pain in bladder."

Kidneys: "Tearing in region of kidneys worse from pressure extending into rectum; pain in region of kidneys in the morning on rising, during menses, so that she could not move."

Ureters and Urethras: "Stitching, shooting, tearing pain in region of urethras and ureters."

Lycopodium is one of the best remedies for the lithic diathesis (Berberis, Lithium carb., and Natrum sulph.). It has been often used for chronic *cystitis* caused by irritation by renal calculi. For *cystitis* and ***urethritis*** of ***infants*** suffering from dyspepsia. The children cry before and during micturition and deposits of red sand are found in the diaper. It often relieves and sometimes cures patients suffering from chronic Bright's disease, when, in addition to the urinary symptoms given above, we have the gastric symptoms, edematous legs and dropsy of the abdomen.

"Penis small, cold and without erections; desire and power diminished; menses variable, too early and delayed; leucorrhea milky or blood red."

Male: For ***impotency*** in men. Nash states that happy results have been obtained from its use by ***old men*** who, on marrying young wives, have found themselves impotent, the result of age. Scores of old men and physicians have verified the truth of the use of the drug for this condition. It is also useful for ***impotency caused by sexual excesses, e. g.,*** a young telegraph operator presented himself at my clinic, sent by his physician who wrote that the boy was hopelessly impotent;

that Picric ac., Phorphorus in several potencies had been used, also electricity, stimulants and even cantharis. The history in brief was that he was night operator and had three young women for assistants whose sexual desires he had tried to satisfy. The result was as stated above. In addition to complete *impotency* he had the atonic dyspepsia of Lycopodium. He was wholly *restored* by the use of the 200th. Gonorrhea and cystitis are also given as causes of impotency in men.

Female: For *chronic* vaginal catarrh with dryness, burning and itching. I had a peculiar case of this kind the first year after graduating. A dark, thick-set, mentally sluggish woman of forty came to my office and after great hesitation said she wanted to be relieved of *vaginal flatulency*. The expulsion of the flatus had become so noisy she could not go away from home. Quizzing brought out the fact that she had the Lycopodium constipation and flatulent dyspepsia. She also stated that she thought she was "passing the change of life," that instead of a liquid flow she passed *large quantities* of something which looked like *dry blood*. She said she was passing some at the time. I asked her to bring me a sample of the dried substance and of her urine for examination. The dried substance was blood and the urine full of brick dust sediment. Lycopodium 30th cured. The stomach symptoms were the first to clear up, the bowels second, and the *vaginal flatulency* third. She never menstruated after that. I have not had much success with it for dysmenorrhea and have never found any benefit from it in palliating the pains of cancer, as is claimed by some.

Mucous Membrane and Skin.

Mouth: "Dryness" is the word most frequently used by provers and patients to express the conditions of the inner and outer skin; and yet the term dryness needs modifying in many sections, *e. g.*, "saliva runs out of mouth at night;" "Saliva dries on palate and lips to a tenacious mucus."

Throat: "Bloody mucus in pharynx and fauces with inclination to swallow it;" also, "cough with hawking of thick, firm yellow mucus from the throat, pharynx and trachea;" finally "skin unhealthy with corrosive vesicles," and "skin scurfy, sticky, clammy." Dryness is more of a sensation than a real condition.

Lycopodium has cured many patients of *diphtheria.* Dr. A. P. Hanchett of Council Bluffs used the 30th as the epidemic remedy in many cases. He would get a smear, send it to the University for a culture and though the report was positive in every case, the patient was convalescing when the report reached the doctor. The exudate first appeared on the right tonsil, thence spread to the left; there was marked swelling of throat, a stopped-up feeling of the nose, albumin in the scanty urine and the general prostration of the patient. It has been successful for *so-called diphtheritic condition following scarlet fever.* With this condition there was much of the bloody discharge from mouth, and edematous swelling of the entire body, most marked about face and extremities.

Blood.

In addition to diphtheritic and *scarlet fever* conditions mentioned above, Lycopodium is occasionally indicated for *typhoid* patients when you find the *red, sandstone deposit* in the urine, great mental and physical depression, constipation and distended abdomen with enlargement and tenderness of the liver. I rarely use Lycopodium below the 30th, often in the 1 m.

GRAPHITES.

Make-up: Fat; greasy; chilly; constipated.

Loc.: Skin; generative organs; mucous membranes.

Sen.: Itching, burning; tearing; of cobweb.

Mod.: Agg. cold; during menses; light.

Amel. walking in open air (Platinum, Pulsatilla).

Leaders: Thick, hard, dry, irritable skin which when

abraded exudes a gluey moisture; fickle, changeable mood (Pulsatilla).

Skin.

"*Hard and cracked in hands;* unhealthy skin, every injury tends to suppurate; proud flesh and fetid pus in ulcer; *eruption oozing out a thick, honey-like fluid;* soreness *high up between thighs* during and after a walk, during menstruation; parts between pudendum and thighs covered with pimples, vesicles and ulcers; *smarting and soreness between nates; itching eruption full of corroding water on many parts.*"

Scalp: "Scales, causing itching and becoming scurf which disappears on washing and then is humid; *eruption* on *vertex painful* to *touch* and *humid.*"

Lids: "*Dry* mucus on lashes; inflammation of margin and external canthi."

Ears: "Moist and sore places behind both ears; sensation of a hard body behind ears."

Face: "*Sensation of a cobweb* (Baryta ac.)."

Extremities: "Nails become black; deformities and thickness of nails."

Among the many skin affections which Graphites will cure I will mention only a few: *Tinea capitis* is the one I have met most frequently. On the vertex you have large scabs (Mezerium), which leave an offensive odor as they come off; cracks behind the ears and at margin of hair from which oozes a thick, yellow exudate which drys into a scab or tetter. With this condition the *glands about* the *ears* and *neck swell* and become very sore, *sometimes ulcerating.* Babies with this condition are usually slow teething and are constipated, with stools covered with mucus.

I have cured three cases of *lupus* with Graphites. Let me give you the record of one to show the connection between affections of the skin and the female sexual organs: Mrs. G. P., wife of a druggist, fat, stout, light, aged 37. She came into my office one hot day in July with a thick veil over her face which she removed with the expression: "I wear this thick veil because I am ashamed to have anyone see me." The entire right cheek was covered with a dark red elevated skin which was beginning to ulcerate at the border and from which broken down tissue came a thick yellow discharge somewhat offensive. On the left cheek and running under the ear was a similar patch and a small one on the neck. She stated her case as follows: "I was up at the Lake last August and went in bathing and swimming one morning when I was menstruating; the water was colder than I thought and chilled me. My menses stopped. For a few days I had a severe, right-sided headache, with a numb, stiff feeling in this right cheek on which you see is a birth mark. . The headache left me after about a week but the birth mark began to spread and has continued to do so till this day. I have not menstruated since that day, now 11 months. I have tried everything suggested by four physicians without help. The last one sent me to you and if you can't help me I'm going back up to the lake and drown myself." Examination revealed the following facts in addition to her story: Her mother had died of cancer of the uterus at the age of 48. One sister had died of t. b. c. at puberty. The birth mark, which, before the checking of the menses, was about half as large as a nickle, became very red a few days before the menses and, if the period was delayed, the spot became redder and burned till the flow began, when the burning and redness began to subside, and were gone by the time the menses ceased for the period. The menses had always been scanty, watery and of short duration. There was a little tendency for the menses to be late, five or six weeks between periods but two or three times she had gone three months. She had never been pregnant. Suffered from a profuse, milky leucorrhea which chaffed the thighs. Perspired easily and the sweat also chaffed the thighs. Her husband had said: "I don't want to know what you give," so I gave him a vial of disks of Graphites 1m B. and T. and ordered five taken on an empty stomach 15 minutes before breakfast and her evening meal. She was to take plenty of water, a little tea, no milk or meat. She was to report in six weeks or before if the menses appeared. She returned in five weeks with the statement: "I've had a slight show but I'm discouraged. You or no one else is going to cure me." I secured her promise to continue the medicine once a week before breakfast and gave her a vial of disks saturated with alcohol. She reported again in six weeks that she was just over menstruating and that she had lost more blood than at any two previous periods in her life. The color of her face was much paler. Again placebo. She came back after two more periods with the report that the last was scanty, more like old times. The face was much improved and she was very hopeful. Again placebo but she returned in five weeks, saying that there had been no menses and that improvement of the face had ceased. I now repeated my first prescription but only for one week. Her next report was menses came on after eight days and flowed for five days. Face greatly improved. At the end of 18 months the face was back to normal and the menses normal except about 30 to 35 days interval. I had to repeat the Graphites once more but only gave one dose instead of a dose daily. I give you this case in full because it is the only one of the kind I have ever cured and for the further reason that in all the cases of *eczemas* of adults I have ever cured by the drug, the "scanty, watery, delayed menses" was the ranking symptom of the group and was always the first to disappear. I have cured *herpes* of the *prepuce* with it.

Nipples: For *cracked nipples* there is no remedy I so often use. I apply the cerate locally and give the 30th internally. *Exuberant granulations* about the nails I treat as I do cracked nipples.

We might leave the study of Graphites at this point with the statement that all these conditions of the skin are but the manifestations of some diathesis, some inner subtle disturbance but for the fact that the diathesis expresses itself by other groups of symptoms in other localities.

As I have stated that *menstrual irregularities seemed* to be the *bases of all skin manifestations in women,* let us take the generative organs for the next location.

Generative Organs.

Female: "*Painful swelling of the ovaries* agg. every time she takes cold or *gets* her *feet wet;* swelling; swelling and hardness of ovaries after menses; menstruation delayed (Calcarea carb., Sulphur, Phosphorus, Pulsatilla); menses too slow, too scanty, too pale; *before and during menses* a *shattering cough; leucorrheas* before and after menses; great aversion to coition."

Male: "Ejaculation does not follow coition in spite of every effort; absence of erection in the morning; emission of semen almost involuntary, without erection."

The first condition we will group symptoms for are: "*delayed menstruation or menses* with eruptions on face and herpetic eruption on other parts of the body, great mental depression, weeping, vertigo and usually indigestion, rancid eructations, constipation though occasionally soft stools."

The leucorrhea is usually milky white, profuse with pain in back, coming in gushes, often taking the place of the menses. A *subacute* inflammation of the vagina and uterus usually precedes and accompanies the leucorrhea.

Indurations and *cauliflower excrescences* which bleed easily and produce severe lancinating pains, have been cured by Graphites. In all such cases which I have met the induration and excrescences were about lacerations of the uterus of women of the Graphites make-up.

Other conditions which follow lacerations are *cystic tumors,* cystic *ovaries.* Of course the first thing is to repair the laceration and then give the drug for a long period of time. The tendency of the Graphites women to get fat about the climacteric period is very marked. The fat is an unhealthy fat. The patient is really anemic.

Mucous Membrane.

As we have already noted that we have nearly all forms of eruptions and other manifestations in diseases of the skin so we find *vitiated secretions* and *excretions* of the M.M., not only from the surface but from the glands. As the symptoms are the same in many respects I will not repeat them but simply mention the conditions of the different sections.

Eye: *Chronic ciliary blepharitis* with swollen, ulcerated, cracked edges of the lids, also *with dry scurf* in the lashes and *burning,* dryness and *itching.*

Tumors of the *lids* (Pulsatilla, Staphisagria) which are apt to be directly on the margin.

Pustules on the *conjunctiva* and *cornea* with an acrid discharge from the eyes during the day but thicker at night so that it agglutinates the lids.

Nose: Useful for *chronic nasal catarrh* with *acute sense of smelling,* cannot tolerate flowers; *ozena;* great soreness of the nostrils which are covered with scabs, crack and bleed easily.

Tongue: Here we find *burning blisters* on lower side and tip (Natrum mur., Nitric ac., Lycopodium) and *aphthous patches;* white, painful ulcers, which, as you know, are *manifestations* of *deep seated trouble* with *digestion* and *assimilation.*

Stomach: The *desires* and *aversions* of Graphites are *many* and *marked.* There is aversion to animal food, the use of which agg. many of the symptoms. *Sweets are disgusting.* and nauseous. They *crave beer, acids* and *cold drinks.*

Many eructations tasting of food (Pulsatilla, Sepia and Sulphur) coming *several hours after* the *ingestion* of the food. This you know indicates slow, imperfect digestion. With or after eructations you have *"necessity to vomit."* We may group the above and call them *chronic gastric catarrh.*

Stools: The symptoms of the abdomen and rectum I have already referred to and will close this location by calling your attention to the *stools.* The first a diarrheic *stool with* particles of *undigested food showing lack of digestion* and assimilation; several formed stools covered with mucus showing functional changes of the mucous membrane.

We have already indicated the changes which take place in the mucosa of the sexual organs showing that you may have all four conditions, viz., irritation, etc.

Respiratory Organs: We have *chronic hoarseness* associated with our skin manifestations, *pertussis* and *spasmodic asthma.* Also *cough* reflex from the sexual organs which I will illustrate by a case: Many years ago a young woman of 17 with a dirty, unhealthy skin was brought to me by her mother for a cough which had attracted my attention while the patient was in the waiting room. It was one of those *hollow, shattering* coughs *coming in paroxysms,* just such a cough as I had cured a short time before with Drosera. So sure was I that Drosera was the remedy that I did not take the case but put up the medicine and asked the patient to report in three days. She did report that the cough ceased the day after beginning to take the Drosera. I ordered the remedy discontinued and recorded another triumph for Drosera. Four weeks later I heard the same cough as the patient came down the hall. After a good deal of hesitation on the part of the patient I got my case, viz., a *menstrual cough.* It began the hour the flow began and ceased the day the period ended. She had had it for three years. The menses were pale and scanty but regular in time. I could not recall the remedy but looked it up and found it and gave Graphites in the 30th three times daily for one week. The cough never returned but the patient and her children have many times.

I call Graphites one of our lesser antipsorics, a great constitutional remedy and use it high and low.

ARNICA.

Make-up: Anemic; rheumatic; hemorrhagic.

Loc.: *Blood;* sore; weak; aching; *sensitive.*

Mod.: Agg. Touch and motion.

Amel. *Hot applications* and food, and elevating the head.

Leaders: For *injuries* such as *bruises,* concussions, *over-exertion* and shock; irritable weakness; cadaverous odor of secretions.

Blood.

Typhoid and Typho-Malarial Fever: "Shivering chilliness over the whole body and head, with heat in head; redness and heat in face; coolness of hands and bruised feeling in back, hips and anterior surface of arms; indifference to everything; low muttering delirium; dusky, red face; involuntary, putrid stools; dark venous hemorrhages from bowels; dry, sore tongue sometimes black; breath fetid; tendency to bed sores early in the disease; great prostration; complete unconsciousness."

You note from the above symptoms that it is indicated for the low, putrid forms of typhoid. It acts best in ten drop doses of the 3x given in a dram of water every two hours.

Septicemia: "*GREAT sensitiveness* of the affected part; *black* and *blue* spots; much swelling; excessive sweat; "steeple-chase temperature."

Useful for those cases where the pus is burrowed deep in the tissues, the result of injuries especially bruises and contusions. The sweat and frothy, yeasty stools, have a cadaverous odor. There is a general tendency to gangrene of all contused wounds. Also a tendency to small, red, exceedingly sensitive boils. The boils do not mature well.

Anemia: The "pale face and mucous membranes;" "the varicose veins;" the "livid color of the skin;" the "hemorrhages from all parts of the body;" the "short panting respiration," all go to show that the blood has undergone profound changes.

Muscles.

Extremities: "Bruised pains in all parts of body; soreness; weakness; excruciating sensitiveness; black and blue spots; fear of being touched; cracking, tearing in joints."

Arnica is useful for rheumatism of the muscles when the soreness and sensitiveness is so great that the patients scream from fear of being touched. The most frequent use I make of it is for bruises when the parts are blue and swollen. For such conditions take one part of tincture and four parts of hot water, saturate a sponge with the solution and apply to the part. I always order it applied to the vulva after a long tedious labor. Give at the same time Arnica 3x.

Respiratory Organs.

Spasmodic Cough: "Cough in children caused by weeping and lamenting; cough caused by anger, with tossing about; cough dry, short, hacking; cough with bloody expectoration; cough with hemorrhages into the nose and conjunctiva; dyspnea with quick inspiration and expiration."

Arnica has been successfully used for a nervous spasmodic cough; more frequently for whooping cough not only to lighten the paroxysms but to absorb the blood which has oozed from the veins broken by the cough. Use the 3x and 6x.

RHUS TOXICODENDRON.

Make-up: Unhealthy skin and scrofulous; tendency to sepsis.

Loc.: *Skin; blood;* muscles; mucous membranes; nerves and *cellular tissue.*

Sen.: *Restlessness; stiffness;* tearing; bruised; burning; chilliness.

Mod.: Agg.: Beginning motion; *rest; overexertion;* chilled when hot or sweating *before a rain storm.*

Amel.: *Change of position; continued slow motion;* heat; rubbing.

Leaders: Dry tongue with *red tip* found in septic conditions. A stiff thick skin; easily chilled agg. by *least uncovering* or *slow motion.*

Skin.

"*Itching* and burning agg. touching or moving the affected parts; *swelling* with white transparent *vesicles* on the inflamed skin; *erysipelatous* swelling secreting a slimy liquid; vesicular and phlegmonous erysipelas of face, head, neck, hands; vesicles between fingers, then over the whole body, with swelling on cheeks; with itching burning; swelling of the face with redness, then scarlet exanthema over the whole body, with itching biting, later back of hands and legs covered with blisters that burst and slowly desquamated."

Rhus shares the honor with Arsenicum in the number and severity of skin manifestations which it will relieve. All forms of *eczemas* which have a *tendency* to *erysipelas* with *vesicles,* burning, tearing pains and extreme *restlessness.*

Scarlet Fever: It has frequently been successful in *typhoid forms* of *scarlet fever* with the Rhus tongue, enlarged glands, marked restlessness, liquid, yellow stools. In such cases of scarlet fever the eruption is never smooth; always irregular.

Smallpox: Rhus has helped many cases of *smallpox* with the same group of symptoms as in scarlet fever except that there were *black bloody pustules.*

Purpurea Hemorrhagica: With the *purpura* you have the *red-tip tongue,* weak tremulous pulse, marked *restlessness,* diarrhea and some numbness of the hands and feet.

Boils, Carbuncles, Abscesses: For *boils, carbuncles, abscesses* and all similar conditions which have a marked *tendency to suppurate,* Rhus will cure if you have the chilliness, the *temperature* and the *prostration* of the drug.

Blood.

"Creeping *chilliness* in the house towards evening; shivering; with warmth of body; *internal* and external *heat* of head without thirst, with stretching, drawing, weakness in limbs; delirium; dull headache with heaviness; vertigo on rising even to falling forward or backward; thirst; *abdomen distended;* a thin, liquid, mucous, at times bloody stool; *dry, red-tip tongue;* eruption similar to *urticaria;* marked *prostration.*" For the above group of symptoms Rhus has been used very effectively in *typhoid.* I have never seen a case calling for it, however, that did not have the *diarrhea* and the *red-tip tongue.* I have found that broths and soups for the diet were better than milk. The exception being junketed milk.

Intermittent Fever: "Creeping chilliness beginning in the lower extremities; a *short, dry cough;* heat as if *blood* circulated *hot through* the *blood vessels* and too violently through the head; redness of the whole body; restless sleep; a slight general sweat in the morning." I have found much prostration in both the intermittent and malarial fever of Rhus.

Sepsis: Rhus is one of the best remedies for *sepsis* I have found. Whether for *prophylactic* or *curative* purposes, where the condition develops rapidly and the symptoms already given appear, especially the *restlessness, diarrhea* and *tongue,* Rhus will seldom fail. Ten drops of the tincture to a pint of water applied locally to a badly swollen arm the result of a cut with the point of a butcher knife materially assisted the internal use of the 6th.

Muscles.

It has been found more frequently indicated than Bryonia for affections of the muscles. The symptoms in this respect are so many, I will give you only a few characteristics from various parts of the body.

Back: "Pain in sacrum when sitting, as after long stooping; bruised feeling in sacrum when sitting with heaviness, amel. moving; stiffness of sacrum with pain on motion."

Upper Extremities: "Swelling of hands and feet; trembling after using them; bruised pain in limbs and joints on which he does not lie; *weakness; stiffness on first moving* after rest; weakness during and after walking, with *paralyzed feeling* in them and weight upon nape; desire to move limbs frequently, which relieves the rheumatic pains; falling asleep of the limbs he lies upon and arm."

Upper Extremities: "Shooting, *drawing*, tearing pains in arms lying still; sprained pain in l. arm in the P.M., 1 to 3, when arm is moved backward and forward; jerking tearing in elbow and wrist; amel. motion; crawling in finger tip as if asleep."

Lower Extremities: "*Weakness;* agg. rest; paralysis with walking difficult, slow and shuffling; tearing in knee and ankle; agg. rest; tension in left knee on rising from a seat; tension as if the *tendons* under knee were *too short;* aching with inability to rest in any position; tingling pain in shaft of the tibia, at night with constant necessity to move legs which prevent sleep; sprained pain in the feet in morning on rising; red feeling of the feet with numbness."

Heart: "Weak sensation of *heart* with *trembling* in it; palpitation when sitting still, so that the body moved with every pulse." When we take in consideration the fact that the rheumatic diathesis is the condition for which Rhus is so useful and the leading modality "worse from getting wet" we see why so many cases of hypertrophy of the heart and rheumatism of the heart have been helped by the drug. It will also relieve the distress of an overtaxed heart such as you find after athletic contests. If you will note carefully you will see that it is for stiffness and restlessness that the modalities "worse from rest, better from motion" apply. You will also observe that it is gentle motion which relieves while violent exertion greatly aggravates all the muscular symptoms.

Mucous Membranes.

Eye: "Inflammation of the eye; redness in the morning with agglutination of lids; soreness around the eye; *swelling* of lids; redness of the white in morning with burning pressure."

It is for *pustular conjunctivitis* of scrofulous patients that Rhus has been most serviceable. The cause in most cases was getting wet. Also useful for granulated lids when there were sac-like swellings of the conjunctiva with the profuse yellow purulent discharge.

Nose: "Tip red and painful to touch; violent *sneezing;* involuntary discharge in the morning; after rising; bleeding when stooping in the morning and at night."

The chronic nasal catarrh is usually accompanied by an offensive, *green discharge* from both nostrils and by severe aching in all the bones. The cause is dampness.

Throat: "Dryness; inability to swallow, with dryness posteriorly." The sore throat of Rhus is always accompanied by "hard *swelling* of submaxillary and parotid *glands,*" and with sticking pains and difficult swallowing due to partial paralysis and swelling of the parts.

Abdomen: "Distention after eating; fermentation; griping; digging; burning; drawing; pains; sensitiveness."

Besides the condition of the mucous membrane and submucosa found in typhoid fever, Rhus produces various inflammations found in appendicitis, typhlitis, peritonitis and enteritis with all of which we find the restlessness, the *red-tip tongue,* the *putrid diarrhea* and prostration.

Brain and Nerves.

Mind: "Restlessness; weakness; stiffness; paralysis."

"Delirium; restlessness."

Eyes: "Closed lids heavy with stiffness like paralysis."

Rhus is one of the best remedies for ptosis and with it you usually find the inflammation of the conjunctiva and cellular tissue.

Larynx: "Oppressed and anxious respiration; obliged to breathe deeply, as if she would suffocate; respiration short at night."

The only use I have made of these symptoms has been for

paralysis of the muscles usually caused by diphtheria. Rhus, Gelsemium and Lachesis are a great trio for post-diphtheritic paralysis.

Cellular Tissue.

There is not time nor is it necessary to repeat the symptoms which can all be explained by the word cellulitis. You will find it in connection with the skin, muscular and even the nervous group of symptoms. You will find it under the general headings of eyes, throat, sexual organs and extremities. Rhus has been used with success in doses varying from ten drops of the tincture to a pint of water for local application to five drops of the 40m.

BRYONIA ALBA.

Make-up: Dark, bilious, sallow, lazy.

Loc.: Muscles, *mucous and serous membranes, blood,* kidneys, uterus, lungs, skin.

Sen.: Stitching, tearing, bursting, throbbing, sharp.

Mod.: Agg.: Motion.
Amel.: Lying on painful side.

Muscles.

"*Aching in every muscle.* Weariness, with *heaviness,* the feet can scarcely carry one on account of heaviness; weakness especially of the lower extremities; *tensive;* painful *stiffness.* Knees *totter* and *bend* under one when *walking; sprained* pain in wrist on every motion; *hot* swelling of instep, with bruised pain on stretching foot; tension in foot on walking; tensive pains on dorsum even when sitting; sticking, tearing pains also swollen sensation of finger joints when writing or on any motion."

The Bryonia pains are *always* worse from motion—the more you move the worse the pain—but the *unsteadiness* of all parts, which is worse on beginning to walk, is better from continued walking. Our most frequently indicated remedy for all affections of the muscles including rheumatism.

Mucous and Serous Membranes.

Meninges: "*Stitching,* tearing, *drawing* pains in the *occiput* and down the *neck and back.* With the above symptoms you also have dryness of the mouth, intense thirst. A white coated tongue and the large, dry, hard, dark stools."

The form of meningitis calling for Bryonia usually results from suppressed eruptions.

Respiratory Organs and Chest: "*Dry cough as if from stomach;* tough mucus loosened only after frequent hawking; cough from mucus in the trachia; mucus causing cough with a feeling that he could not get out enough; *cough worse when coming into a warm, close room; stitching* in the *sternum* when coughing causing him to hold the chest with his hand, stitching pain in sternum, *worse from motion,* so severe he must hold his breath or cry out; pleuritic pains in chest; *friction murmurs* in pleura."

Whether in bronchitis, the first stage of pneumonia, pleurisy simple or with effusion; peri-, endo- or myocarditis the Bryonia patient *sweats* easily and *profusely.* His pains may be greatly relieved by bandaging the chest tightly. Heat applied to the chest will help Bryonia reduce the inflammation and help absorb any effusion or exudate. Plenty of pure cool water will not quench his thirst but relieves the constipation.

Stomach: "Excessive thirst for *large quantity of cold water* which does not distress but rather *refreshes;* desire for acids; longing for coffee; sensation as if a stone lay in the stomach, after eating, making him fretful. Pain in the epigastric region on pressure with anxiety; soreness in the pit of stomach when coughing; sour or bitter eructations after eating; nausea; vomiting of food but not of drinks; distention with sensitiveness to pressure."

The condition for which I have found Bryonia most frequently indicated is what the patients call "a bilious attack". These patients are in the habit of taking calomel "to jog the liver." When they do without calomel for some time, the bowels become constipated, the tongue heavily coated, the appetite greatly increased and they have a dull or bursting headache. Then comes vomiting of food and bile, sometimes bitter sometimes sour. The stools become diarrheic and putrid. Bryonia 3x given four times daily for two or three weeks will cure our patients of these attacks.

Nose: "Swelling with *bleeding;* bleeding for a quarter of an hour in *morning* after rising; bleeding *daily.*"

I have often verified this "bleeding" in those conditions, viz., the prodromal stage of typhoid; from vicarious or suppressed menstruation and with congestive headaches, reflex from congestion of the liver, kidneys or stomach. The *epistaxes* always *relieves,* temporarily, this bursting, splitting *headache.*

Intestines: "*Distended; sensitive;* distention after eating *relieved* by emission of offensive flatus; sudden cutting, digging pains compelling him to bend double, relieved by profuse pasty stools; sensitiveness and pain, in the hepatic region and in right side below the false ribs, worse from deep inspiration or motion of any kind; griping, pinching about umbilicus."

Abdomen: Bryonia is frequently indicated in *appendicitis* when you have constipation, extreme pain and tenderness locally; the thirst, headache and temperature of the drug. Notwithsanding the fact that many practice to the contrary, I feel we get the best results from heat locally when Bryonia is the remedy. I feel sure many a patient has been saved an operation by the use of Bryonia.

Dr. W. H. Dickinson claimed that in seven out of every ten cases of typhoid for which Bryonia was indicated, it would be the only remedy indicated, because the symptoms of the drug correspond to those of every stage of typhoid. If we take the dull morning headache, the mental confusion, the nose bleed, the delirium, talking about his business, the white coated tongue, later becoming brown, the thirst, abdominal soreness; the hard, dry, dark stools, we have the symptoms showing the condition of the mucous membrane of stomach and bowels during typhoid fever. The extreme soreness, thirst, coated tongue, high temperature call for Bryonia in peritonitis, enteritis, typhlitis, etc.

Blood.

I have already given you the various symptoms which indicate its use for *typhoid*. You will find it useful for *scarlet fever* when the *eruption* is rough, elevated in clusters and slow making its appearance. In such case the temperature is high, the thirst intense, the bowels constipated, the child slightly delirious, and there is a tendency to "stiffness of the muscles of the neck" (meningitis). In a few cases I have found it useful when there was recession of eruption.

Female Generative Organs.

"Menses suppressed; menses too early, too profuse, with dark red blood; metrorrhagia of a deep red blood with pains in the loins and in the head; suppressed menses with bleeding of nose; swelling of labia; lumps, indurations and inflammation of mammæ, with diminished or suppressed flow of milk."

Bryonia has helped many cases of *vicarious menstration* with the headache of the drug better after a profuse and *long continued nose bleed.*

The most frequent and satisfactory use I have made of Bryonia has been for *engorement* of the *breast* of the parturient woman. The breasts are enormously distended, hard and sore; the temperature is from 99 to 101; stools dry and hard, and the patient complains of a bursting, splitting headache. *Bryonia 3x* five drops every few hours internally with one part of tincture of poke root to three of water applied to the breasts *will* in most cases like the above *prevent suppuration. Puerperal metritis* with *cessation* of the *lochia,* the headache, heaviness of the legs, intense thirst, and marked *soreness* of the *uterus* will often yield to Bryonia. The first sign of success will be establishment of lochia and flow of milk. If this does not take place within twelve hours change the remedy. Use Bryonia 3x every half hour at first, then every hour. Finally for pelvic peritonitis where the agg. from motion is marked; great soreness; hard, dry stools; and the Bryonia headache.

Kidneys.

"Urine almost brown, red, reddish yellow with white sediment."

It is for functional disturbances that Bryonia is so often indicated, especially in such places as Iowa where *hard water* and *sudden changes of weather* cause *irritation,* pain in loins, general stiffness of the muscles and the conditions stated above. The only help for chronic nephritis I have ever secured from Bryonia was when there was an acute agg. of the chronic condition. The climate makes Bryonia the leading polychrest in Iowa, first because of its action on the respiratory organs and muscles and second upon the kidneys.

Skin.

I have already called your attention to its use in certain forms of scarlet fever helped by Bryonia. These cases are uncommon but the cases of measles needing the remedy are numerous. Next to Pulsatilla I use Bryonia most frequently for measles when the cough is very painful, more dry than the cough of Pulsatilla with soreness in the chest, the eruption delayed or receded.

There are a score of conditions for which Bryonia is a leading remedy. I use it from the 3x to 1m but most frequently the 3x.

HEPAR SULPHURIS CALCAREUM.

Make-up: Suppurating; sensitive.

Loc.: Glands; nerves; connective tissues; skin.

Sen.: Sharp; splinter-like, sticking; sore.

Mod.: Agg.: Cold air; drafts; part becoming cold; least touch or exertion; lying on painful side.

Amel.: Warmth, especially warm wraps; damp weather.

Leaders: *Every injury suppurates;* the patient sweats easily; the *agg. of every symptom from a draft of air* causing chilliness and nausea. As *Kali iod.* is called the "*liquid knife*" because it *absorbs* certain forms of *tumors* so Hepar is called "*the homeopathic lancet*" because it either *hastens* or *prevents suppuration.* You note I stated hastens or prevents suppuration. Many cases of inflammation have been prevented from suppurating by giving the 30th of Hepar. On the other hand cases where suppuration has begun are hastened, *i. e.*, prepared for the evacuation of pus by giving the 3rd and thus tissue has been saved, for as you all know pus means loss of tissue.

Not only have attacks of *tonsilitis* been aborted by the 30th or hastened to suppuration by the 3rd, but Hepar has cured many cases of suppuration when after the evacuation of pus the suppuration and swelling still continue. Also useful to prevent repeated recurrences of the disease. The leading symptoms of the group are *fetid odor of the saliva* which saliva is very profuse, the *splinter-like pains agg.* by swallowing and the marked sensitiveness to air, especially *drafts* of *cold* air.

The *inguinal glands* next to the tonsils seem to be mostly affected (Bubos). The same conditions, sensations and modalities exist. Abscesses of the labiæ often call for Hepar. Rarely abscesses of the lungs will present Hepar symptoms.

Mucous Membranes.

Eyes: "Inflammation and swelling with redness of white; pain from daylight; in any bright light if he moves them; sore *agglutinated* at *night;* hard mucus; pain in balls with bruised pain on touch; *pressing*, sticking pains in lids."

For many conditions of *scrofulous patients, e. g., blepharitis, corneal ulcers, chronic catarrh, kerato-iritis,* erysipelas, eczema. In all cases the patients are anemic, sluggish, have low vitality, sweat easily—worse at night. Quite a large per cent. of the patients have suffered from the ill effects of Mercurius (salivation). The ulcerations of the cornea involve the deeper layers and the amount of pus is large in the anterior chamber. The chronic catarrhal conditions are also accompanied by much pus which is hard and lumpy. The erysipelas is of the purulent form.

Ear: "Sticking pains on blowing nose; external ear red, hot and itching; purulent discharge."

For *otitis* and *otorrhea* following overdosing with Mercury. The discharge is mucous, bloody, purulent or mixed. In many cases particles of bone may be found in the discharge. The pains are generally severe, sharp, sticking and burning. The agg. is from cold.

Nose: "Coryza with inflammation, swelling of the nostrils; mucus from the posterior nares mixed with blood; bleeding; smell sensitive or lost."

We have two conditions here, viz., *chronic catarrhal* and the *result of mercury*. With both we find *ulcers* with soreness, sharp splinter-like pains; swelling; profuse *greenish-yellow,* offensive discharge (Pulsatilla, Kali iod., Graphites); and the *agg.* by cold air and touch.

Mouth: "White aphthous pustules on inside of lips and cheeks and on tongue; offensive odor; bitter taste."

For *stomatitis* when the ulcers bleed easily and when there is an offensive odor from them (Kali chlo., Muriatic ac.). For *abscesses at* the *roots* of *teeth* when the teeth have mercurial fillings.

Throat: *"Sticking as from a splinter on swallowing, extending towards ear on yawning;* soreness beneath the larynx after eating; smarting agg. swallowing with rawness and scraping; feeling as if he had to swallow over a swelling."

Useful for *follicular pharyngitis* with the sensations and modalities of the drug.

Stomach: "*Desire for vinegar;* appetite only for pungent things; frequent odorless, tasteless eructations after eating; nausea in morning; vomiting of bile in morning after long retching; gnawing as from acids, rising into throat."

The best remedy for *acid dyspepsia* following the abuse of mercury or quinine, when the ranking symptom is the desire for *spices* or *acids.*

Rectum, Anus and Stools: "Urging, but large intestines are wanting in peristaltic action and cannot expel even soft feces, only a part can be forced out by aid of the abdominal muscles; soft, difficult, scanty stool with much urging; clay colored."

The secretions of the intestines together with the weakness gives us a condition peculiar to Hepar, *i. e.,* by straining the stool is partially expelled, but owing to its sticky, putty-like character a part remains and is drawn up as the intestine goes up when straining ceases (Silica). This stool is light-colored, showing lack of bile.

We also find a diarrheic stool, sour, light-colored, undigested, containing undigested food and mucus; also green, and of decayed odor. We also have *sour sweat* which with the *sour stools* are the ranking symptoms of the group.

Sexual Organs: "Ulcers externally on prepuce, similar to chancer."

For *venereal ulcers* with very profuse *offensive discharge.* Also for *venereal warts* with offensive odor (Thuja).

Respiratory Organs: "Loose cough agg. by deep breathing so as to cause vomiting; *paroxysmal cough, if slightest portion becomes cold, with sensitiveness of nervous system;* a suffocative cough from tightness of breath *agg. talking, stooping,* and *late in evening;* frequent deep breathing as after running; dyspnea."

Chest: "Oppression, with burning; feeling as if hot water moved about in it; sticking pains in sides."

For *subacute laryngitis* with profuse secretion of thin mucus.

9

For *membranous croup,* the last stage, *when* there is a *large accumulation* of *pus* which *increases* the *dyspnea* and *hoarseness.* For this condition use the 6th and do not repeat too often. If given too low and repeated too often Hepar will only agg. the condition you wish to relieve. It does so by drying the purulent secretions and adding that much obstruction to that of the membrane. With all conditions of this section, Hepar patients sweat profusely and are weak. You never find much temp. nor do you find a hot, dry skin. (Aconite, Bromine, Spongia, all have temp. and dryness of the skin and *usually precede Hepar in croup.*) For the last stage Hepar is second only to Kali bich.

Hepar is also frequently called for in *chronic bronchitis.* Here again we have large collection of pus, a loose rattling cough and respiration with agg. from *cold air* and in the early morning, with the same profuse sweat on least exertion.

In the *last stages of pleurisy with exudation* when you find the above conditions and modalities. Finally for *chronic pneumonia* with free purulent expectoration and threatening abscess. Notice that the symptoms are directly opposite those of Sulphur for this condition. With Sulphur everything is tight and dry and the temp. high and going higher.

Skin: "Yellow; *unhealthy; slight injuries suppurate* (Silica); red itching spots, soon covered with yellow blisters, which change to scurf (Staphisagria); soreness and moisture in fold between scrotum and thigh (Sulphur); cracking and smarting of hands and feet; ulcer bleeding on slight wiping (Nitric ac.); ulcer sensitive to touch (Asafœdita); agg. by cold of every kind (Silica).

For *eczemas* of all varieties with the above symptoms, especially the bad odor, and agg. by cold. For *boils* and all *injuries* with *tendency* to *suppurate* (Echinacea). I have found that the use of Hepar internally and a solution of 1 to 500 of the tincture of Echinacea locally act nicely together.

Thermic Centers.

Hepar has chills and chilliness very marked. The temperature is never very high accompanying the catarrhal and septic conditions. The sweat is a constant factor agg. at night, is sour, offensive and greatly agg. by exertion.

NUX VOMICA.

Make-up: Dark; firm-fibered; excitable; ill-humored.

Loc.: Brain and nerves; digestive organs including the liver; respiratory organs.

Sen.: Dull; sharp; twisting; *urging;* nausea.

Mod.: Agg. in early morning; *uncovering;* cold, open air; *coffee;* liquor; draft; sedentary habits; noises; odors.

Amel. from free elimination; wrapping up warm and dry.

Leaders: Excitable; sensitive; impatient; *vertigo; sour taste* and *eructations;* ineffectual urging.

Brain and Nerves.

The most pronounced characteristic of Nux is spasm of all muscle fiber whether voluntary or involuntary. These spasms are tetanic. They produce irregular, perverted, peristaltic action of the muscles thus affecting digestion and nutrition as well as elimination and so laying the foundation of many diseases. The spasms acting on thermic centers produce well defined paroxysms of chill, fever and sweat. There are very few changes in structure such as we find in Phosphorus and Argentum nit., nor is there marked inflammation, but the irritation and changes of function are marked. Let us now observe the symptoms of these two conditions in the brain and nervous system.

Trunk in General: "*Spasms* with *tetanic rigidity* of nearly all *muscles,* with interruptions of a few minutes during which muscles are relaxed; convulsions brought on by *slightest touch* or draft of *cold air; contractive pains through* whole body; *opisthotonos with inability to move but wants to be held* (case of poisoning); weakness; paralysis."

Stomach: The most frequent *cause* of *convulsions* which Nux will cure *is indigestion,* the result of partaking of all sorts of food and drinks in a hurry, when tired and at improper intervals, as is the habit with us Americans. For the above reason Nux is our most frequently used remedy. To illustrate: A bright, active boy of seven years was having one convulsion after another. I could not find any cause till I saw in the pockets of a younger brother some haws. I gave the patient two drams of mustard in water. The boy vomited over a pint of the haws. I did not think anything more was needed and left the boy only to be recalled after an interval of two hours because the convulsions continued. Nux 30th stopped them. Emptying the stomach and bowels is one of the essentials to success when using Nux for acute indigestion. *Chorea* is often *helped* and sometimes *cured* by Nux. *Epileptiform convulsions* are palliated by Nux if the *cause* is *indigestion.* Regulation of *diet* is *important* in these cases and some other remedy will usually be needed to complete the cure.

When treating convulsions with Nux, keep your patient dry, covered, quiet and warm.

Mind: "*Quarrelsome even to violence; ill-humored; sensitive* to impression on senses; *intolerance* of talking, music, singing, bright light, and strong odors; *hypochondriacs after eating* (just remember how you felt after your last debauch); *dread* of *literary work* at which one must think, *in morning;* taciturn; impatient."

Most of the above mental symptoms are reflex from the stomach. It is also useful for *brain fag* of *students,* bookkeepers, *persons of sedentary habits* who do not get proper exercise. Such patients are hypochondriacs; have fiery tempers, are passionate, jealous, have a sluggish liver and suffer from alternating *constipation* with the *ineffectual urging,* and diarrhea.

Head: "*Aching in morning in bed,* as if beaten with an axe; *aching* in morning on waking even *before opening the eyes;* aching *worse from eating with* nausea and *sour vomiting; stupefying,* aching on waking, better from rising; *dizzy heaviness* in morning with *intoxicating confusion; vertigo; tensive* pain; pain as if he had not slept enough; *intermittent pain* as if a nail were forced deeper and deeper into the parietal bone."

One of our best remedies for *nervous, sick headache,* the "American headache" (Sanguinaria, Spigelia and Iris), usually the result of gastric disturbances. If the attack comes on soon after a meal, empty the stomach. If it comes later give the patient half pint or pint of hot normal salt solution. For *congestive headache,* worse in the morning, *with* marked *vertigo,* foul breath, bloated face, bad taste and the contemptible mental state of the drug. With the congestive form the patient suffers from hemorrhoids, worse from walking. For a *recurring headache, i. e.,* one coming on after sleep or after a period of close application of the mind. *Neuralgic* headache, generally supra-orbital (Cedron, Spigelia, Nartum mur.). With all forms of headache you find the mental symptoms, the nausea and vomiting and the *agg. from* the *use of coffee.*

Eyes: "Lachrymation in morning; *photophobia* in morning with *obscured vision;* vision sensitive, cloudy; jerking, sticking pains through the l. hemisphere of the brain, towards the parietal bone and occiput."

For *neuralgia* ciliary and supra-orbital; *amaurosis* from tobacco and alcohol with a restricted field of vision; *asthenopia* due to retinal hyperesthesia; *photophobia* worse in morning, better later in day; *atrophy* of the *optic nerve.* For the last condition the active principle of Nux, Strychnia is better. One of our eye specialists in Des Moines, who had gained a wide reputation for successful treatment of atrophy, told me his method was to use strychnia $\frac{1}{50}$ grain hypodermically about the orbit two or three times per week and the tincture of Nux vomica, five drops before breakfast, each day. Remember all you can do for such cases is to arrest the progress of the disease.

Ears: "Ringing; hissing; roaring (China, Belladonna) in the morning after rising; sticking, sharp thrusts."

"*Otalgia* with *intermittent pains,* worse in bed and in a warm room; *deafness* with the roaring, ringing, etc., with great sensitiveness of the nerve."

This condition usually comes with the headaches.

Jaws: "Drawing in the masseter muscles with stiffness; tetanic rigidity; drawing, tearing *pains* in the muscles of the jaw; *contraction* of the jaws *like lockjaw.*"

Useful for *prosopalgia* agg. in morning, stiffness and spasms of the jaws, the result of exposure to cold and wet.

Mouth: "Pain in hollow tooth, if cold air enters mouth; drawing, boring, tearing pains in teeth, even sound teeth, *agg. cold air* and *thinking about them.*"

The odontalgia is better from warmth, worse from cold, especially cold air and after eating. It is the result of taking cold or ulceration. With the latter you have a *sensation* as if the *teeth,* even the healthy ones, were being *wrenched out.*

Stomach and Abdomen: "*Scraped sensation* in pit; *pain* in pit in the morning, then cutting in abdomen and nausea; *cutting as from a stone* in epigastric region worse from walking, better from sitting; feeling in epigastric region as if overloaded; seems as if esophagus were constricted by spasm; *flatulent distention of abdomen; rumbling* and *gurgling* in morning in bed with spasmodic and griping flatulent colic and heat in hands and soles (Sulphur). "Gas rising and becoming incarcerated under short ribs; *weakness* in ring *as if hernia would form* (Cocculus); *pain* in *ring,* in morning *as if hernia* would become *incarcerated;* cutting and pinching in the hypogastrium with fermenting rumbling, then watery diarrhea; *cutting* as if *flatulence* were *forcing out* the *bladder, perineum, rectum* and *anus.*"

This irritation of the nerves of the stomach and intestines

resulting in perverted peristalsis is the beginning if not the cause of seven tenths of all the ills for which Nux is useful. Besides reflex conditions in other locations, such as the headaches, it produces marked *gastralgia* and *enteralgia,* nausea and *vomiting;* acid, atonic, and flatulent *dyspepsia,* etc. All this causes mal-nutrition with its long train of disorders.

What causes the *irritation?* It *is caused* by the use of *alcoholic beverages; coffee;* highly seasoned, rich foods; mixed diet; over-ripe and *unripe* food (Arsenicum) and excitement. Nux is also very useful for *hernia* (Cocculus, Lycopodium, Veratrum) caused by the abnormal peristalsis.

Urinary Organs: "*Urging;* frequent, *ineffectual,* difficult micturition."

Nux is the best remedy I know for irritability of bladder or urethra *caused by the use of the catheter.* You may have any of the symptoms mentioned above plus *inability to void,* or inability alone. The patient seems to wait for the use of the catheter. I have used Nux 30th for this condition more often than for all the others of the urinary organs. In such cases the use of the catheter has been painful. Aside from this cause *retention may* be due to *spasmodic closure* of the *neck* of the bladder, the result of irritation by calculi (Berberis). It is useful occasionally for *strangury,* also for *paralysis* with dribbling of urine.

Sexual Organs: "*Erections* in morning, also after naps; *menses* too early *with cramps.*"

For an intense, agonizing *dysmenorrhea* with constant desire to defecate and urinate, also with nausea, pain in sacrum as if it would break, red face and ill-humor; for *irregular labor pains* which go down the thighs, accompanied by urging to stool. With the uterine conditions the patient is always cross (Chamomilla, Nitric ac.).

Respiratory Organs: "*Dry cough* from midnight till daybreak; dry, *fatiguing* cough about midnight if she lies upon back, worse lying on side."

For *cough* of public speakers, especially *from talking* in the *open air* (Alumina), better from warm drinks; *reflex cough* associated with indigestion worse after eating, with soreness over stomach. I cured a patient of asthma, the attacks coming towards morning, always worse after eating a heavy meal in the evening. Nux 30th every four hours and fasting after the noon meal cured. Whether one would have cured without the other I do not know.

Back and Extremities: "Burning, bruised, tearing pain along the vertebræ, bruised pain in lumbar region in morning, with pain as from gas low down in the hypogastrium; tottering, unsteadiness in lower extremities; stiffness in the hollow of the knee with tension; paralytic drawing in the muscles of the thigh and calf, painful on walking."

For *spinal irritation* with partial paralysis of the extremities; *lumbago* worse at night in bed (Rhus), with stiffness and inability to turn over; the back feels stiff, lame and bruised. For *multiple sclerosis* and palliative for locomotor ataxia.

Liver: "*Stitches* in *region* of *liver* worse from contact or motion; throbbing in hepatic region, agg. by the slightest touch and by every movement, with pulsations, shooting, pressive, and tensive pains; pressure and stinging in the region of the liver; throbbing in and below the hepatic region as if an ulcer would form."

For *hob-nail liver* which, as you know, is one result of the excessive use of alcohol. With this you usually have the *constipation, hemorrhoids,* and *yellow* sclera and *skin;* for *congestion of* the *liver* with *engorgement,* extreme soreness and yellow skin. The cause of this form of liver trouble is often fits of anger.

Heart.

The symptoms of the *heart* are not many and will be reserved for study and grouping when we take up Strychnia. The *condition* is mostly *due* to *portal obstruction; angina* due to suppression of hemorrhoids, with constriction, agonizing pain, vomiting and in some cases opisthotonos with protrusion of eyes.

I have seen good results from different potencies from five-drop doses of the tincture for atrophy of the optic nerve to the 1m for insomnia.

The above are a few, the most important, of the many conditions for which this great polychrest is used. I use all potencies from the 3rd to 1000th.

MERCURIUS.

Loc.: *Blood; bones;* all tissues to some degree, *glands.*

Sen.: All the sensations.

Mod.: Agg. *drafts;* cold, damp weather; *NIGHT sweating;* lying on right side.

Amel. moderate temperature.

Leaders: *Sweat without relief; free secretions;* increased saliva; metallic taste; *flabby tongue.*

Blood.

Mercurius produces in general *profound anemia,* with *degeneration* of the *red blood corpuscles,* loss of albumen and fibrin and *diminished coagulability* of the blood. There is also a marked tendency to destructive action and the *effete* matter is *retained* in the *system.* Sore mouth, salivation, decayed teeth are among the first symptoms to appear. The drug produces irritation, inflammation, functional and structural changes of nearly every tissue of the body. The *most frequent fever is* the *catarrhal; rheumatoid arthritis.*

Brain and Nerves.

"*Trembling of hands* (Argentium nit., Platina) and tongue. T. of limbs agg. *night,* excitement, attempting to hold anything; amel. walking and standing, sleep in bed; *involuntary motion of hands and head; hastiness in all motions;* jerking; *weakness;* restlessness towards evening: he could not remain sitting."

Hysteria with restlessness, the agg. at night; hurried talking (Hyoscyamus); easily agitated; *chorea* when dependent upon some diathesis. There is nothing characteristic about the aura or convulsions.

Mind: "Delirium like *delirium tremens,* muttering (Hyoscyamus); believes he is losing his reason, thinks he is dying. *Illusions, e. g.,* sees water running where there is none; *anxiety;* apprehension, with feeling as if he had not control over his senses, without heat (Ignatia, Veratrum); sadness; *slow answering questions* (Lycopodium phos., Aconite, Opium); *memory weak.*"

The mercury patient in most conditions is *disgusted* with himself and *talks suicide.* He is *morose* and *mistrustful.* There is restlessness and fear of some impending evil.

Head: "Aching in brain just beneath the scalp, as if heavy and tight; *tensive pain encircling head above the eyes and ears;* weakness like a dullness and as if there were a vibrating in forehead and turning about in a circle; drawing; jerking pain in temple."

For a *catarrhal headache, syphilitic,* agg. at night. The *most marked sensation* being the sensation as if the head were bound tight by a band. Also for subacute *meningitis.* With these two conditions you will usually find bone diseases, especially of the skull.

Face: Neuralgia of the face from taking cold, when the tearing, shooting pains are agg. at night, when you have profuse saliva and the flabby tongue.

Speech: "*Stammering* (Stramonium); speech *difficult, on account of trembling of mouth and tongue;* tremulous; impeded; unintelligible."

Bones.

Head: Mercurius is occasionally indicated for *ulceration* and caries of the bones of the skull, about the *eyes* and in *jaws.* You get the *agg.* from *touch,* also the agg. at *night.*

Teeth: "*Decayed and became loose in succession;* fell out at slight touch; those that remained were ***black, bare, loose*** and ***carious; denuded*** gums, with nightly pains in teeth, jaws and head; jerking pains agg. at night."

Gums: "*Swollen* and ***separated from teeth; bleeding*** from slightest touch; spongy; ulcerated; suppurating; ***sore pain on touch*** and from *CHEWING;* agg. hard food."

A remedy of the highest rank for ***dental periostitis*** with marked ***soreness*** and ***pain from*** the least ***touch,*** agg. at night by warmth of bed, also offensive saliva. For ***inflammation*** and ***ulceration*** of gums with the same symptoms.

Back and Extremities: We have symptoms of caries of the spine but it is for the long bones of the extremities that Mercurium has a ***marked*** "Elective affinity." Here we have ***caries*** of the bones, ulceration of the bone and periosteum, also of the muscles and skin above the diseased bone. The discharges from the ulcers are sanious and very offensive. The ***aching*** is severe at night and there are sharp pains whenever the ulcers are dressed. The ulcers bleed readily when touched (Nitric ac., Asafœtida).

Mucous Membrane.

Eyes: "***Inflammation,*** with swollen, inverted torsi and ***sensitiveness to light*** agg. open air; ***forcibly drawn together;*** heat and biting as from horse radish, with redness; chronic conjunctivitis with fine injection around the cornea."

A very ***valuable*** remedy *for all forms of OPHTHALMIAS; CATARRHAL* with muco-purulent, excoriating discharge, agglutination of lids, marked photophobia, ***agg. at night*** with rawness and ***redness*** of the ***margin*** of the ***lids;*** *SCROFULOUS* with the ***agg.*** at ***night*** and still more from ***heat of fire;*** rarely *SYPHILITIC* when the inflammation is caused by working with a bright light, *e. g.,* automobile works, glass blowers, etc., Mercurius has also helped *ULCERATIONS* of the ***lids, tear ducts, cornea.*** The ***corneal*** ulcers are usually ***serpiginous*** with ***turbidity*** and marked tendency of sloughing of the entire cornea, photophobia, nightly agg.

Ears: "*Bloody and offensive* matter flows from ears (Tellurium), internal ear sore and denuded; feels inflamed internally and externally, with pain partly cramplike, partly sticking and feeling as if stopped by a swelling."

Has cured many persons suffering from *acute* and *chronic catarrh* of the *tympanum* extending into the eustachian tube, causing deafness. The cause may be an ordinary cold but often after measles; also for sufferers from *suppuration, ulceration, herpetic* and *furuncular INFLAMMATION* of the auditory canal. The *otorrhea* of Mercurius is composed of *blood, pus, mucus* and *serum.* The agg. at night and cold is marked, also agg. by extreme heat.

Nose: "*Offensive odor from the nose as in coryza* (Aurum); frequent sneezing agg. morning without coryza; *acrid flow* with the odor of old cheese; bleeding during sleep."

Useful for *ozena* when in addition to the bad odor there is marked soreness of the bone, *i. e.,* ulceration of the membrane has extended to the bone; *catarrh.* I remember a man about 40, who came with the statement that he must leave the climate unless his nasal catarrh could be cured. There was marked soreness of the nose and a profuse discharge of mucus, pus and blood, which was adherent to the nostrils. He had tried everything. He had decayed teeth, the craving for acids and a loose mucous stool. He had the teeth cared for, used glycothymoline for a wash and took Mercurius sol. 3rd before each meal and at bed time. It took two months to cure him.

Mouth: "*Tongue black* with red edges; white; tremulous: *coated and showing the imprint of the teeth in edges;* swollen. and ulcerated."

I will not give you all the symptoms of the highest rank but condense them into the following conditions; *aphthous stomatitis* with broad, shallow ulcers, undermined; profuse saliva; the bad odor; the sharp sticking pain and agg. at night. The pillow is often wet with saliva after sleep.

Throat: "Redness of soft palate, tonsils and uvula with

ulceration; *suppuration of tonsils with sharp sticking pains* (Hepar); inability to swallow liquids below region of the larynx; it returns through nose."

One of our most frequently used remedies for *catarrhal* and *ulcerative* conditions of the *throat*, also for suppurative tonsilitis. The pains on swallowing are sharp and sticking (Hepar, Nitric ac.).

Stomach: We find some peculiar desires and aversions, *e. g.*, *aversion to bread and butter*, also to *wine* and *brandy*, to which he was accustomed; ravenous appetite but she feels it is not genuine hunger. For *catarrhal* gastritis with burning pains agg. at night and after eating.

"*Hard and distended from gas;* griping with constant desire for stool, but little is evacuated (Nux); intestines sore as if pressed so that he cannot lie on the right side (Magnesia mur.)."

It has served me for *catarrhal enteritis* with *cutting, tearing* pains and *discharge* of *mucus* with slight *tenesmus*; for appendicitis after the acute symptoms have subsided and you have tenderness in the region, with stools of blood, mucus and soft fecal matter. One case of *subacute colitis* with marked tenderness and profuse mucous stools followed by a sensation as if there still remained large quantities, yielded to Mercurius 3rd.

Rectum: "*Constant ineffectual urging with tenesmus of rectum, with protruding, painful, sore hemorrhoids.*"

Stools: "Diarrhea in the evening, at night; *stools streaked with blood;* of green mucus (Argentum nit., Ipecac, Gamboge) *with burning* and protrusion of anus and tenesmus after stools; green, slimy, acrid excretions from the anus."

One of our best remedies for *diarrhea* when the stools are mostly mucus and when there is some tenesmus. Also for a mild form of dysentery.

Urinary Organs: "*Constant desire, but little urine is passed;* must urinate at least every hour, day and night with *burning* in the *urethra* on beginning to urinate; *involuntary micturition* if he does not hurry; a *greenish, painless discharge* agg. at night from the urethra; swelling of the forepart of urethra with pus between gland and prepuce which is hot, red and painful."

First for *cystitis* with discharge of mucus which burns, with dribbling, tenesmus; for *gonorrhea* with *profuse discharge and swelling of the inguinal* glands, and balanitis. Finally *albuminuria of pregnancy* but Mercurius cor. is better suited for that condition.

Sexual Organs: "Prepuce swollen as if distended with air or water to a blister, at the *end* of the *penis; under* the prepuce at first *vesicles* which *become* large, *bleeding ulcers* with *margin everted like raw meat, caseous coating on base of ulcers; leucorrhea greenish causing biting* in *forepart of genitals,* so that she must scratch, when the *biting turns* to *burning,* agg. evening and night; menses too profuse."

Mercurius has been used with success for *abscess* of the *vulva; pruritus; subacute ovaritis,* generally with a tendency to suppurate, *specific* and *nonspecific vaginitis* with the greenish *excoriating discharge;* herpes of the prepuce and *venereal ulcers.* A young man presented himself with the following symptoms: "Ulcers beneath the prepuce, bleeding freely, warts over the skin of the penis which he had been clipping with scissors; a profuse discharge from the urethra with burning during micturition and painful buboes. He also had gonorrheal conjunctivitis. Treatment was five grains of Mercurius sol. 3rd every three hours, bathing the parts with 1 to 2000 mercurial solution and then sprinkling powdered Mercurius sol. 3rd over the entire surface. The parts were dressed twice daily. The condition cleared up in three weeks.

Respiratory Organs: "Violent night cough which rings and feels as if everything in the chest were dry, with pains in the chest and small of back."

Aside from *chronic bronchitis* and *laryngitis* with a spasmodic cough agg. night and lying on the right side. I have used Mercurius a few times for *lobar pneumonia* of infants of the right side with jaundice; tenderness of the liver; and a loose nocturnal cough without expectoration. A few cases of *chronic pleurisy* with the *sharp sticking* agg. night.

Gland and Glandular Organs: Mercurius acts upon all glands, causing any of the four conditions: Ir., itis, functional and structural changes. The glands most frequently affected are those of the neck and groins. The glandular organs are the parotid, tonsils, *liver,* spleen and kidneys. We use Mercurius sol. more than any other form of Mercurius for liver troubles, especially for *chronic inflammation* with *marked tenderness,* yellow skin and sclera; loose, mucous stools and agg. night and lying on right side.

Skin: "*Jaundice* with biting, itching on abdomen; *TETTER* with superficial ulcers on the tetter which became covered with *yellow scabs;* heat; *round pimples* especially on thighs and legs, becoming round ulcers, at last scurfy; *ulcers* with whitish-gray bases and *margins* which *bleed easily.*"

Useful for *eczema; herpes;* intetrigo with the agg. night and a marked tendency to ulcerate, with severe sharp, burning, lancinating pain.

The symptoms and conditions which we have considered above are those of pure quicksilver or of Hahneman's black oxide (Mercurius sol.).

There are many compounds of Mercurius which differ from the pure quicksilver in the intensity of their action, also in causing new symptoms and conditions. We will not enter into their action as fully as we did that of Mercurius, but simply take up the different members of the family and compare them with the original. The first we will study is *Mercurius corrosivus* (corrosive sublimate).

Mercurius Corrosivus

Its *action* is very similar to that of Mercurius sol., only *much intensified*. Mercurius cor. has much less moisture; it has the highest temperature of any of the Mercurius group; also more pain. Its action is most severe on the mucous membranes and kidneys.

I cured one of the worst cases of *gonorrhoeal conjunctivitis* I ever saw with the 6th, three grains every three hours. The mucous membrane hung in threads so great was the destructive inflammation; the swelling was marked and the photophobia such that she could not keep the eye open. The pain was expressed by the child as, "It burns like fire."

Many of our oculists consider it one of the best remedies for the *retinitis* of Bright's disease. Numerous cases of pustular *ophthalmia* and *ulceration* of the cornea, *choroiditis,* and *kerato-iritis* with adhesions. *Note* the *intensity* of the *inflammation* and destruction of tissue.

Mouth: "*Violent stomatitis, large aphthous patches* which are *often syphilitic.*"

Throat: Now and then for *diphtheria* with little membrane, hot, dry throat, high temperature, scanty albuminous urine.

Rectum: I have found it the *best remedy* for the *most severe form of dysentery* when you have a high temp., great thirst and severe chill after drinking, stools almost clear blood, with shreds of the mucous lining of the intestines, constant urging to stool and also to micturition and terrible tenesmus.

Urinary and Sexual Organs: Although it is highly spoken of for violent cystitis, I have never used it with success except for most *severe specific urethritis* (the so-called "dry clapp") with violent erections, discharge only drops of blood; almost constant urging. I use the 3rd for this condition.

Mercuric Sulphide (Cinnabaris).

We would expect that a compound of Mercurius and Sulphur would produce more groups of skin symptoms than any remedy in the Materia Medica, but the contrary is the fact. One case very similar to the one mentioned under Mercurius sol., which did not yield to Mercurius sol., did improve very readily under the Mercurius sulph. It has also helped me in one or two cases of *gleet.* I can only vouch for its use for warts and condylomata of sycotic origin excited by gonorrhea infection.

Mercurius Cyanatus.

The only help I have ever had from this member of the family was for *diphtheria.* You will find very *little* or no *membrane* (exudate), *little inflammation* of the throat; drowsy; urine albuminous, scant, in some cases completely suppressed. These are the cases one dreads. Allen has the following under throat, in the highest rank: "*Necrotic destruction of soft* parts of palate and fauces." Use it low and repeat often.

Mercurius Dulcis.

This is pure calomel triturated for our use. The abuse of this drug is what has brought the entire mercury family into disrepute. My old preceptor used to have me make the famous "blue mass pill" usually 15 grain doses. He used to say: "We must give enough to touch the gums," Nowadays it is used in 1/10 gr. doses given every hour till you get the desired result, *i. e.,* diuresis, and free evacuations of the bowels.

The only use I ever made of the drug is for "diarrhea of infants." The symptoms are: *Stool greenish,* rarely dark gray, some straining, a little excoriating, liver enlarged and tender, mucous membrane of mouth pale, sometimes covered with aphthous patches, foul breath, much saliva. Use 6th.

Mercurius Iodatus Flavus.

We usually speak of this as "Mercurius protoide." Bear in mind that the "elective affinity of Iodine is for the glands, so when added to Mercurius we may see why the compound acts most profoundly on the glands and M.M. *Follicular tonsillitis* is the condition for which it is most frequently used. The tonsils are large, tender, covered with follicles; the tongue is coated yellowish white on the base; the breath is bad; the servical glands are swollen; there are often sharp pains in the Eustachian tubes; occasionally suppuration of the middle ear and rupture of the ear drum.

It is better than Mercurius sol. for syphilitic iritis, but not as marked for photophobia as Mercurius cor.

It is better than Mercurius for chronic post nasal catarrh involving not only the Eustachian tubes but the frontal sinuses. The peculiar coating of the tongue is always present in these cases.

Mercurius Iodatus Ruber.

The two conditions in which this Mercurius excells is for *sore throat* and diseases of the *sexual organs*. It differs from the "protoxide" in that it acts on the left side and has more temp. The other symptoms are the same for this group. Many physicians claim that for all conditions due to syphilis, such as erosions, ulcerations, inflammations, discharges, etc., of the sexual organs the ruber is the most effective of the group.

Mercurius Nitrosus.

One of our prominent oculists told me once when I took a patient to him who was suffering from *conjunctivitis* which I thought Mercurius sol. should cure but did not, that if we homeopaths would use the nitrate of Mercurius for such conditions of the eye we would have less failures. I have since verified his statement many times.

ARGENTUM NITRICUM.

Make-up: Nervous; dyspeptic; anemic.

Loc.: *Mucous membrane; nerves;* blood; liver; kidneys.

Sen.: *Trembling;* weakness; aching; boring; splinter-like; rawness; soreness; distention.

Mod.: Agg.: *Emotions,* anxiety and suspense; *sugar;* close room; brain fag; night; bright light.

Amel.: cool air; cool bath; tight bandaging.

Leaders: Craving for sugar; flatulence.

Mucous Membrane.

Eye: "*Blood red,* with swelling of caruncula lachrymalis and with *clusters* of *red vessels* extending from inner canthus to cornea; gray spots and bodies in shape of serpents moving before the vision; redness of conjunctiva, of eyeballs and lids; puckering and interstitial distention of conjunctiva; increased secretion of tears; *filled with mucus* causing *blindness;* neuralgic pains."

The use of Argentum as a *prophylactic for ophthalmia neonatorum* is so well known that most states make its use compulsory in all cases of newborn babies. For its curative effects it is used when you have *violent* inflammation, great swelling, *large quantities of pus* and mucus. Most frequently used for *purulent ophthalmia,* also for chronic ulcerations of the margin of the lids with thickening of the lids. Combine local application with the internal use of the 30x and keep cold applications to the eyes.

Stomach: "*Irresistible appetite* (desire) for sugar; violent *eructations,* insipid or tasting of ingesta; *nausea* worse during and after meals; faintish, nauseated feeling in P.M. with palpitation of heart; retching; *vomiting* which *tinged* the cloth *black;* painful swelling of pit; sensation of *lump* in pit with *tremulous feeling* in and *sensation* as if the *head* were *in a vice;* trembling and throbbing."

The best remedy we have for the *gastritis* of *drunkards.* There is always a large quantity of gas and marked distention which is somewhat relieved by the eructations. For *disordered stomach* especially of *children who crave sweets.* Such children have thick, white coated tongue, nausea, eructations, diarrhoea and much flatus; with stool of green mucus like chopped spinach. For *ulceration* of the stomach when the *pains extend* into the *chest,* shoulders, and down into the *abdomen.* With this condition you find nausea and the *vomiting* tinged with blood. There is marked agg. of the stomach symptoms from food or water. Use the 12x or 30x.

Throat: "Redness of valeum palati, posterior nares and isthmus; *dark redness of uvula and fauces; sensation* of a *splinter* when swallowing; *thick, tenacious mucus* obliging him to hawk; *rawness* and soreness; roughness; scraping."

The sore throat which Argentum nit. will cure is usually caused by smoking and drinking. There is dryness and the splinter-like pain is marked. Catarrhal conditions with the sensation of a hair often causes a cough agg. by smoking.

Urethra: "*Inflammation* with pain; *priapism; burning* in urethra during micturition with swollen feeling and *difficulty* in *passing* the last part of *urine; ulcerative* pains between the acts of micturition; ulcerative pains as from a splinter during the act of micturition; *painful erection;* chordee; ineffectual urging."

The best remedy for the early purulent stage of gonorrhea when there is a profuse discharge; *terrible cutting, burning pains* and frequently *bloody urine.* Use the 3x or 6x internally with the local application.

Female Sexual Organs: "Ulceration of vagina, os and cervix, with frequent bleeding from points of ulceration; copious, yellow, corroding discharge." The same treatment as for the Urethritis.

Rectum: "Urging, sudden with copious, liquid stool; burning with bloody mucus."

For *dysentery* with the bloody, slimy mucous stool, also for chronic diarrhea with the copious stools containing shreds of mucus and undigested food with vomiting and the emission of much flatus.

Brain and Nervous System.

Mind: "*Does not undertake anything lest he should not succeed;* memory impaired; ill humor; excessively merry; delirious rage; *easily excited or angered;* always in a hurry; complete loss of consciousness; *apprehensive* of some incurable disease."

Nearly twenty-five years ago a prominent physician was sent to me for treatment. He had been treated in a Chicago hospital for progressive paralysis of the insane. He had had and still was having repeated attacks of epilepsy. He presented the following symptoms: silly; easily excited; jolly one minute, mad and sullen the next; mind so weak he could not write a sentence. (I still have four pages of scribbling without one complete sentence. He gave it to me to mail his wife.) His bowels were loose, frothy, at times involuntary. He craved candy of all kinds. His *epileptic attacks* were as follows: A sharp cry; fall; violent muscular twitching of all the muscles, especially marked of the throat; complete unconsciousness; frothing at mouth; often bit his tongue; then a deep sleep for about three hours. The silly and sullen *moods* were *worse after* an *attack*. He had used tobacco to excess, and alcohol to some extent. He was deprived of both, put upon Argentum nit. 30x and a regulated diet. He was so improved after four months that he went south for a short time and then home in Iowa. He resumed his practice; afterwards was mayor of his city, president of the Hahn. Med. Assoc. of Iowa, and wrote a book. His epileptic attacks never returned. I have *cured* two other *epileptic patients* with the remedy.

Head: "Headache from mental exertion, better from binding the head tightly; *aching* with *enlarged feeling;* drawing in bands over surface of brain *or* sinuses; apparently congestion with throbbing of carotids; heaviness and stupefying dullness of the head; weaknes of mind and inability to express himself suitably and coherently; vertigo with weakness of limbs and trembling; *boring* in left frontal eminence; aching in one side with *enlarged feeling* in the corresponding eye; intermitting, cutting, *motion* in *occiput* extending *through* left *hemisphere* to frontal protuberance, increasing and decreasing rapidly."

The president of a large investment company who worried a great deal and worked hard came to me with the following symptoms: "sharp cutting pains through left side of head with vertigo, nausea and vomiting;" "head feels as big as a bushel basket;" "weakness and trembling of the limbs." Was in such condition he could not attend to his business. I gave him Gelsemium in different potencies without much benefit for about one year. One day he came in and said "I am going to New York and want you to give me something to stimulate me." I gave him some Picric ac. and an introduction to T. F. Allen, in which I stated that Gelsemium had done him a little good. When the man came back he brought me the following from Prof. Allen. "You forgot the complement of Gelsemium, give it in the 30th." I did and cured the patient. I have also used it for *gastric headaches,* for headaches caused by fright and excitement, also for brain fag.

Alimentary Canal: Diarrhea with the characteristic colors and consistency of the remedy with the enormous distention of the abdomen has been cured. The *cause* in such cases being *emotion* such as fright, anger, or excitement.

Vocal Cords: Argentum nit. has cured patients of hoarseness and *aphonia* when the cause was the same as that of the nervous diarrhea.

Extremities: "Weakness; trembling; chorea-like motions; jerking; paralysis." A few cases of *chorea* the result of fright have been cured by the 30th.

Skin: "Discolored from a blue gray to violet or bronzed; skin brown, tense and hard."

This Argyria has led to its successful use in a few cases of Addison's disease.

Argentum is used in all strengths according to the conditions and susceptibility of the patients.

The use of no other remedy has brought me so many patients as has Argentum nit.

AURUM.

Make-up: Sanguine; black hair; dark eyes; olive-brown complexion; exceptionally for light haired, scrofulous persons.

Loc.: Brain and nerves; bone; *circulatory system;* glands; sexual organs.

Sen.: Suicidal anguish; tearing; sharp; sticking.

Mod.: Agg.: *Affections;* depressing, disordered *emotions; cold; night.*

Amel.: Cool open air; bathing.

Leaders: *Intense* and *hopeless* mental depression; disgust for life; suicidal tendency.

Aurum has a destructive action on bones and the connective tissue in parenchymatous organs. It is a *grand remedy for* patients suffering not only from *syphilis* but from the *maltreatment* of *syphilis* by *Mercurius.* Bear these facts in mind as we study the symptoms of the different locations.

Brain and Nerves.

Mind: "*Disgust for life, suicidal tendency* (Arsenicum, Nitric ac.); *peevish* and *vehement* wrath at least contradiction (Bryonia); *quarrelsome* (Platinum, Nux vom.); imagines that he is not fit for this world and longs for death which he contemplates with delight; imagines he cannot succeed in anything (Argentum met.); *weeping,* because he imagines he has lost the affections of his friends (Pulsatilla); *apprehension* and anxiety from a noise at the door and fear lest some one would come in; anthropophobia."

Aurum is our *greatest remedy* for *settled melancholia.* It is most useful for the *melancholia of which syphilis is* the cause. The patient is so disgusted with his life that he even contemplates suicide but rarely attempts it. In this group you will find most *violent pains* in the bones, worse at night;

especially caries of the nasal bones which are sore to touch. The offensive odor from nose and mouth are also important symptoms of the mental group.

The *melancholia* often takes a *religious* turn. The patients think they are to be damned for something they have done. They weep, cry and bemoan their imaginary fate.

Bones.

Head: "Tearing, aching in bones, on lying down, as if broken, so that all his vital energy seemed affected; bony tumors on the upper part of left forehead and on right vertex with boring pain agg. touch."

For exostosis and bony tumors also ulcerations of the bones of the skull.

Nose: "*Ulcerated nostrils*, agglutinated (Nitric ac., Thuja, Phosphorus, Mercurius); *sore feeling internally* agg. touch; putrid odor of discharge from the nose when blowing it out (Kali bich.)."

Caries of the *nasal bones* which are very *painful to touch*, boring pains agg. night. With the caries you also have ulceration of the mucous membranes and submucous tissue causing a profuse, bloody, mucous, purulent discharge which is very offensive to the patients and others.

Face: "Swelling of cheeks with drawing and tearing in jaws; burning and tearing in zygoma; drawing tearing in the left side of the face."

Caries of the bones of the face including the mastoid with the same kind of discharge from ears and nostrils as mentioned above.

Extremities: "Aching, drawing pains in the bones agg. at night."

Helpful for bony tumors and caries.

Sexual Organs.

Male: "*Swelling* of *right testicle* several days at 6 P.M. and towards 11 P.M. with *aching when touched* or *rubbed;*

testes swollen and *hard* (Pulsatilla, Rhododendron); tensive pain in right testicle as if bruised; testes mere pendent shreds."

Female: "Menses too late and scanty or absent; prolapsus of uterus with induration; leucorrhea, profuse and corroding, white, yellow, thick, not offensive, agg. walking."

Useful to *prevent* or check *atrophy* of testicles of boys who masturbate. In this condition the testes may be mere shreds and you have as additional symptoms of the group, listlessness, poor appetite, low spirits, coated tongue, poor memory and obstinacy. Also for *chronic enlargement* of *testicles,* with induration, sensitiveness and severe pain agg. night. Occasionally for *hydrocele.*

For *chronic metritis* when the uterus is large and heavy; and sensitiveness of the vagina. For sterility especially when the woman broods over the condition. With the latter condition you may find hysterical spasms, hysterical paralysis, palpitation of the heart and ovaritis.

Circulatory System.

Heart: "*Attacks of anguish, with tremulous fearfulness,* anguish coming from the precordial region and driving one from place to place; palpitation at night when lying on the back."

Aurum is a valuable remedy when the compensation of an hypertrophied heart begins to break causing the wandering pains, the irregular pulse, the palpitation, the feeling as if the heart would stop beating and the mental symptoms.

Veins: "Orgasm as if the blood were boiling in all the veins; heat in vertex; burning in arms, heat in face, feet and hands."

These symptoms may be found in any group.

Use the 30th and higher.

CUPRUM METALICUM.

Make-up: Neurotic; fair-haired; the carbo-nitrogenous constitution.

Loc.: Nerves; muscles; digestive tract.

Sen.: Cramps; cold; colic; convulsive, choreic; confused, lancinating, lightning-like.

Mod.: Agg.: Suppressions; vomiting; hot weather.
Amel.: Warm drinks.

Leaders: Cramps in calves of legs; convulsions.

Nerves and Brain.

Mind: "Deathly *anxiety in attacks,* with tossing about, without heat; obliged to think a long time before they can answer; *delirium* in attacks, with incessant, disconnected talking; full, hard pulse; inflamed eyes; wild look, *ending in sweat.*"

For *mania* with foolish gestures, mimicry; shrinking from every one, with fear and attempts to get away (Belladonna); with marked chilliness not amel. by heat.

Head: "Drawn backward; aching agg. motion; lancinating pains; bruised sensation in brain and eyes on turning the eyes; vertigo on looking up (Plumbum) with vanishing vision as from a veil before the eyes; intermittent lancinations in forehead and vertex, sometimes in temples and vertex, agg. pressure."

For *headaches* of various forms when you have the sensation as if cold water were poured over the head. The pains are very violent, usually reflex, accompanied with vomiting of all food and drink taken. We also have an extremely violent *catarrhal headache* over the *frontal sinuses* (Kali bich.).

Cuprum is also indicated in *meningitis,* generally *cerebral,* rarely *spinal,* sometimes *both.* The cause is suppressed eruptions. The symptoms of this group are: *loud* screams, convulsions with clenched thumbs, blue lips, unconsciousness. I have often found it helpful for *hemorrhage* in the brain *caused by* severe convulsive attacks of coughing in *whooping cough.*

Face: "*Blue,* with *blue lips;* sticking, drawing pains; spasmodic and tetanic contraction of jaw."

The "blueness" belongs with the convulsive group. Cuprum is also used for neuralgia of the face when the pains are stinging, burning agg. by touch (Arsenicum).

Throat: "*Audible gurgling of drink; constriction* of pharynx making swallowing difficult."

For *spasms* of the *esophagus* (Zinc.) and *pharynx;* also for a *paroxysmal cough* with intense pain behind the sternum on attempting to swallow.

Stomach: "Appetite lost; *hiccough* with spasmodic contraction of pharynx; ineffectual *retching* with constriction of esophagus and across chest in direction of diaphragm (Cactus); *cramp and pains* in *stomach* and bowels; *griping* and *pressure,* then *vomiting.*"

Abdomen: "*Tense, hot* and *tender* to touch; *spasmodic* motions of *muscles;* contracted; sore; *colic.*"

For *cholera morbus, infantum* and asiatica.

In addition to the *horrible, crampy pains* and *convulsive vomiting* you may have hiccough and watery stool. There is intense thirst for warm drinks and warm liquid food which produce the gurgling sound when swallowing. Frequently you have the general convulsion followed by unconsciousness.

Stools: "*Violent diarrhea;* stools watery with flakes."

Nothing marked in this section. These two symptoms are found in several of the Plumbum groups.

Respiratory Organs: "Hoarseness as though he cannot speak; fatiguing *cough* with *interrupted,* almost *suppressed respiration;* short, violent, dry cough at night between 11 and 1, agg. by sitting; *respiration difficult;* suffocative loss of breath; spasmodic dyspnea, with constriction of chest, then spasmodic vomiting; much bloody mucus, purulent expectoration."

For *pertussis* and *laryngismus stridulus with* both of which you are liable to have *convulsions* and when you do you will also have the "*clenched thumbs*" and "*blue face* and lips." For *spasmodic asthma* with which you have the blue face, constriction of the throat, marked dyspnea, retching and vomiting. For *pneumonia* when there is *want* of *reaction;* you have a jelly-like, mucous expectoration, much rattling in the chest, marked dyspnea, coldness of the surface and cold sweat (Tartar emet., Cuprum ars., and Arsenide of antimony). Many cases of pneumonia in the septic cases of Flu were saved by Cuprum.

Back and Extremities: "Cramps; convulsive movements; periodic, painful contractions of fingers and toes, often so that the fingers could not be extended by force; drawing and tension, often with shuddering and chilliness though skin was not cold; jerking of arms and hands; *cramps* especially in *calves of legs;* cramp from ankle to calf; weakness; painful weakness of ankles."

For *spinal irritation* when there is extreme *sensitiveness* along the entire length of the spine, and *violent* spasmodic *pains.* Chorea of the most violent type has been cured by Cuprum. The *grimaces,* the *fearful cramp* in the *calves,* the *jerking of the extremities;* the *attacks* of *suffocation,* the inability to swallow *are* all symptoms found in the choreic *group.*

Allen puts it down as useful for *intermittent fever* with the following symptoms: "Icy coldness of the whole body, predominating cramp in the limbs, blue surface, collapse and suppression of the urine." I have never met such a case.

Use 30th.

CUPRUM ARSENICOSUM.

Make-up: Nervous.

Loc.: Nerves; thermic centers.

Sen.: *Icy coldness;* burning; *cramping;* spasmodic; vertigo; nausea.

Mod.: Agg. from motion and damp weather; better from rest.

Nervous System.

Cholerine and Cholera: "*Icy coldness* of the *whole body* with *cramps* and obstinate *hiccough;* haggard face, intense thirst; nausea and vomiting worse after eating; burning, cramping, spasmodic, colicy pains in the abdomen; marked tenesmus of bladder and rectum; pulse small, weak, compressible; tremulousness; entire body covered with cold moisture."

For *Asiatic cholera, cholera morbus, cholera infantum,* with all these conditions, hot drinks and injections will relieve the pains and help save life. Give injections of equal parts of milk and water of the temperature of the body for cholera infantum. Also hot fomentations to abdomen; hot drink and injections if there is extreme vomiting and purging. If convulsions occur put the child in a tub of water with temperature 105. Give the 6x or 12x in hot water.

Alimentary Canal: "*Burning* along *esophagus* from stomach to mouth; burning, cutting in stomach while eating; obstinate hiccough; nausea and distress at epigastrium; cramping pains in lower bowels with tenesmus of rectum and bladder; vomiting and purging, with cramps and collapse."

Occasionally for *enteralgia* from blood poisoning and also from excitement.

Chorea: "*Trembling* of the whole body, very noticeable on *attempting to WALK; SPASMS in* the *extremities;* quivering, impossible to control."

Useful for *chorea, caused* by *shock* or fright *with* great *prostration.*

Thermic Centers.

I have always considered the nerve centers the location for cholera infantum, asiatic cholera, etc., but Cuprum ars. seems to have a separate action upon the thermic centers for I have found the "whole body" alternatingly moist and dry in two cases of uremic poisoning and one of diabetes, amel., when the amount of urine had suddenly changed from very profuse to very scanty, the ascetomes in abundance, patient drowsy, and coma threatening. This patient's skin was cold and moist. The other patient was a child with acute nephritis, following scarlet fever. The symptoms were scanty, albuminous urine; repeated general convulsions; great restlessness; loose, dark stools, marked thirst, icy cold skin which was dry. The temperature in the axilla was only 98 but in the rectum was 104.8. There was one other peculiar fact about the diabetic patient, viz., varicose ulcers of the legs, which had a tendency to become gangrenous, healed under the continued use of the remedy. For the first condition the 3x was used but after a few days the 18x was substituted. The remedy should be more thoroughly proven.

FERRUM.

Make-up: *Anemic.*

Loc.: *Blood;* circulation; brain; nerves; mucous membrane.

Sen.: *Hammering; beating; weakness; sensitive.*

Mod.: Agg.: *Night;* repose; violent exertion.

Amel.: Gentle motion.

Leaders: *Face,* which is usually pale, reddens on the *least revocation.*

Brain and Nerves.

Mind: "Excited by the slightest opposition; anxiety from slight cause, with throbbing in pit of stomach; desire for solitude."

Ferrum has been used for *hypochondriasis* also for *melancholia depending upon* profound *anemia,* the patient wants to be alone and brood over her sorrows.

Head: "Sick headache after menses, with hot head and cold feet, *hammering and beating, so that she must lie* down; pulsations; confusion; rush of blood to head; swelling veins of head; flushes of heat to face; vertigo when descending as if everything went around with her; bursting, sticking pain with chilliness."

Ferrum is *only* useful for *anemic headaches*. It is often given when Belladonna is indicated and vice versa. Both remedies are used for so-called *congestive headaches*, with *flushed face, throbbing,* beating pains in the *head* greatly agg. noise, bright light, odors, sudden motion or excitement. With both the head is very hot and the feet cold. If your patient is anemic as shown by the pale mucous membrane and anemic murmurs give Ferrum, if plethoric give Belladonna.

Back and Extremities: "Bruised pain in the sacrum; soreness in small of back on rising; shooting and tearing down through upper arm also from hip joint down tibia; cramps in soles of feet and toes."

Ferrum is useful for *neuralgia due* to *anemia*. For *lumbago* amel. walking slowly. For rheumatic condition about the insertion of the deltoid muscle (Bryonia) with very severe pain about the entire shoulder, making motion almost impossible. Also for neuralgic pains along the nerves from the hips to the toes, pains which are always amel. by moderate motion (Rhus).

Stomach: "Appetite variable; meats disagree (Pulsatilla); *anorexia,* dislike for all food (China); A. without bad taste or thirst. *A. for he always feels full;* eructations of food as soon as he eats (Antimonium crud., Pulsatilla, Phosphorus); vomiting of food after midnight; after eating (Pulsatilla, Lycopodium); cramp-like pains in the stomach."

Let us add the symptoms of this locality under the heading of stools as the two should be grouped together.

Stools: "*Watery with flatulence, more frequent after taking food or drink* (Colocynth, Croton tig.); watery without pain or smell, constipation.

The *indigestion* of Ferrum is due to anemia. The *juices* of the digestive tract are all *vitiated* hence we have *slow digestion* with *eructations* and *diarrhea*. Let me cite you a typical case which I observed 35 years ago. A fair haired baby boy 16 months old, who had suffered from severe attack of cholera infantum accompanied by meningitis. He had a ravenous hunger, which vanished at sight of food; there were frequent attacks of vomiting, when the normally pale face became paler, there was a thin, watery, painless, odorless stool whenever he could be induced to take nourishment, with a flushed, scarlet red face just before and during stool. If he ate anything like bread and butter, particles of undigested food appeared in the stools. The stools were not only after eating, but came on at night, 10 to 2 even, if he did not eat. The child sweat freely and was very weak. One day the mother asked: "What remedy is it that has a crimson face during stool?" From this hint Ferrum 30th was given every four hours with prompt improvement and complete recovery. It has often cured babies suffering from the above group of symptoms during detention (Podophyllum, China).

Female Sexual Organs: "Milky corrosive leucorrhea; swelling and induration of the vagina; smarting pain like that of excoriation during coition."

I have found it very helpful for the *leucorrhea* mentioned above *in chlorosis* of girls and young women, with profuse watery menstrual flow; the diarrhea. some *cramping* in *legs* (Cuprum ars.); the *diarrhea,* face of a pale almost greenish hue but which flushed scarlet red under excitement. Marked palpitation of the heart and dyspnea on going up stairs. Use the 30th for this group.

Blood.

The *first action* of Ferrum is to *produce* more rapid oxidation causing an *increase* of *red blood corpuscles* with a rise of *temperature; then* comes a *reaction with a marked diminution* of the *red* blood *cells* and *PROFOUND ANEMIA.* Therefore you will find Ferrum useful for the anemic persons who have suffered from some condition in which there was high temperature and an increase of red blood cells but in which there now is a marked decrease in the number of red cells and a normal or perhaps sub-normal temperature. Your cause may be hemorrhage, or loss of some of the other fluids of the body (China). Next to general anemia, *chlorosis* is the form calling most frequently for Ferrum. In chlorosis as in other conditions calling for Ferrum the *watery stools,* the *pale menstrual flow* are *ranking symptoms.* I have purposely omitted speaking of the heart and lung symptoms of Ferrum because they are more prominent under Ferrum phos. In closing just a word about the potency and repetition of dose. For the acute conditions use the medium or higher potencies and repeat often; for the chronic conditions and for anemia itself the medium or lower and do not repeat so often. I will always remember the statement of an old French physician when he regretted that he had hastened the death of so many young women suffering from incipient t. b. c. by giving too large doses of iron. For that condition I never use Ferrum below the 30th. Do I not believe in iron as a food? Yes, most assuredly yes, but give it in the patients diet in the form nature has provided it, but never as a potentized drug.

PLATINUM.

Make-up: Haughty; neurotic.

Loc.: Brain and nerves; sexual organs.

Sen.: Crawling; cramp-like; sticking; jerking; *numbness.*

Mod.: Agg.: Touch; emotion; sexual; chagrin.

Amel.: Walking in cool air.

Leaders: *Hauteur;* eroticism; disordered sense of proportion.

Platinum has a narrow field of action but it is unique in its field. Probably due to the fact that it is closely related to so many remedies having nearly the same action but larger fields, Platinum is not used as often as it should be and Ignatia, Stramonium, Plumbum, Stannum are prescribed when not so well indicated. Platinum acts promptly and thoroughly, rarely needing an intercurrent or other remedy to help complete the cure.

Brain and Nerves.

Mind: "*Arrogant; proud; contemptuous;* pitiful *looking down upon people* usually venerated with a kind of casting them off, in paroxysms and against her will; illusions as if everything were too small, all persons physically and mentally her inferior, but she herself physically large and superior; *lively* so she could dance one hour, weeping the next; for two days everything seemed joyous, could laugh at the saddest thing, then the third morning and evening sadness with weeping, even at joyous and laughable things if spoken to (Ignatia); weeping mood after slight reproaches. Weeping agg. in evening, amel. in open air; out of sorts with the whole world, everything seems too narrow (Pulsatilla); it seems that she did not belong to her own family; thought she was not fit for the world, *weary* of *life* but great dread of death, which she believed was near; sensitive, morose, discontented."

Every one of this long list of symptoms is of the highest rank. Note that they run through the whole scale of emotions. Most of the symptoms are reflex from the sexual organs. *Hysteria* is the most frequent condition, generally the result of excitement. In this group you have the alternating laughter and weeping; the arrogance; spasmodic action of any or all muscles; constriction of the esophagus; globus hystericus; alternating anesthesia and hyperesthesia in various parts of the body. Second for *melancholia* of the *religious form*. The patients want to get off by themselves, are *afraid* of death for which they are not prepared, weep and howl and are sleepless. Sometimes helpful in *puerperal mania* with suppressed lochia, extreme sensitiveness of the parts (Plumbum); and unchaste talk and action. You will find the last two symptoms most marked in *nymphomania due to suppressed menses* (Hyoscyamus). Never in all my experience have I heard such coarse, vulgar, at times profane, language or seen such disgusting actions as I heard and saw in a superintendent of schools who was drenched by rain while out riding during the time she was menstruating. The menses stopped, then followed a severe chill, high temperature, wild delirium and finally the symptoms mentioned above. I told her physician that for the suddenness and violence of the attack I suggested Belladonna. He replied that he had used it in several potencies. Being informed by her mother that she was often *hysterical* and "*hard to get along with*" *during* her *menstrual periods* we decided upon Platinum 30th. But the only potency we had being the 200th we gave that, five drops every two hours. The menstrual flow returned after 12 hours and she was normal after about one week. I was informed later that her condition at the menstrual period was also greatly improved.

Head: "*Intermittent cramp-like drawing constriction,* agg. about the forehead, *beginning slight, increasing till violent, ending slight;* cramp-like, as if screwed in; wave-like, benumbing, about right orbit; numbness in sinciput as if constricted, in a warm room full of people, with fretful impatience and heat in the upper part of body; *numbness* through the head *as if bound;* numb pain on top of the head as if scalp would be contracted, and as if weight were on it; crawling on right temple, afterwards extending down along lower jaw with coldness."

Platinum is most frequently used for *periodic,* usually *menstrual headaches.* The numbing paralyzing pains gradually increase till they become violent and then as gradually decrease. This process is repeated. The pain is agg. stooping and amel. walking quietly in the fresh, open air. The headaches usually come at the time of the menses which are always profuse. You will also find other symptoms from the sexual organs and many mental symptoms in this group.

Face: "*Painful,* cramp-like *numbness* in left malar bone; tense, *numb* sensation in zygomata and mastoid processes as if the head were screwed together."

Sometimes helpful for facial neuralgia when the sharp, pinching, shooting pains leave the parts *numb* (Verbascum).

Abdomen: "*Constriction;* pressure in hypogastrium during profuse menstruation with ill humor; pressure downwards toward genitals, as during menses (Belladonna)."

Frequently *palliative for dysmenorrhea,* rarely for *painter's colic* in women.

Sexual Organs: "*Sensitiveness* and *pressure* in mons veneris, with internal shaking chill and external coldness; voluptuous crawling in abdomen with anxious oppression and palpitation, then painless pressure downwards in genitals with sticking in sinciput and exhaustion; erections in sleep with amorous dreams."

Menses: As the female generative organs are the only section of the M. M. location I will give you the symptoms in connection with those of the brain and nerves. They are: "Leucorrhea like the white of an egg (Alumina); *menses* too *early* and *profuse;* too early, lasting eight days with drawing pain in abdomen the first day; much clotted blood the first day of menstruation."

Allen gives the following conditions for which Platinum has been used: *Puerperal nymphomania, satyriasis; sexual melancholia* of both sexes; pruritus of the vagina; prolapsus uteri; chronic ovaritis, dysmenorrhea; sterility; albuminous leucorrhea and fibroid tumors."

I mention this long list of conditions to show you the intensity of action of the drug in this location. You will note that the *symptoms show irritation, inflammation, functional* and *structural changes.* Let me in closing emphasize what I have already said or intimated, viz., that most of the *symptoms* given under *mind* and *head have* their *origin* in *disturbances* of the sexual organ, which explains their frequent appearance together in the various groups of both locations.

PLUMBUM.

Make-up: "*Dry* skin; bilious constitution"; jaundiced; neurotic.

Loc.: *Brain and nerves; parenchyma* of *organs* especially the *kidneys;* uterus.

Sen.: "*Griping, twisting, cutting colic;* weakness; restlessness; hyperesthesia and anesthesia; shooting, lighting-like pains.

Mod.: Agg. from exertion and excitement.

Amel. hard pressure and rubbing.

Leaders: *Wrist drop;* enteralgia; atrophy of muscles; undeveloped uterus.

Brain and Nerves.

Mind: "Slow of perception; memory lost, so that when talking he was often unable to find the right word (Lycopodium, Phosphoric ac.); delirium; coma."

Many of the conditions of Plumbum have anxiety and restlessness, then sadness and dejection; in some cases delirium followed by coma.

Head: "Aching; heaviness; vertigo; throbbing, tearing pain."

While there are not many symptoms of first rank in this section these few form the center of a group which includes symptoms from all parts and locations of the body. The first condition we may call *cerebral paralysis.* In this group we find, in addition to "aching and heaviness," deficient memory, impaired speech, because *neither* the *brain* nor the *tongue work well, e. g.,* "unable to find the proper word" and "partial paralysis of the tongue;" also blunted consciousness; partial paralysis of the face, eyes, throat and extremities.

Face: "*Expression anxious* and of suffering; spasmodic contractions; muscles almost immovable."

Tongue: "*Trembling;* cannot be put out; *articulation imperfect,* sometimes only confused sounds."

These *face* and *tongue symptoms* are only *manifestations* of the general *paralysis*.

Throat: "Swelling of tonsils, with induration; swallowing difficult."

You will sometimes find it useful for *granular sore throat*, but the important symptom is *"Swallowing difficult,"* which *indicates paralysis* of the *pharyngeal muscles*.

Stomach: *"Hiccough;* eructation; nausea; *vomiting, constant* of food, of everything taken into stomach, of fecal matter, blackish liquid streaked with blood; pain in pit extending to loins and down legs; tightness in epigastrium; *feeling* in epigastrium as *if ball ascended* to *throat*, where it caused suffocation, preventing speaking and swallowing, with anxiety."

Plumbum will sometimes be found *useful* for *gastralgia* when the *pains* are very *sudden* and *severe, better* from *hard pressure* (Colocynth) and eructations. The vomiting of "fecal matter and brownish liquid streaked with blood," accompanied by cramps, indicate *hernia* and *painter's colic;* rarely *gastralgia* due to emotions.

Abdomen: *"Retraction,* with hardness and *pain* at the *umbilicus radiating* to the lumbar region and iliac fossæ; *retracted* with hard knots over it, worse along median line; paroxysmal *tearing* worse at umbilicus, better from pressure; *colic radiating* to all *parts* of the *body*, worse from cold, eating, at night, from light pressure or touch; better from hard pressure, warmth, emission of flatus; *umbilicus* seems to adhere to the spine with pain so violent at times that he was almost wild, tossed about and pressed his fist into abdomen."

The above, as you know, is a complete picture of "painter's colic," and I told you how to treat it when we were discussing Colocynth. When such a picture is the result of *incarcerated hernia, syphilis, infantile paralysis*, the abuse of Mercurius, Colocynth, or other poison, Plumbum 30th is the homeopathic remedy.

The sensation of the intestines being *"spiked to the back-*

bone," the "***pulling in***" of the ***umbilicus*** and constipated stool of ***hard, dry, black balls*** are usually found in every group *except* that representing ***hernia,*** when you have complete obstruction of the bowels and the violent vomiting. How does Plumbum relieve strangulated hernia? By restoring the harmony of peristalsis. Nux does the same but there is this difference, the Nux quiets the irritation while Plumbum stimulates the paralysis, thus restoring harmony. In the chronic hepatitis group you have the "*feeling of a string pulling the liver backward*" and the constipation, nausea and yellow skin. When the *gastritis* or *gastralgia* is the result of poisoning *from Colocynth,* you will find *diarrhea* with the same "pulling up" of the rectum; when the poisoning is that of *Mercurius* you also have *diarrhea* and ***tenesmus.*** Constipation is found in all the other groups.

Urinary Organs: "Tenesmus, ineffectual urging or passing only drop by drop after great effort which increases the pains; ***micturition difficult,*** impossible; involuntary."

Paralysis of the bladder.

Sexual Organs: "Jerking, paroxysmal pains along the spermatic cord into the testicles which are retracted (hanging down under Pulsatilla); ***hyperesthesia of genitals*** in females: spasmodic dysmenorrhea, increased desire and restlessness; *vaginismus.*"

The spasmodic *dysmenorrhea,* which is often the first of a series of symptoms ending in abortion, belongs to this location. The others are found in the *nymphomania* and *vaginismus.*

Neck, Back and Extremities: "Neuralgic pains in spine extending into occiput; pain in lumbar region, usually lancinating, and in nates, posterior part of thigh, knee, sole and toes worse from stooping, better from pressure and rubbing; trembling of legs and hands; spasmodic contraction of joints worse at night; paroxysmal pains more in muscular parts of the thighs; worse evening and night; cramps, acute and paroxysmal pains; lightning-like pains of lower extremities."

The above are the symptoms found in *infantile* and *spinal paralysis;* also of *multiple sclerosis, posterior spinal sclerosis* and *rheumatism.*

The symptoms of the group most commonly found in infantile paralysis are those of *weakness;* smooth, shiny, cold skin; *atrophy* of the muscles; *alternating hyperesthesia and anesthesia.* We have a few pains usually neuralgic in character. The constipation of the drug also belongs in this group.

The shooting, lightning-like pains are most frequently found in locomotor ataxia and the two varieties of sclerosis (Thallium). The other forms of the Plumbum neuralgias are always severe, generally cramp-like in character. The trembling and weakness felt in nearly all groups are the result of paralysis caused by changes in the nerve centers, also atrophy of the muscles.

Female Sexual Organs.

Uterus: "*Undeveloped uterus;* premature birth; abortion: menorrhagia; metrorrhagia."

Plumbum not only produces neuralgic dysmenorrhea but abortion due to lack of development of the uterus. I remember one case in which the depth of the uterus was only a little over one inch. She suffered terribly at every menstrual period which was somewhat irregular. *Plumbum* cured the dysmenorrhea. She afterwards married, became pregnant and miscarried at the end of the seventh week of gestation. We then began the use of Plumbum, giving the 200th three times a week. The use of Plumbum and the effect of miscarriages (seven in four years) resulted in her giving birth to a four-pound child. Since then she has borne two children but she has had no miscarriages.

Hypersensitiveness of the vulva and vagina is a marked symptom of Plumbum, often amel. producing many other nervous symptoms. The least touch of clothing produces vaginismus. In one case was this so marked that a local anesthetic was necessary to make an examination.

The 30th is the best potency.

Parenchyma of Organs.

Kidneys: "Nephritis with fever, *albuminous* urine without edema, without urea; sp. grav. 1002; brownish-red, turbid. acid, flocculent sediment consisting of red blood-corpuscles and many short, thick, turbid cylinders beset with red blood-corpuscles; all the symptoms of acute, diffusive nephritis."

No remedy has been as often used for *chronic, interstitial nephritis* as Plumbum. It has *arrested* progress in many cases after other remedies had failed *and* has *permanently cured* not a few cases.

The same may be said of chronic *Bright's disease* with *hypertrophy* and *dilatation* of the *left ventricle, dropsy,* numbness and paralysis of the lower *extremities.* I found it helpful in a few cases of *hemorrhage* of the kidneys when bleeding was profuse and accompanied by excruciating pain along the ureters. You find *mental depression* present in *all* kidney troubles. The *skin* is usually *dry* and *yellow* with the chronic varieties.

I never use Plumbum below the 30th, often in the 200th and occasionally in the 1m.

SILICA.

Make-up: Clear skin, suppuration; sensitive.

Loc.: *Brain and nerves;* glands; bones; M.M.; skin.

Sen.: Chilliness, sharp; sticking.

Mod.: Agg. *cold drafts; damp;* checked perspiration; *excitement.*

Amel. *warmth;* wrapping head and neck.

Leaders: *Tendency to suppuration* and of all injuries to head; *chilliness* agg. at time of new moon. Silica has an especial affinity for the cartilages and hence we find it most useful for suppuration and fistulas of joints and of the vertebras.

Brain and Nerves.

Mind: "*Sensitive* (Nux vom., Ignatia) *to noise and anxious therefrom;* even lachrymose; easily startled, gloomy; irritable: *peevish,* difficult to fix attention."

Silica is the remedy for those "who lack sand." The patient is exceedingly irritable and at the same time lacks ambition to undertake anything (Argentum nit.). He is easily disturbed by any little excitement and tires easily. The cause may be the chronic effect of shock but more frequently the condition is due to drainage of the vital force by suppuration (China).

Head: "*Bruised pain above the eyes, so that he could scarcely open them*, pain agg. opening eyes. *Tearing* in *vertex as if* it would *burst* extending through the head, with *throbbing* and *chilliness*, necessity to lie down and toss about, *amel. binding head* tightly; *tearing* in the *occiput* extending upward and forward over side of head; *stitching* in forehead with chilliness in nape and back, amel. warm wrapping of the head, scalp sore to touch."

For severe headaches due to nervous exhaustion which in turn is due to drainage of fluids (China). The pains are neuralgic and come in shocks. They usually begin or end in the occiput and the relief from wrapping the head warm is very marked; cold agg. to an equal degree. Some good and nourishing diet helps.

Eye: "Vision dim; flickering; blackness before the eyes after the headaches; letters run together when reading."

The only condition in this section is *ciliary neuralgia.*

Heart: "Orgasm of blood on movement, also when sitting, with throbbing of whole body."

This symptom is caused by spinal irritation and belongs in that group.

Neck and Back: "*Stiffness of the nape with chilliness;* pain in curved spine on beginning to move, weakness in back with paralyzed feeling in lower limbs, difficulty in walking; stitching in coccygeus on rising; *pain in coccyx as after a long carriage ride;* bruised pain at night in lumbar region and hips agg. stooping."

Whereas some of the above symptoms may belong to the

bone location most of them are caused by anemia and irritability of the spine, again caused by loss of fluids, injuries, and even the diseases of the bony spine which passes the cord and its meninges. You may call the conditions *neuritis, neuralgia, spinal anemia* or irritation, in either case warmth and rest will relieve while cold, motion, and pressure will agg. Some cases of spinal *sclerosis* have been palliated by it.

Bones.

Eyes: "*Swelling* in region of *lachrymal gland* and *sac*, redness around the eyes."

Ears: Often helpful for canthus of the orbit with ulcerative pains, amel. warmth. "Tearing, sticking pains above the ears agg. behind them; pain in ear and down the neck; difficulty in hearing due to roaring in ear (Capsicum, Tellurium)."

Silica has cured many cases of *otorrhea following mastoid* abscesses. You find a *thin watery* discharge in which are *particles of bone*. Extreme soreness to touch of mastoid region and *sharp sticking pains* greatly *agg.* by *cold* and pressure but equally *amel.* by *wrapping* the whole *head warm*. Deafness may result. The discharge may contain blood.

Nose: "Discharge of blood, mucous without much coryza; dryness of nose; marked soreness."

Caries of the bones of the nose as shown by particles of bone in the discharges (Mercurius).

Mouth: Necrosis of jaw and abscesses at the root of the teeth especially *if you have the Silica 6,* thin discharge with bony specks coming from a fistula. The same soreness and modalities as elsewhere.

Neck and Spine: We have already hinted at *Pott's disease, curvatures* of all kinds when other symptoms point to *suppuration*, especially when there are *fistulas* from the spine. Do not forget your splints and curettes but bear in mind that *Silica* will materially *assist* these *other means to a cure*.

Glands.

I have mentioned glands as one of the locations. You see by this time that any or all glands of the body may become inflamed, breakdown, suppurate, and discharge having the modalities of Silica. I have never known it to abuse suppuration as Hepar and Mercurius will but it is more frequently indicated than either after suppuration. Glands of the labia are often affected. I have had two cases of abscess of the liver, one discharging through the lung, the other through chest walls, neither of which healed completely till Silica 30 was used.

Mucous Membrane.

Rectum, Anus and Stools: "*Stinging; cutting; frequent, ineffectual* desire to stool, but *discharge of* only *mucus* with *chilliness* of body; stools remain in the rectum as if there were no power to expel them; *hemorrhoids* sensitive though protruding but a little; *moisture with* sticking and *itching* about anus; constriction during stool; burning after dry stools; in spite of straining, hard, difficult, unsatisfactory stool; *stool that has protruded slips back again,* after urging and straining the abdominal wall is sore."

The key to the constipation of Silica is found in the symptom "stool that has protruded slips back again" (Hepar). Why does the stool slip back? Because of the contraction of the sphincters, which are irritated by pressure. As the stool presses down it opens up the fissures and as you have hemorrhoids and ulcers the condition is agg. These are the cases which the orificial surgeons help by paralyzing the sphincters under an anesthetic but the relief will only be *temporary* unless you use Silica. The hemorrhoids and fissures are conditions which should be included in the constipation group and treated in the same manner.

The *diarrhea* with the offensive odor, agg. by cold air with the cold, offensive perspiration on head, etc., I have found in only one case, a case of general sepsis.

Sexual Organs: "Itching and swelling of the scrotum, violent erections; emission at night; itching of pudenda during the menses, with soreness and eruption on the inner sides of thighs (Alumina, Kreosotum); bearing down pains in the vagina; leucorrhea of white, watery fluid. Pain in labia; menses increased with attacks of chilliness on their appearance."

Silica has helped sores of *elephantiasis* of the *scrotum* (Kali bich.), and *balanitis*. The symptom *"seminal emissions" calls* for *special attention, as* it is both a *cause and* an *effect* of conditions. *Recall that* I have several times stated that *loss of fluid* was one of the *causes* of the condition. This is especially true of the loss of semen. On the other hand a *brain easily affected by emotions* together with the hemorrhoids, fissures, ulcers, etc., about the pelvis will cause *erections* and *emissions.*

Abscesses of the labia with the fistulous openings I have mentioned under glands. The *acrid excoriating leucorrhea* and the *excessive menstruation* greatly *increase* the *irritability and weakness* of the patient.

Respiratory Organs: "Hoarseness agg. morning with tickling in larynx and cough; cough with purulent expectoration with vomiting of masses of purulent mucus agg. morning and H.M.; lumps of yellow, thick expectoration after violent coughing; expectoration which makes water turbid, heavy expectoration which sinks in water."

We make use of these symptoms in *two classes* of *patients,* first those suffering from *phthisis,* second the *bronchorrea* of old people. Use the 30th and higher.

STANNUM.

Make-up: The t. b. c. diathesis.

Loc.: *Lungs; mucous membranes;* female organs; nerves.

Sen.: *Weakness* of *chest;* anxious, heavy.

Mod.: Agg. using the voice; after motion.
Amel. expectoration.

Leaders: *Pains* gradually *increase,* then as gradually *decrease; weakness,* especially of the *chest.*

Before taking up the locations I will call your attention to the mental symptoms. They are the unexpected (Ignatia), *e. g.,* the t. b. c. patients are sad, depressed, hopeless; the *weakness* is *felt* much *more* on *going down stairs* than going up, etc.

Lungs.

"*Hoarseness* on beginning to sing, with *weakness* and *emptiness in the chest* so that she must stop constantly and take a deep breath, at times the H. is *relieved by cough;* mucus in trachea in A.M. easily expelled by forcible cough, with *weakness* of *chest* as if *evicerated,* with weakness of the whole body and of limbs; irritation to cough on breathing as from mucus in trachea; *cough shattering,* deep, short, weak, hoarse as from weakness in the chest; *fatiguing, paroxysmal* cough so that the epigastric region was painful as if beaten; *expectoration salty,* of a globular, grayish lump of *thick* mucus *containing* a *clot* of *black blood;* E. greenish, *offensive,* yellow, thick and viscid; respiration short, difficult from weakness of respiratory organs, with emptiness in stomach; *dyspnea* amel. opening clothes, agg. on motion with want of breath."

For acute and chronic *bronchial catarrh.* The *agg.* from noon till midnight in the acute is very marked. In both forms the cough is dry during the night. There is a salty expectoration, either loose or of balls of mucus with blood in the center in *pulmonary t. b. c.* with which we have the *weakness* of the *chest* and entire body, sweat every morning at 4 A.M., rapid emaciation but *not hopefulness.* In addition to the cough and expectoration peculiar to the drug, warm drinks will amel. the cough; profuse expectoration will amel. both cough and heaviness. You also have the knife-like pains in the chest, either neuralgic or pleuritic.

Mucous Membranes.

Mouth: "*Tongue coated yellow.*"

This symptom is found with all conditions of Stannum.

Throat: "Sticking in upper part of fauces, causing dryness and swallowing; rawness and scraping in the morning agg. deglutition, with dryness but without thirst."

For *chronic catarrhal pharyngitis,* usually tubercular, with the above symptoms plus the hawking up of hard lumps of mucus.

Sexual Organs: "*Menses too profuse; leucorrhea* of a transparent or yellowish mucus; *prolapsus* of *uterus* and *vagina;* itching of vulva agg. evening."

The leucorrheal discharges sometimes become thin and watery. The prolapsus is always accompanied by the leucorrhea, the weakness of the chest and the mental symptoms.

Rectum and Stools: "*Frequent ineffectual urging;* sticking pains in rectum with itching about anus; stools soft, scanty, with mucus towards the last."

Although Stannum had been used for and had produced wonderful results at the hands of the ancients, the only use made of it in Hehnemann's time was as a *vermifuge.* Besides the symptoms found under rectum and stools we find: Sinking, empty, all-gone feeling; stomach and abdominal pains; pale, sunken, sickly countenance with dark rings beneath the eyes; the yellow tongue, bad breath and restless sleep (Cina).

Brain and Nerves.

Mind: "*Sad;* fretful; anxious; discontented; discouraged; aversion and dread of people; restless, distracted; not persistent in work; fruitlessly busy."

Note what a gloomy mental picture the provers and patients have painted! Also recall what I said of the mental symptoms in the t. b. c. group, and you will get a proper conception of the rank of "*hopefulness*" in other t. b. c. groups. The symptom "anxious" is agg. before the menses (Actea rac.). Most of the other mental symptoms, especially the hypochondriac and tearful mood, also belong to the menstrual groups.

Head: "Pain as if constricted by a band; pain as if brain were forced asunder and tense; heaviness; vertigo; pressure and constriction of the whole upper head slowly increasing and slowly decreasing; tearing, intermittent, sharp jerking pain agg. stooping."

For *neuralgic headaches* with the characteristic *pain, increasing and* then *decreasing slowly.* The time of the headache is from 10 A.M. to 4 P.M. for several days before menses.

I use Stannum in the 30th and higher.

N.B. For the t. b. c. conditions I always use Stannum iod. 3rd and 6th.

ZINCUM METALICUM.

Make-up: *Neurotic.*

Loc.: Brain and nerves, mucous membranes.

Sen.: Restless; trembling; sharp, shooting, lightning-like.

Mod.: Agg. *when exhausted;* noise, touch, *wine.*

Leaders: Restlessness especially legs and feet, twitching of muscles. *Agg. from wine.* Amel. camphor; Agg. in P.M.

Brain and Nerves.

Mind: "*Cross;* impatient; fretful, peevish humor (Chamomilla, Antimonium crud.); child cries towards evening; fickleness (Pulsatilla); *weakness of memory;* difficult conception; absence of ideas; very variable moods, *alternating sadness and hilarity.*"

We find *delirium* in low fevers with subsultus tendinum, trembling of hands and coldness of the extremities. Sometimes useful in *general paresis.*

I had one patient who presented the following symptoms: *very forgetful, restless,* wanting to walk about all the time and exceedingly *irritable* if his whims were not gratified; tottering gait and general coldness. Alcoholic liquors, especially *wine*, agg. the mental symptoms but for a time seemed to amel. the muscular. The man, a brilliant attorney, had used alcohol to excess and been cured of syphilis. Zincum phos. 30th with regular massage and regulated diet rich in phosphorus restored him but it took over a year.

A second case cured at our hospital was one of *melancholia.* She was a dark, firm-fibered (Nux) woman who had lost her husband through an accident some six months before. She would sit in her chair or lie in bed and stare. If the attendants tried to rouse her she paid no attention at first but if they continued she would become very angry, the only exception was when roused for her meals. She ate readily and seemed to enjoy her food. The stools were loose and she seemed weaker both mentally and physically after stools. *Her legs were never still.* Under Zincum val. she made such improvement that she was considered cured by her family but the tendency to sit or lie for about 36 hours and stare would recur about once a month. Note that the restlessness was confined to her legs and feet. She also had hysterical convulsions with alternating laughing and weeping for about five weeks after the death of her husband.

Head: "*Aching* in *head* and *eyes* after a glass of accustomed *wine,* and in open air, and washing in cold water; vertigo so that he could not stand, in attacks preceded by sharp pressure at the root of the nose and a sensation of drawing together of the eyes as by a cord, followed by nausea, faintness and trembling of the hands; tearing, stitching, pinching pains in head; *heaviness* and *dullness* with vertigo as if he would fall to the left."

I have used it in several cases of *neuralgic headache,* mostly of school children who worked too hard at their books, but did not get exercise or sleep enough. The pains were always very severe, came in the P.M. and frequently accompanied by eye trouble, *e. g.*, blurring of vision (one half of the object) and photophobia, and a strained, tired feeling. Fitting of glasses in these cases, while not able to completely cure are a great help to Zincum in completing a cure.

For hydrocephalus, I used it in two cases which had been helped but for some reason could not be cured by Apis. Both were cases following severe attacks of "summer complaint." The head was hot especially in occiput; the eyes staring, in one case strabismus; marked restlessness in both, of the feet in one, of the entire body in the other; both had had convulsions which Apis had controlled; both were cutting teeth; both received Zincum met. 30th.

Eyes: "*Dim vision; photophobia;* objects appear elongated, sometimes double."

The only use I have found for Zincum in this section is the disturbed vision in connection with the hydrocephalic headache. With these few cases I have also found neuralgia, the pains about the orbit extending into the occiput are sharp and shooting. The neuralgia is often found with the headache of school children.

Mouth: "*Salivation* with *crawling* on *inside of cheeks;* drawing, sharp, jerking pain in teeth."

I have found it useful in a few cases of *difficult dentition.* The *constant* motion of first *one foot* then the other (Helleborus); the rolling of the head (Podophyllum) sometimes boring it into the pillow, the soft pulse; weakness; coldness; and twitching of muscles (Belladonna) are the symptoms of this group.

Throat: "*Spasmodic pressure upward* in pit or upper part of *esophagus;* constriction in esophagus during deglutition. with spasm."

This means *globus hystericus.* I found the two symptoms quoted in a young student who came to consult me for dyspepsia with the *sensation* as if the "*stomach would collapse*" coming in her last hour in the A.M. 11–12. Frequently the sensation was accompanied by *blurring* of *vision,* rarely she also had the *headache.* The globus hystericus is often found in the other groups of Zincum, but is of minor importance.

Abdomen: "Distention; cutting, sticking, gurgling, rumbling and tearing pains agg. walking and standing, amel. rest of body and mind."

You will find *colic* whether *flatulent* or *lead* with the retraction of the abdomen (Plumbum) frequently associated with the Zincum groups. I have frequently used it for *enteralgia* of *alcoholics* (Nux) when the stools were small, hard and the stool accompanied by pressure and clawing in anus. *Reflex symptoms* of *floating kidney* are *palliated* by Zincum.

Urinary Organs: "Retention of urine *when beginning to urinate;* sitting with legs crossed, bending, cannot pass but feels as if the bladder would burst."

I have used it a few times for *hysterical retention* of the urine when the bladder was greatly distended and when the patient finally voided a large amount of clear urine (Ignatia). Partial paralysis of the bladder is a condition produced by Zincum and symptoms of dribbling or retention are found in several groups of the drug.

Sexual Organs: "Drawing up of testicles with pain and swelling; *emissions* at night *with* lascivious *dreams;* excitement at night before and during menses."

In the cases I have used it for *neuralgia* of the testicles there was marked pain but no swelling. I relieved *pruritus* and marked *sexual excitement* in two school teachers. Both had thick, *bloody,* mucous *leucorrhea before* the *menses.* The *itching* and *excitement* were *so great* during the menstrual period as to *interfere with sleep.* One obtained some relief by bathing with hot water. Both were extremely nervous. I gave Zincum 30th and ordered douches of Carbolic ac. 1 to 5000 every night for 10 days before the menses. You usually find the mental and sexual symptoms grouped together.

Respiratory Organs: "*Dry, spasmodic cough morning* and *evening.*"

The only use I have ever made of Zincum for the above symptoms was in *whooping cough.* The symptom which called Zincum to mind in these cases was not the one usually given, viz., "during the spasms of cough child grasps the genitals" but the *red,* blood-shot appearance of the eye. The patients were babies, the attacks were severe and I gave Zincum because I feared rupture of blood vessels of the brain (Plumbum, Mephitis). I used the sulphate 6th.

Back and Extremities: "*Sticking* pains along spine when sitting and walking; bruised pain when walking in open air, with weakness; sharp, cutting pains in region of kidneys often forcing him to stand still, amel. continuing walk; stiffness, trembling in limbs; uneasy feeling in extremities (fidgets) so that patient cannot keep still; boring pain in head after drinking wine."

The only condition for which the above would be the ranking symptom is *spinal irritation caused* by *anemia.*

The above are the conditions for which I have used the metallic Zincum. I have also given one group of symptoms for which I prescribe the *valerianate.* The symptom of the *highest rank* is "*fidgety feet.*" The conditions in which it is found are *in hysteria,* melancholia and "epilepsy without aura."

ZINCUM PHOSPHORICUM.

This member of the family has proven itself the best of the group *for* an *exhausted brain,* whether *of business men, student* or those who have been the victims of *epilepsy* and *its maltreatment.* Let me give you the record of one case of the latter condition as an illustration of many: Mr. A. J., age 36, married, father of three children, farmer. He had been bright and normal till gored by a bull when in addition to the shock of the encounter he had lost a large amount of blood. Soon after, attacks of epilepsy set in. They were severe, and nearly always in the P.M. The attacks were suppressed by large amounts of Bromides but his mind began to deteriorate.

This was first noticed in his inability to figure and make change, then in planning his work and finally inability to do any work. His wife led him into the clinic room by the hand. He took no note of anything. When asked a question, he either paid no attention or slowly turned to his wife. He ate well, slept well and the bowels were in fair condition. When asked about his sexual condition his wife answered: "He has been no good since he was hurt." When we ordered the Bromides discontinued the wife said: "If we do, we'll have the spell awfully." However, the Bromides were discontinued and Zincum phos., 3x two grains night and morning, substituted. We cut all meat out of his diet, making it mostly fish, fruit and cereals. The wife reported in two weeks that he was having attacks every day but that they had not been so severe for the past three days. No mental change. Two weeks later report was: "attacks fewer and lighter and knows a little more." At the end of the second month there had been a little more improvement in the attacks and great improvement in his mental state. He could do a few chores now. We changed the potency to the 6th under which he continued to improve more rapidly. At the end of 18 months he was doing his work as before the injury. However, he still has two or three attacks a year brought on by overexertion or excitement, once after intercourse. This was the only case where loss of blood was recorded as an etiological factor. I have always been in doubt as to which was the more important factor, the loss of blood, the fright or the Bromides. All I can say is that many cases of epilepsy have been helped and some cured by substituting Zincum phos. for the Bromides or even when the attacks continued after the Bromides had been discontinued. I have not cured many cases of grand mal but Zincum, Phosphorus and Lachesis have cured more for me than all the other remedies.

ZINCUM SULPHURICUM.

This member of the family seems to have a stronger "*elective affinity*" *for* the *skin* than any of the others. We have the following symptoms: "Skin pale yellow; deadly palor, skin milky white, blisters on neck, discharge first of bloody water, later a thin, green, ill-smelling pus; frightful prurigo."

Useful for many skin affections when used either internally or locally or both. Zincum lotions and ointments are too frequently used to allay the itching and burning of the skin. However, they are less harmful than preparations of sugar of lead used for the same purpose. I always give Zincum sulph. internally when I apply it locally.

The *sulphate* is also most frequently *used* when the mucous membrane is the location and the eye the section. The symptoms are: "inflammation of the eyes during menses; pain as from sand evening and night with lachrymation; *burning* in the P.M. in eyes and lids in morning and evening with dryness and pressure; biting photophobia and lachrymation with agglutination of lids in morning, agglutination of the inner canthi in the morning with a pressing soreness; itching; and cloudy vision."

Zincum sulph. is one of our best remedies for both *acute* and *chronic conjunctivitis*. The mucus is profuse and sometimes the dim vision is due to its presence, rarely to pus (Argentum nit.). Generally the cloudy vision is due to trouble of the optic nerve.

ZINCUM PICRATE.

Aside from the preparations of Zincum already mentioned the picrate is the only one I have ever used. It has been found useful in affections of the *sexual organs* and *prostate gland* (Ferrum pic.), *e. g.*, a man of dark complexion, firm build, a lawyer, 36 years of age came to me for *seminal emissions*. He had been given to excessive venery from 22 to 28 when he married. His wife had been dead about one year. He said he had lived a proper life while she lived and since. These emissions came towards morning, always accompanied with dreaming that he was having intercourse with his wife. Although this left an unpleasant impression when awake the reason for his coming was that the *act* and *dream* unfitted him for business the following day. He dreaded to go to his office and was unable to plead a case before a jury. I first tried Argentum nit., but it did no good so I changed to the Picrate of zinc, which completely restored his mental condition and reduced the number of emissions to one or two per month.

BROMIUM.

Make-up: Scrofulous patient, children with enlarged paratoids and subject to croup.

Loc.: Larynx; heart; respiration; *paratoid glands;* ovaries.

Sen.: Weak; spasmodic constrictions, burning; suffocative fits.

Mod.: Agg. *warm damp weather;* overheating; drafts.

Amel.: motion; nosebleed relieves the vertigo, headache, and chest symptoms.

Leaders: The suffocative, wheezy croupy cough.

Mucous Membrane.

Respiratory Organs: "*Scraping in* the *larynx, in* the *evening producing cough* (Pulsatilla) and *rawness* provoking hawking; stitching posteriorly on swallowing saliva with feeling of *constriction;* cold sensation, with a cold feeling when inspiring; spasmodic closure of the glottis; contracted sensation in the trachea or feeling as if the throat were pressed against the trachea; hoarseness; loss of voice; cough on deep inspiration with paroxysms of suffocation suddenly on swallowing; respiration oppressed, difficult; patient cannot inspire sufficient air; amel. walking even rapidly."

I have quoted many symptoms in this section because I have verified them all many times.

For *croup* either *diphtheritic, membranous* or *idiopathic*, not in the first stage but after the temperature has subsided, the patient is prostrated, perspires easily, has a tight, hard spasmodic cough with rattling of mucus in larynx. The suffocative attacks (Spongia) are prominent in this group. The *spasms* the ranking symptoms.

For *spasmodic croup* when the patient starts up as if choking and wants a drink of water which amel. the condition. Every intake of air provokes the cough; agg. if the air is hot and damp.

For *idiopathic asthma* which seemed to be caused by constriction of the trachea. The asthma is amel. while on water especially salt water.

Glands.

Submaxillary: "Parotid glands swollen and sensitive."

Used for *inflammation* and *suppuration* of the *parotid* and other submaxillary *glands* following diphtheria.

Female Sexual Organs: "Dull pain in the ovaries; stitching pain from mammæ to axillæ, cannot bear pressure on mammæ."

It has been used for *chronic ovaritis with spasmodic contractive dysmenorrhea,* menses too early and too profuse. Sometimes loud emissions of flatus from the vagina during the menses. The 6th, 12th, and 30th.

IODIUM.

You are all familiar with its use in the operating room. Did the surgeons ever explain why the part was painted with Iodium before an operation? Have you ever been told why so many doctors paint all kinds of swellings with Iodium? The answer is found in the *power* the drug has *of producing absorption.* Its primary action is to close all absorbing vessels of the skin. Its secondary action is to stimulate all absorbents to greater activity. By taking advantage of the first action and sealing all absorbents you prevent infection; by taking advantage of the secondary action you check the excessive waste of gland, muscle and fat tissue and ***prevent emaciation*** which is the ***ranking*** symptom of the drug.

Make-up: "Dark hair; dark yellow, tawny skin; excitable; restless."

Loc.: Glands, thyroid, mesenteric, mammary; testicles; M.M. of larynx and lungs; heart, skin.

Sen.: Hungry; dry; pulsating, heat.

Mod.: Agg.: *Heat* of ***room*** wrapping part; exertion; night; rest.

Amel.: *Cold air;* bathing; eating.

Leaders: *Always too hot;* affections of glands; choking hoarseness; ***emaciation.***

Brain and Nerves.

Mind: The mental condition of Iodium is irritability and sensitiveness.

Glands.

Throat: "Swelling of tonsils and uvula which is elongated." *Acute tonsilitis* which involves the *Eustachian* tube and upper part of the throat, causing deafness.

Many cases of ***goitre*** have been cured by Iodium. The ***dark complexion*** of the patient and the *firmness* of the ***gland*** are the leading symptoms.

Let me put in a word of warning at this point about the external use of Iodine for goitre. Never use Iodium externally unless you are giving it internally. I have known many cases of rheumatism and pulmonary troubles develop on the dissipation of goitre by the external use of Iodium. Many cases of mumps have been helped by Iodium.

Stomach: "*Ravenous hunger;* appetite lost; cramp-like gnawing, burning pains in stomach; frequent nausea; vomiting bile after eating."

Abdomen: "Abdominal pains which return after each meal; enlargement of the abdomen which renders it impossible to lie down without danger of suffocation; *swelling and inflammation* of the mesenteric glands (Calcarea iod.); pancreas enlarged; hard swelling in the inguinal glands; *region* of *liver, sore* to *pressure;* hard painful swelling of the spleen (Ceanothus)."

You find the nucleus of several groups in the above. *Chronic enlargement* of the *spleen,* with marked hardness and tenderness, profuse saliva, and soft, frequent, whitish stool.

Both *acute* and *chronic pancreatitis* also with salivation, vomiting and the profuse watery stool (may be constipated with chronic). With the chronic you may have melancholia as well as irritability.

For the cirrhotic liver especially when due to excessive doses of Mercurius, you will find tenderness in region of liver and the whitish colored, soft stools, also the dingy livid skin.

Stools: "Diarrhea, *soft, whitish,* frequent *stools; constipation.*"

I mention the stools of Iodium under this location because the condition is usually caused by functional diseases of the liver and pancreas.

Urinary Organs: "Involuntary micturition; also frequent and copious; urine at times turbid, dark, at others milky; sp. gr. 1025 to 1038."

Some cases of *diabetes* have been reported cured when in addition to urine of high sp. gr., and a reaction for sugar there was *canine hunger.*

It helped me in one case of degeneration of an enlarged prostate with alternating retention and dribbling of the urine.

Sexual Organs: "Testicles diminished in size; double its former size; priapism; impotency; menses too late; menses too early."

Please recall what I said at the beginning about increasing and decreasing the activity of the absorbent vessels and you will understand the dual action here.

It has been used for *hydrocele* more than for any other condition in this section. Insert your needle and draw out most of the fluid and then through the same needle, without withdrawing it, inject the solution of Iodium. Be sure at the same time to give Iodium internally in the 6th or 12th. Many cases have been cured by the internal use, without the injection.

Many cases of *orchitis* have been cured by it. I advise painting the diseased organ and giving the 6th internally as we did for goitre. I would always advise a suspensory for the testicle and see to it yourself that it is properly adjusted. If you do, this will relieve the exasperating dragging pains which extend up into the abdomen.

For the other sex Iodium has been used for *ovarian cysts, chronic menorrhagia* and *metrorrhagia.* With both of these conditions you get agg. warmth and *after stool.* Also *with* both you get *atrophy* of the *mammary gland.* For *chronic ovaritis* where you have a thick yellow, *acrid leucorrhea,* atrophy of the mammæ, goitre. Sometimes *induration of* the *cervix* may *accompany* the *ovaritis* and again we may have the induration without the ovaritis but with the other symptoms of the ovaritis group.

Again we may have a very painful *metritis with* nervousness, increased desire to urinate with *heat* and *dryness of* the *vagina.*

Many claims as to its use for *cancer of* the *uterus* are made. I do not think it has ever cured cancer but I do know that the use of Iodium internally and the use of it locally has decreased the discharges whether of blood or pus and mucus mixed with blood and by so doing has relieved much of the odor which makes such patients a sore trial to themselves and their friends. With many of these conditions I wish you would remember the *rapid emaciation,* the *ravenous hunger* and the *wedge-like pain between* the *uterus* and *ovary.*

Respiratory Organs.

"Pain in larynx with desire to cough; frequent pain in region of larynx and sublingual glands, with stitches, smarting and rawness in air-passages; *hoarseness;* croupy cough amel. expectoration of mucus; respiration tight; difficult, especially inspiration." Rapid, short respiration agg. slight exertion: breath lost; sighing.

"Constriction of chest; *sticking, tearing, burning pains in chest.*"

Iodium has a wide, well-defined field in this section. *Laryngitis* whether *simple inflammatory* or *fibrinous* has been cured by it again and again. Also *chronic catarrhal laryngitis.* The ranking symptoms are: make-up of patient, the dry skin, the *dry cough,* the high temperature; the *dyspnea* indicate it *for* the *simple laryngitis.* For *membranous croup* it follows well after Aconite. Your temperature is still high, the cough dry and sawing; the dyspnea marked, the skin dry; the pulse rapid and full. Stop the Iodium if the pulse becomes weak, the skin moist, the cough loose, the fever gone, and give Kali bich. or Hepar.

It will help you for your *whooping cough* patients of the Iodium make-up if the emaciation is great, due very often to the fact that the child vomits so much of its food (Kali bich., Ipecac). Here again you have the *ravenous appetite* as a ranking symptom.

Iodium belongs to the *pneumonia* group. It is a hybrid of Aconite and Bryonia. It lacks the restlessness and anxiety of Aconite and the sharp sticking, stitching pains of Bryonia, but you have the high temperature of both; you also have the dry skin of Aconite, which belongs only to the very first stage of Bryonia. Hepatization has taken place; the dyspnea is marked. Again your make-up ranks first, *i. e.,* the scrofulous or t. b. c. diathesis is especially prone to give us the above group of symptoms. Finally for *phthisis pulmonaris,* apices are affected, the skin is dry, the emaciation is rapid, the appetite ravenous, the cough dry, the voice rough, the dyspnea marked and agg. by the least exertion. Occasionally the patient is despondent (Stannum iod.).

Heart.

"Precordial anxiety causing constant change of position; *palpitation* agg. movement."

Before we proved Strychnia phos., I considered Iodium the head of the trio of remedies for fatty degeneration of an hypertrophied heart (Iodium, Arsenicum, Phosphorus) and used it in the 6th. Now I put the S. P. at the head of the quartet and use it as much as I do the other three. Iodium is second. You ask if the symptoms are not different enough to guide you? Yes, in a few cases; No, in most cases. You take a patient with a very large compensating heart, and let him have a severe run of typhoid, or diphtheria, and when the "break in compensation" comes and your muscles rapidly change to fat cells the symptoms are very much alike. Arsenicum and Iodium are more rapid in their action. Phosphorus and Strychnia phos. more stable, slower and more permanent. My experience is that you seldom have a break in compensation following any condition for which either Iodium or Phosphorus have been used. Iodine is useful for *pericarditis* complicating pneumonia. It shares the honors with Bryonia for that condition but ranks below *Colchicum* when the pericarditis complicates rheumatism.

Extremities and Muscles.

"Pain in muscles and bones at night preventing sleep (Mercurius); convulsive startings and twitching in muscles (Actea, Cuprum); shortness of the tendons (Rhus); erratic pains in joints. Emaciation (Plumbum)."

Iodium has helped *articular rheumatism*, also *gonorrheal* and *wandering rheumatism*. The latter sometimes attacks the meninges and heart. With the articular you have *hot swollen joints* much pain and the *agg. at night.* For *sinovitis* after the abuse of mercury in scrofulous patients, whether in the first stage or after suppuration has taken place and you have a bloody serous discharge.

It is said of the Chinese that no matter with what people they intermarry the offspring is always Chinese. So with Iodium, no matter with what drug it is combined the symptoms of the compound bear the characteristics of Iodine.

SPONGIA TOSTA.

Make-up: The croupy; light-colored.

Loc.: Larynx; heart; glands.

Sen.: Anxious; suffocative; of a plug; soreness.

Mod.: Agg. cold, dry wind (Aconite); awaking (Lachesis); exertion.

Amel.: lying down; warm foods or drinks.

Leaders: The *light; croupy, ringing, crawling,* sawing, *barking cough; surging of blood and heat to face and chest,* and the rapid, pounding heart.

Respiratory Organs: "Region of *thyroid gland* seems *indurated* (Iodium, Conium); pain in region of larynx, when singing; scraping in larynx with burning and constriction; dryness of larynx agg. by hawking (Belladonna); *hoarseness* (Phosphorus, Iodium, Bromium); cough from low down in the chest, with soreness (Sanguinaria); dry cough day and night agg. eating and drinking, with burning in the chest chest (Carbo veg.); respiration difficult as if a plug were sticking in the larynx and the breath could not get through on account of constriction of larynx (Lachesis)."

One of our leading remedies for *simple goitre* (Iodium, Calcarea iod., Bromium, Thyroidin) when the *patient* is *fair* with *brown hair, staring eyes;* hoarseness and *SUFFOCATIVE SPELLS* at night. Occasionally for *Exophthalmus* when in addition to the above you have the *rapid, beating heart* and *tremors* of the hands.

Laryngitis with sensitiveness of the part of the larynx involved, with harsh, croupy cough and *suffocative spells* at night. In the conditions above named the temperature is not high as in Aconite or Iodium and usually it follows well after them.

Occasionally for *phthisis* or *diphtheritic* croup of the larynx. For chronic *inflammation* of the *vocal cords* with hoarseness and when the voice gives out on using it (Phosphorus).

For *bronchial catarrh* when you have the wheezing, asthmatic breathing and cough amel. eating and drinking, agg. cold air. Rarely, with the bronchitis, you have profuse expectoration, if so, you will have the suffocative attacks agg. at night and when lying with the head low. Also agg. in a close, warm room.

Occasionally helpful for *whooping cough* agg. after midnight and by cold air.

For *pulmonary tuberculosis* following pneumonia with the chronic *hoarseness*, the profuse expectoration, and the suffocative attacks at night.

The most frequent use you will make of Spongia is for croup, the second most frequent will be for goitre. Use the 6th and 30th.

ACTEA RACEMOSA.

Make-up: Dark; nervous; muscles well developed; overworked.

Loc.: *Nerves;* female generative organs; belly of muscles.

Sen.: Twitching; trembling; jerking.

Mod.: *Agg. before the menses;* cold; wet.

Amel. in open air; gentle, continued motion.

Leaders: Fear of going crazy; *gloom and dejection.*

Nerves and Brain.

Spinal Cord: "*Drawing, tensive pain* at points of spinous processes of the three upper *dorsal vertebræ* (China, Sulphur) in the morning on bending neck forward."

It is frequently called for in ***spinal irritation*** of women who have been disappointed in love, of business men who have failed, women who have borne children too rapidly, men who have overexerted either mentally or physically and of children who have been frightened.

Mind: "*Grieved; troubled* and sighing, miserable, dejected feeling alternating with joy and playfulness; vision of all sorts of animals; fear of death; mania after neuralgia."

Very useful for delirium of all forms including tremens; the patient sees all sorts of forms, most frequently dark objects (Stramonium), talks all the time on all kinds of subjects, constantly changing from one subject to another. His body is as restless as his mind. She is constantly changing from one position to another. One minute she fears she is going crazy, the next she fears she is going to die and the third she threatens to commit suicide. For *insanity* or *mania,* most frequently puerperal mania. With the insanity you have the melancholia of the drug, with insomnia. The patient constantly sighing and moaning with the mania. I have found that most of these cases come at the time of the menopause and are accompanied by hot flashes and chills.

Head: "*Drawing pain* and *soreness* in the *occiput* extending to the vertex, pressing outward and upward in upper part of cerebrum as if there were not room enough, *soreness in* the *occiput* caused by the pain through the whole brain, worse from motion."

The headaches of Actea are mostly neuralgic. You find a neuralgic headache, reflex from uterine troubles, also associated with meningitis. Then we have the climacteric headache and finally the headache of the debauchee. With all uterine and meningeal forms there is a sensation as if the cord were too short. The pain is relieved by dropping the head back on the shoulders and greatly agg. by bending the head forward. With all headaches you have the insomnia.

Eyes: "*Pain in balls,* in center and between ball and orbital plate of frontal bone; eyes congested during the headache; vision of black specks."

Useful for *ciliary neuralgia* when the balls feel too large and sharp pains shoot up into the vertex.

Uterus: "Pains in the uterus shooting from side to side and upwards."

With these *neuralgic pains* of the *uterus and ovaries* we have found heaviness and bearing-down sensations, also great sensitiveness. The spasms are occasionally epileptiform, the woman frequently hysterical. Used for *after pains* when there is *great sensitiveness* and intolerance.

Chest and Lungs: "*Lancinating pains* along the false ribs worse from motion; tickling in larynx causing a dry cough worse from speaking."

Actea has cured *rheumatism of the diaphragm, pleurodynia,* and the cough described above which is usually reflex and purely nervous.

Heart: "Stitching, catching pains in region of heart followed by palpitation; pains extend down the left arm (Spigelia), which feels numb."

For *angina pectoris* in women suffering from rheumatism or some uterine trouble. You will find the pulse weak, irregular, and palpitation from the least motion.

Neck, Back and Extremities: Let us include under this subdivision of brain and nerves the *muscles.* "*Rheumatic pains of neck and back with stiffness and contractions;* drawing tensive pain at points of spinous processes of three upper dorsal vertebræ on bending the neck forward; excessive muscular soreness; constant irregular motion of arms worse from motion; rheumatic pains in joints, with heat and swelling; severe aching pain in lumbar and sacral region, down the thighs and through the hips; violent lightning-like pains along the spine."

For *chorea.* When we recall the causes of chorea and bear in mind that Actea is most suitable to women at the age of puberty and the menopause; also that it irritates the nerves and muscles and is agg. by wet, motion and excitement, we readily see why Actea is more frequently called for in chorea than any other remedy. *Spinal irritation* often yields to the remedy and occasionally *spinal meningitis*. Muscular rheumatism when the belly of the muscles is affected. The "*obstinate insomnia*" of the drug comes in the rheumatic group. The patient cannot sleep because of pain; he tosses about; is extremely restless and should he fall asleep it is full of unpleasant dreams, never is the sleep restful or refreshing.

Female Generative Organs.

In addition to the symptoms mentioned under the other locations we find: "*Menses* profuse, early; scanty, delayed; *irregular;* suppressed; bearing-down pains during pregnancy." The irritation of the uterus which produces the menstrual colic mentioned above sometimes becomes severe enough to *produce miscarriage*. I once asked a woman who had called me for hemorrhage after producing a miscarriage upon herself what she had used and she replied, "Tea from black snake root." I have in many cases *prevented miscarriage* by using five drops of the 3x every three hours and enforcing absolute rest. The history of these cases always shows symptoms of *endocervicitis accompanied by profuse menses*. I have found the scanty delayed menses more frequently with the pure neuralgias. The reputed use of Actea given for a few weeks before childbirth to make labor easier has some foundation in facts. I made a special study on about 500 cases when in charge of the Benedict Home and am convinced that its use shortened the time and lightened the sufferings of labor. I gave five drops of the 3rd or 6th night and morning for about three weeks prior to delivery. With all the conditions of the female generative organs you will find the mental and nervous symptoms in varying degrees of severity from mild insomnia to epileptic convulsions.

PULSATILLA NIGER.

Make-up: Catarrhal; weak; changeable; tearful; emotional.

Loc.: Mucous membrane; sexual organs; veins; brain.

Sen.: Burning; itching.

Mod.: Agg. *warm air, room or bed;* evening; lying; rest; beginning motion; rich, fat food; puberty; pregnancy.

Amel. *cold, fresh air;* erect position; after a good cry.

Leaders: Emotional disposition; chilliness; foul breath; aversion to fats and pastry.

Mucous Membrane.

Eyes: "*Burning and itching; lachrymation* with deeply sunken eyes; *inflammation* of margin of the lower lids; agglutination of lids in morning; itching; biting."

For *catarrhal conjunctivitis* when the cold, open air and wind agg. the itching and burning, and increase the discharge of thick mucus and pus which not only cause agglutination of lids but dimness of vision; *blepharitis also* agg. in the cool, open air; *tumors* of the lids; *granular lids* with the itching and burning; *inflammation* of the *tear ducts,* also fistula with profuse, thick, bland discharge; *hyperemia* and *ulceration* of the *choroid; ophthalmia of infants* either catarrhal or *after* the *misuse* of *Argentum nit.*

Ear: "*Pain* as if *something forcing out; stopped* sensation with distant *roaring; hearing difficult,* as if ears were stopped; sound of wind or rushing of water at 4 P.M."

Otitis, external with *redness* and *swelling* of concha; *otalgia* darting, tearing pains amel. by cold applications, the pains often extend into the face and teeth; *otorrhea* with the thick, *purulent discharge* occasionally blood, but as a rule *non-excoriating; deafness* with a feeling as if the ears were stopped, sometimes as if the pulse were beating in the ear. The deafness and otorrhea often follow scarlet fever. When this is true you usually find that the *pernicious habit of greasing the child* during the fever has been practiced. The *ear pains,* like the cough of Pulsatilla, are decidedly *worse* at *night.*

Nose: "*Stoppage* in evening on going to bed, and blowing out of thick, yellow, opaque mucus in the morning; *sneezing* and *discharge* of green, *offensive mucus* with smell as in old catarrh; *coryza* with loss of smell and taste; bleeding with stopped catarrh; blowing blood out of nose in the morning."

Pulsatilla is the best remedy for what the laity call "a ripe cold." So aptly does the term express the totality of the symptoms of Pulsatilla that I have many times prescribed it with success for this condition in the last stage of acute influenza, without seeing the patient.

Also useful for *chronic catarrh* of the nose with one modality to which I will call your attention, viz., "better in fresh, cold air." That refers to stopped up condition of the nose. When the Pulsatilla patient goes out into the cold, fresh air the nasal discharge becomes thinner and freer. This relieves the "stopped up" condition and the headache caused by it (Kali bich., Hydrastis).

Catarrh of the *antrum* has been cured by Pulsatilla even after it refused to yield to drainage. The discharge in these cases is orange-yellow and thinner than the nasal, though subject to the same modalities.

Mouth: "*Aching of teeth* as soon as anything warm is taken into the mouth; jerking pain in teeth *better* when *cold water* is taken into the mouth, worse when the water becomes warm; *tongue covered with* a tenacious *mucus* as with a membrane; *dryness* of tongue, palate and lips on waking in the morning, soon changing to much tenacious mucus (Kali bich.); *taste* bitter, slimy, foul, insipid, disgusting especially in morning."

For *neuralgia* of the teeth especially of pregnant women. The other symptoms of the mouth are for the most part reflex, *e. g.,* dryness of all the parts in the morning is due to mouth breathing during the night because the nose is occluded.

Throat: The same "dryness in morning" with "rawness and scraping to get rid of the tenacious mucus."

Stomach: "*Eructation* of *food* (Lycopodium, Phosphorus) of *gas* tasting of food: E. of bile, bitter, in the evening; E. of bitter fluid; E. tasting of rancid tallow after eating cakes, or of bad meat after dinner; the taste remains; ***nausea*** and vomiting ***with chilliness, gnawing; heaviness;*** sensation as if one had eaten too much."

Pulsatilla is more frequently called for in disorders of the stomach than any other remedy except Nux vom. There is ***not much irritation, no inflammation*** and very rarely ulceratoin *or* other ***structural changes.*** You have all forms of ***dyspepsia,*** acid, atonic, flatulent. The ***aversion*** to *fats* and ***pastry, and*** the ***craving*** for ***fruits and acids*** are *very* ***pronounced.*** The ***causes*** of the troubles are the use of *ice cream,* ice water, ***bad milk*** or ***meat,*** etc. The *tendency* of Pulsatilla patients to catarrh is marked, especially so to catarrh of the stomach.

Intestines: "*Distention* after eating (Lycopodium) with intermitting colic, rumbling and gurgling in the evening agg. in bed; ***moving*** of ***flatus*** from one part of the intestines to another with griping, pinching and frequent diarrheic stools; ***drawing, tensive*** pains like labor pains; drawing pains in upper abdomen, extending along spermatic cord into the testicles."

Anus: "Painful, ***protruding, bleeding hemorrhoids,*** agg. in the evening with itching; ***frequent evacuations*** of only *mucus.*"

For ***intestinal catarrh*** of ***infants*** with nausea, vomiting, colic about navel and diarrhea, chilliness worse in the evening. The ***colic*** and ***diarrhea*** are ***caused*** by taking cold, ***eating fruit,*** ice cream (Arsenicum), ***fats*** or ***pastry.*** With the intestinal catarrh the diarrheic stools are covered with mucus.

For ***hemorrhoids*** associated with gastric troubles which ***bleed*** profusely ***after stools. Rarely*** for ***dysentery,*** stools of blood and mucus with ***burning*** in the anus, no tenesmus.

Urinary Organs: "*Micturition involuntary at night in bed;*

frequent desire; *spurting of urine* when coughing or laughing; dribbling of urine when walking or sitting" (Causticum).

The three conditions for which I have frequently used Pulsatilla are *catarrh of the bladder, incontinence of urine* and *gleet*. The *incontinence* is most frequently found in young girls who have leucorrhea. The desire comes on suddenly and they wet their clothes or bed. The catarrh of the bladder is generally due to exposure to cold. The urine in this condition is very turbid. Sometimes the cause is an enlarged prostate. There is no inflammation, no irritation with the gleet, only a profuse, milky or slimy discharge.

Vagina: "*Leucorrhea* with burning pain, *painless; thick,* of the color of milk, worse lying down; *leucorrhea* thin, acrid with swelling of pudenda; milky, painless."

I have never seen a case of Pulsatilla leucorrhea which was *acrid.*

Respiratory Organs: "*Tickling* and *scraping* in larynx causing lachrymation, and dry cough; hoarseness, inability to speak a loud word; *cough from dryness* and *scraping in* the *trachea; constant* cough at night, after lying down, preventing sleep; *dry* cough at night better sitting up; dry cough with expectoration of yellow mucus; respiration short after dinner, want of air on attempting to breathe through nose."

The cough from "tickling and scraping in larynx" is the *cough of measles.* It comes at the time the eruption is in the M.M. The dry, night cough is also of measles. Note that the first cough causes lachrymation. There is no other remedy so often useful for measles as Pulsatilla. Under respiratory organs, eyes, skin, sleep, stomach and stools you find symptoms just like those caused by measles, a complete picture of the uncomplicated case of the disease. For *bronchitis* with cough better sitting up and in open air, worse from warmth of bed and cold water.

Sexual Organs.

Male: "*Testicles swollen;* right side of the scrotum swollen; *drawing pain in spermatic cords; soreness of* testicles so that clothing seemed too tight."

One of the *most frequently* indicated remedies for *epididymitis* and *orchitis.* The pains of both are usually associated with pains in the small of the back, *chilliness* especially in the P.M., nausea, etc., but never relieved by hot applications. It is *here* that the *mental symptom* of the drug, *i. e.,* melancholia, *applies to men.* Useful for *hydrocele* with the mental symptoms. The cause of the orchitis is most frequently metastasis during measles.

Female: "*Menses suppressed,* delayed, with coldness of body, chilliness and trembling of feet. Drawing pain extending towards uterus in the morning with nausea; contracting pain in left side of uterus like labor pains, forcing her to bend double; swelling of breasts with tensive pains as if milk rushed into them when not nursing."

Let me explain that last symptom first. Under normal conditions there should be no pain when a woman nurses her babe, but irritation will often cause this abnormal condition. I have also found this symptom in a few cases of young women, school girls. The methods of irritation were by tight clothing for the purpose of concealing the developing breasts or by carrying their books. In three cases I have found milk in the breasts from such irritation. And while speaking of young girls let me remind you that Pulsatilla is *one of* the *four* great *remedies for incipient tuberculosis when menstruation* is delayed. With this *amenorrhea* group you will find all the concomitant symptoms but the two which rank highest are the *cough* and *loss of weight.* The *dysmenorrhea* of Pulsatilla is *caused* by *getting* the *feet wet* and by fits of *anger* (Chamomilla, Colocynth). The pains are severe, colicky, the menses are late and scanty. The *suppressed menses* of the drug are also caused by fits of anger and getting feet wet.

There is no remedy whose symptoms emanating from the mind and sexual organs are so marked and closely related to each other as are those of Pulsatilla. One of the results is phantom tumor. I have had two cases of *imaginary pregnancy*. One woman was extremely anxious to become a mother; the other, who had an idiotic child, equally anxious not to have another child. With both all the usual changes of gestation took place and the baby clothes were made. With both labor pains began and I was sent for. Now for the part Pulsatilla played. The cause of sterility in the first case was a profuse, chronic leucorrhea which our remedy and proper adjuvant treatment cured and she afterwards bore two children. The only thing Pulsatilla could do for the second woman was to relieve her mental condition.

Circulation.

Heart: "*Palpitation* from talking after heavy meal; *rapid* if she lies on the left side, with anxiety and want of breath; anxiety in the precordial region in the evening with impulse to commit suicide."

For palpitation when you have general sluggish circulation and the *chilliness* which you have noticed in all groups. The pulse soft and rapid with attacks of suffocation. The *symptom* of *highest rank in* this group is also the *mental.*

Veins: Often indicated for "*varicose veins* and *ulcers*" with which you have the "*smarting, itching*" and the "chilliness" though warmth aggravates. The most frequent condition calling for it in this section is phlebitis, especially of the lower extremities, *phlegmasia dolens* of Pulsatilla women.

Sleep: It will reward you to study the sleep symptoms of Pulsatilla. You find them in nearly every group. The patient is always "*late in falling to sleep.*" The *sleeplessness* is *due* to "*anxious heat*" or "from *fixed ideas.*" When she does get to sleep at midnight the sleep is "*restless,*" full of dreams, she is too hot, the dry cough wakes her. The child with stomach trouble starts from sleep frightened and screaming from some unpleasant dream. I use Pulsatilla low. I also get a fresh preparation frequently as it deteriorates rapidly.

SEPIA.

Make-up: Thin; weak; relaxed; sallow; craving excitement.

Loc.: *Female generative organs;* thermic center; circulation; skin; liver; M.M.

Sen.: Weakness; of prolapsus, as if a lump, dragging.

Mod.: Agg. cold air and weather; during pregnancy; sexual excesses.

Amel.: Violent exercise; warmth.

Leaders: Pain and weakness in lumbar region; faint sinking in the epigastrium; bearing-down feeling.

Female Generative Organs.

Vagina: "Dryness after menses; and of vulva causing discomfort when walking; yellow acrid leucorrhea before menses with soreness of pudenda with burning pain and excoriation between the thighs; leucorrhea *looking like milk, pus,* lumpy; discharge bloody, slimy; of a few drops of blood fifteen days before menses."

Uterus: "Beginning to prolapse; congested; and a yellowish leucorrhea pouring from it (Lillium tig.), prolapsus causing pain in the lower half of body with pain in the pelvis and lying especially on right side; feeling as if clutched and suddenly released at 7 P.M., causing nausea; pressure as if everything would issue through the vulva in the P.M.; pressure downward as if everything would fall out, with oppression of breath and pain in the abdomen; she must cross her limbs to prevent protrusion of vagina, yet nothing protrudes; but there is an increase of gelatinous leucorrhea; menses too early, too late. scanty, appearing only in the morning scanty, lasting only one day."

Nearly all of the above are found in black type in Allen's Hand Book and have been verified again and again. They are all first rank symptoms and appear in many conditions, and yet no group made up exclusively of them could be complete even if it included all of them. Let us take for illustration the condition "*prolapsus uteri.*" All the dragging and *pressing* symptoms are in the group and *in addition* the *knotty, difficult,* scanty *stool,* the frequent *urging to urinate,* complete *indifference* to her affairs and *desire to be alone; yellow spots* agg. on face with a general *sallow skin.* These are all what I call "reasonable" symptoms, the result of pressure on the rectum, bladder, veins, etc. What caused the prolapsus which is the cause of all this trouble? There are two causes. The *uterus* is *heavy,* often due to some disturbance of the portal circulation. The *supports* of the uterus are *weaker than usual* besides trouble with the portal circulation, *subinvolution* or *tumors* may be the *cause of* the *increased weight* of the *uterus.* I have often met the above group during the first three months of *gestation.*

Sepia has helped many cases of *induration* of the uterus. Also for *chronic endometritis* with tenderness over the uterine region, pain in the lumbar region, sinking in the epigastrium and constant desire to urinate, it is one of our best remedies.

Many cases of *amenorrhea* and *dysmenorrhea* have been *relieved* by Sepia. *With* the amenorrhea you have more of the nervous symptoms, *e. g., flushes of heat,* chronic dyspepsia, *nausea* and *vomiting,* relieved by eating and lying down; *longing for acids.* The Sepia *leucorrhea* is always present with both the amenorrhea and dysmenorrhea.

For *disorders of* the menopause like the *chills* and *hot flushes,* irregular periods, a flow at one period scanty, the next profuse; one time delayed at others early, severe pain in lumbar region agg. standing or stooping, amel. when lying down, a tremulous feeling about the heart, unrefreshing sleep, *cold, damp feet* with neuralgic headache of Sepia. Occasionally *swelling* and *tumors of* the *breasts* come and go with the menses *at* the *climacteric period.*

Mucous Membranes.

Eyes: "*Redness* of the white in morning on waking, with *burning,* smarting and *pressure;* swelling with burning and lachrymation which amel. the swelling; pain as from sand (Natrum mur., Zinc phos.), agg. by pressing the lids together and rubbing."

Helpful in scrofulous conjunctivitis with the *head* and *liver group.*

Nose: "*Stuffed;* nostrils inflamed, swollen, scabby; *dryness* (Natrum mur.) in *nostrils* and *fauces* with a swollen feeling, yet without coryza."

Nasal polypi and a dry nasal catarrh.

Stomach: "Craving hunger; desire for vinegar; aversion to meat; *nausea;* amel. eating, before breakfast, on washing mouth, on walking, with blackness before the eyes; nausea in the evening with weakness even to fainting; vomiting of food and retching; nausea as if everything in the abdomen were turning around, with watery salivation, bitterish sour; vomiting during pregnancy straining her so that blood comes up; *empty feeling* (Podophyllum, Ignatia, Pulsatilla) with *nausea;* as *soon* as she *thinks of food* she would have *pulsations* in pit, ebulations in chest like palpitations, then internal heat of face and body without redness or thirst but with sweat; burning in pit."

Sepia has *cured acid dyspepsia* with *sour* or putrid *eructations,* bloated abdomen, *nausea* and vomiting and *diarrhea.* Also *atomic* dyspepsia, generally *associated with amenorrhea* and *pregnancy,* occasionally at the climacteric period. The *headache* and *hypochondriac mood* of the drug are important symptoms of this group. The nausea and vomiting generally amel. lying down and sometimes by eating are of minor importance but present in most cases. The *depression* and *weak-*

ness, the *result* of *overwrought brain* or sexual *excesses,* occasionally appear.

Gastric catarrh will claim most of the remaining *symptoms* of this section, such as longing for acids, soreness over stomach and hepatic region, feeling as if something were turning about in stomach or rising toward throat, the bad taste, sallow complexion, etc.

Liver.

"*Sticking, cutting, sore, jerking pain* in hepatic region; full sensation in the hepatic region on lying down."

Sepia has relieved the condition known as *torpid liver* which *includes any* or *all* of the *symptoms* I have just *quoted, plus enlargement* of liver, "pain between shoulders and down the back," "sallow complexion," "white-coated, blistered tongue," "hemorrhoids."

This group is very often associated with the pelvic, the cause of the two being the same.

Thermic Centers and Circulation.

Let us first consider the *portal circulation.* Please recall the liver and pelvic symptoms especially the hemorrhoids. To these add "palpitation of heart with beating in all the arteries," "orgasm and congestion of the chest as if hemoptysis would follow," "faintness," etc., and you will get a good idea of Sepia's action on the circulatory apparatus proper, more especially the venous. From *disturbances* of the *thermic centers, result "hot hands"* and *"cold feet,"* "flushes running upwards," *"hot flushes followed* by *chills."* I have met a few cases in which a hot wave would come from the extremities or pelvis to the heart and be followed by syncope. I first thought it was an aura and that the "faint" was an epileptic convulsion, but being present when the attack came on showed me that there were no spasms or other symptoms of epilepsy except the unconsciousness. The cause was disturbed circulation.

The heart's action was very violent, following the attack. The only time I ever prescribed Sepia to a man was for this condition following intercourse. The man had been a "rounder" and was over 65 years of age. The Sepia helped.

Skin.

"Red, roughness on face; round, red spot on hand not amel. by scratching; red, herpetic spots above hips, on side of neck with itching; brown spots on elbows, surrounded by a herpetic looking skin; yellowish brown spots about the neck scaling off when rubbing; itching pimples on chin; *itching* on elbows (Rhus tox. and Sulphur), on face, hands, back, feet, abdomen."

Although *brown "liver spots"* is the symptom most frequently quoted by our authors, I have rarely met one. Patients with *hang nails* and ulcers about unhealthy finger nails I have often cured. Herpetic and eczematous eruptions with the other conditions are frequently cured, *i. e.,* disappear as the other condition is cured. I remember two cases, sisters, who came to the clinic to be cured of herpes who were suffering from *chronic catarrhal* metritis. They were cured by Sepia. Use the 30th and higher.

CHAMOMILLA.

Make-up: *Neurotic,* rheumatic.

Loc.: *Nerves,* mucous membranes, sexual organs and joints. including all tissues of joints.

Sen.: *Peevish,* impatient; sad; *changeable;* cross; sharp; shooting; cramp-like; jerking; pains seem intolerable.

Mod.: Agg. lying in bed; at night; warmth; music; cold, damp, windy weather.

Amel.: *Being carried about.*

Nervous System.

Mind: "Whinning; *snappish;* restlessness; the child wants this and that, but when given it angrily pushes it away; *pitcous* *moaning* of a child *when refused* what he wants; the child will *only be quiet when carried* on the arm; moans on account of trifles; heat of one side of face when moaning; *peevishness* about everything, especially about pain with dyspnea; impatience; intolerance of being spoken to or interrupted, worse after sleep; anxiety; *excitement;* confusion; weeping; *uncivil.*"

Ears: "Drawing, tensive, shooting pains extending into ears, worse on stooping with a disposition to be angry at trifles; tinkling and buzzing in the ears; hearing acute."

Face: "Convulsive movements of the muscles of the face and lips; spasms of the jaw; stretching jaw extending into inner ear also into teeth."

Mouth: "*Aching* in teeth agg. *by warm drink amel. by ice water;* intolerable pains in molars making him peevish."

Stomach: "Eructations; stitching, griping pains in pit of stomach and beneath the short ribs, impeding respiration."

Abdomen: "Cutting, sticking pains from flatulence, extending into the chest; griping tearing in region of navel and lower down on sides, with pains in small of back as if broken."

Uterus: "Labor-like pains with frequent urging to urinate."

1. The mental symptoms of Chamomilla are very marked. The *emotions* are most *profoundly affected.* The *patient* is *easily angered* and the effect is felt in nearly every part of the body. The result may be suppression of the menses, of the lochia, of the milk. Anger may bring on acute indigestion, diarrhea or puerperal convulsions. I remember one case of most *unbearable after pains* brought on by the patients becoming angry at the nurse, promptly cured by the remedy. Threatening miscarriage and menstrual colic both caused by anger have yielded to Chamomilla. The peculiar modalities of the odontalgia have been verified many times. The best remedy for people who have used Opium, Bromide, also tea and coffee to excess.

2. The nervous conditions covered by Chamomilla vary from the slightest algia to a profound convulsion of children.

The causes of the latter are excitement and the irritation of dentition. With the convulsions you have one cheek hot and red, the other cold and pale. The head is covered with hot perspiration.

Sexual Organs.

Male: "Excited sexual desire; sycotic swelling of the prepuce; itching, stinging pains at the meatus; burning in neck of bladder when urinating."

Female: "Drawing from anterior part of small of back, griping and pinching in uterus, then discharge of large clots of blood; profuse discharge of clotted blood, with labor pains in uterus and tearing in veins of legs; acrid watery discharge from the vagina after dinner; profuse yellow, biting leucorrhea; menses suppressed."

Chamomilla has been used with succes for both *menorrhagia and metrorrhagia,* when the flow is irregular, dark, clotted with much pain; or for constant oozing of dark foul blood with occasional gushes of bright red blood. It has *prevented miscarriage* when there were the *irregular pains,* which were *caused* by *excitement,* especially *anger.* Many times it has helped to hasten a protracted labor when the pains were unbearable extending into the thighs or any direction except bearing down as they should. At such cases the os is usually rigid.

Mucous Membranes.

Respiratory Organs: "Larynx raw; scraping on account of tough mucus in larynx which is only detached by violent hawking; whistling, wheezing and rattling in trachea when breathing; dry cough at night from irritation low down in the trachea; cough in paroxysms at midnight with which something seems to rise in throat and suffocate him."

Nose: "Irritation compelling one to sneeze, with crawling, dry heat; stopped sensation, and feeling as if coryza would appear, also with pressure in forehead."

Joints.

"Cracking in joints, especially those of lower extremities; soreness of all joints as if bruised and tired out, no strength in hands and feet, though without ordinary weariness; pain in the periosteum with paralytic weakness."

The importance of the joints pains is the marked effect they have in bringing on and agg. the mental condition.

Chamomilla is the most frequently used remedy, for children, we have in our materia medica. For the many abnormal conditions during the period of dentition no remedy is so successful. It regulates the bowels, quiets the nerves, produces sleep and improves the disposition. The ranking symptoms of this group are "*only satisfied when being carried, one cheek red and hot, the other pale and cold* and the teasing for something only to reject it when he gets it."

The 30th potency is the best for most patients. However the 200th helped in two cases when the 30th failed. One was a patient who had suffered from a long attack of neuritis for which a good deal of morphine had been used; the other a case of dysmenorrhea for which morphine and other anodynes had been used.

SECALE CORNUTUM.

Mak-up: Thin; spare; scrawny; dark.

Loc.: Involuntary muscular fibers; blood; nerves; uterus and M.M.

Sen.: Twitching; cramps; burning; too hot.

Mod.: Agg.: *Warmth;* during menses and pregnancy.
Amel. *cold;* forcible extension.

Leaders: *Icy cold feeling externally; burning hot internally* so that patient objects to covering and the bluish color of skin below the eyes (Ipecac).

To help interpret the symptoms of *ergot,* bear in mind that it *acts upon* the *involuntary muscular fibers* of the *arterioles causing* violent and persistent contraction thereby cutting off the blood supply to the parts the arterioles nourish and causing *dry gangrene* (*Lachesis moist gangrene*). This contraction is what causes emptying the gravid uterus. Our fathers in medicine abused this power of the drug, but at present we understand that we should use it for its physiological action only after the uterus is emptied of all its contents. The most frequent use is in putrescent diseases with the external coldness, the threatening collapse and irregular weak pulse.

Brain and Nerves.

Mind: "Delirium; raving; *anxiety with fear of death* (Aconite, Arsenicum) and with difficult respiration; stupor; consciousness till last breath."

There is nothing marked about the mental symptoms of Secale and they are of second rank in the uterine group. We might call the condition *puerperal mania*. With the delirium there is the symptom "feels too hot" and the patient throws off the clothes and orders the windows opened.

Back and Extremities: "Pain in the back amel. stooping, agg. in lumbar region; *extremities pale, cold and wrinkled, as if they had been long in hot water;* trembling, agg. exertion; spasmodic, drawing pains with crawling; weakness agg. upper arms; *coldness and insensibility of fingers and toes.* Fuzzy feeling (Phosphorus); sensation as if asleep with formication."

Ergot has been used for *cramps* of the extremities with the numbness and coldness also cold sweat. For *paralysis* with the same cramping coldness, formication and numbness. The *modality* amel. *from uncovering* is the ranking symptom of the group.

Sexual Organs.

Vagina: "Gangrene of vaginal mucous membrane, with a dark slate color; discharge almost black, fluid and fetid; hemorrhage from the uterus (Ustilago, Carbo veg.); irregular contranctions of the uterus; Ustilago, descended so that it almost protruded from the labia, was hot and painful, or was open; urging to urinate and labor pains, amel. by wet bandages or by pressure upon the abdomen; *expulsive pains;* cessation of lochia, with fever, inflammation of uterus and later an abscess which opened through the vagina."

Many *cases* of *abortion* have been produced in women and cattle who have eaten bread made from spurred ryė or from eating the rye from the shock. One of the best proofs of our law is that many cases of *threatened abortion* from other causes have been arrested by the use of *ergot.*

It has expelled fibroid tumors of the submucous variety by causing contraction of uterus and forcing the tumors through the mucous membrane. The contraction of the blood vessels has also *arrested the growth in the mural fibroids,* and caused degeneration. The continued use of Secale has brought the *subinvoluted uterus* to its *normal size.*

For *puerperal METRITIS* with *putrid discharges* cold, clammy skin, *tympanitis* (Terebinthina, Carbo veg.) suppressed urine (Stramonium) and tendency to collapse. The modality "*intolerance from covering*" is a ranking symptom in this group also.

For *dysmenorrhea* with the *bearing down forcing pains* and the modalities. The internal heat comes in flashes.

Let me caution you about the use of large doses for uterine hemorrhage, also for expelling fibroids. Always watch the kidneys, as albuminuria, hemorrhage and suppression of the urine have been caused by it.

For the physiological action use the ampules.

Mucous Membranes.

Stomach: "*Appetite unnatural;* appetite ravenous; *thirst,* with dryness of the mouth and throat; violent vomiting of food, water, blood; *cramping pain in the epigastrium* which is tender."

The above symptoms are partly of the nerves and partly of

M.M. I have never used it for gastritis or gastralgia but the above symptoms are prominent in other groups.

Rectum, Anus and Stools: "Anus wide open (Apocynum can., Phosphorus); hemorrhage from the bowels; blood does not clot (Phosphorus); diarrhea amel. by hot bath; an exhausting, *thin, olive* green, dark-brown stool; stool involuntary."

For a pernicious *diarrhea* with stools like the above, plus the *unquenchable* thirst; vomiting after drinking (Arsenicum) suppression of urine, *skin shriveled* and *very cold, aversion to heat,* especially being covered. For the *last stage* of *dysentery,* the stage of collapse with the thin stools plus some blood and mucus. *Coldness* and *collapse* are the ranking symptoms.

Lungs: "Expectoration of blood during violent efforts to breathe, respiration difficult as from a weight on chest (Phosphorus), so that he must take deep and forced inspiration; sighs (Arsenicum); anxious respiration."

Secale is useful for *hemorrhage* of the *lungs, dark venous blood* with bad odor (Capsicum, Phosphorus) and for a *cough* with pains all through the chest agg. by pressure on the chest. The cough of spinal anemia.

Face.

The expression of the Secale patient is so marked I would impress it on your mind. Bear in mind what I told you of the general make-up and add the following: "Face *drawn, sunken, hippocratic, pale,* agg. in morning, anxious, collapsed; lips blue sometimes in the collapsed stage; *risus sardonicus.* For its homeopathic use give from the 3rd to 30th.

SABINA.

Make-up: Sycotic, plethoric women with hemorrhagic tendency.

Loc.: Sexual organs; extremities; blood.

Sen.: Pulsative; constrictive; digging; tearing; burning.

Mod.: Agg. stooping; cool open air; motion; *warm air,* room, or bed; touch.

Leaders: Amel. lying flat on back with legs extended; cold applications; pain from sacrum to pubis; metrorrhagia with sexual excitement and *intolerance of music.*

Sexual Organs.

"Burning, sore pains in gland and fig warts agg. touch; os tincæ is open; discharge is red, profuse, paroxysmal; agg. motion; constrictive pain in region of uterus; menses profuse for nine days, passing clots of blood after rising."

Dysmenorrhea with *aching pains extending through from sacrum to pubis,* shooting down the thighs, pains in small of back extending around the pelvis.

Uterine hemorrhage of plethoric women with gouty tendency, with bright, red flow, agg. by every motion accompanied by shooting, cramping pains *from sacrum to pubis* and from small of back to the genitals and down the thighs. Rarely the flow is dark and clotted. Occasionally the flow ceases on patient's walking about (Magnesia mur.).

For an *offensive, acrid leucorrhea* with itching, biting and burning, during pregnancy. Finally for *threatening miscarriage* with the pains from back to pubis. With the hemorrhages, the flow is hot and usually comes in gushes.

Back and Extremities.

"*Drawing pains in the back extending into pubic region;* uneasiness and dragging forward like weak *labor pains;* sprained, tearing, paralytic pains in the joints and muscles of upper extremities; *bruised pain in middle of anterior surface of the thigh;* sticking in heels extending outward, tearing in metacarpal bones; *painful drawing in phalanges,* agg. walking."

Sabina has relieved *chronic arthritis and gout* in fleshy,

plethoric women when the pains are agg. by warmth and amel. in cool, open air. The pains are sharp, sticking, tearing and may appear in any muscle or joint in the body. For *arthritic nodes.* The *ranking symptom* of this section if the *make-up* of the patient, *i. e.,* gouty plethoric. In addition the *patient* is usually *depressed.* Use the lower potencies and repeat frequently.

TRILLIUM.

Make-up: Hemorrhagic diathesis.

Loc.: M.M.; female genital organs; urinary organs.

Sen.: *Sensation as if hips and back were falling to pieces;* sharp; cutting.

Mod.: Agg. sitting erect; motion; after eating.

Amel. bending forward; exercise in open air.

Although most of our authorities give Trillium as a remedy for profuse bleeding, blood either red or dark and clotted, from nose, kidneys, rectum and uterus; I have never verified the statement except for *hemorrhage from the uterus,* and that limited to hemorrhage caused by *fibroid tumors.* In several *inoperable cases* of *fibroids* the use of the tincture of Trillium or the 1st of the Trillin has checked the hemorrhage, reduced the size of the tumor and made the patient comfortable. In one case in which the tumor had been the cause of premature birth its use carried the patient to full time.

ARSENICUM ALBUM.

Make-up: The nervous, restless, debilitated.

Loc.: All tissues and organs of the body; has a special "*Elective Affinity*" for the mucous *membrane* and *skin.* Arsenicum produces all conditions from a simple irritation to the most profound tissue change, like fatty degeneration, epithelioma.

Sen.: One of our *chief burners,* sharp, splinter-like, cramping, stitching, profound *weakness,* extreme *restlessness,* fear, throbbing, anguish, etc.

Mod.: Agg.: 12 to 3 A.M., cold, damp, at night lying on the affected side.

Amel.: Heat, warmth, hot drinks, hot food.

Brain and Nervous System.

Mind: Everything from a slight algia to complete paralysis. Our mental symptoms are: "Delirium worse at night; with carphologia; restlessness; anguish; with tossing about the bed; despair; driving him from place to place for relief; despairs; weeps."

Fear: Sees ghosts day and night, *dread* of death and yet a disposition to suicide.

Our nervous symptoms are: "*Burning, tearing, lancinating, shooting* (like a small red-hot wire along the course of the nerves) pain about the face, the eye, the teeth, the tongue, the stomach, the intestines, etc." These pains are relieved by heat, especially radiated heat, are worse after midnight and from cold.

Membranes.

Eye: "Intense *burning, dryness* and pain, with *suffusion* of eyes. The membrane is minutely injected, much swelling externally, with hot excoriating tears."

Nose: "Much swollen, very sore, secreting a profuse, watery acrid mucus or mucus and blood."

With this discharge there is violent sneezing. Useful for *hay fever*. Acute and chronic rhinitis. The fluent coryza may alternate with a dry.

Mouth: The membrane of the tongue may be white, red, blue, brown or even black according to the different conditions from which the patient suffers. It is always dry. A red streak down the center with a silver color on either side is the most common Arsenicum tongue. Not only on the tongue but in the mouth, in general, we have blisters, *vesicles, aphthæ*, and *ulcers;* the latter frequently cancerous.

Throat: "Dryness, *burning*, difficult deglutition, constriction, soreness, swelling, inflammation, ulceration, diphtheritic exudate."

The latter is dark and thin; if detached bleeding often follows. It is in the latter stage of severe cases of diphtheria where you have profound prostration, irritable stomach and acute nephritis with albuminuria that you find Arsenicum indicated.

Stomach: "Irritation; inflammation; ulceration; intense thirst for cold water but the water does not refresh the patient; on the other hand it irritates and causes "distress," "nausea" and "vomiting."

For this reason the patient drinks only a little at a time. Violent nausea, retching and vomiting, vomiting of the contents of stomach first, then of mucus, blood, mucus and blood mixed, coffee grounds. The vomiting brings no relief. Fear of death is the mental symptom which usually accompanies the vomiting. Burning, soreness, constrictive, cramping are the leading sensations.

Intestines: Again, "irritation; inflammation; ulceration; functional and structural changes." "*Burning;* cutting; stitching; tearing pains," also "distention and soreness." With these you have the "*anguish,*" "*anxiety,*" and "*fear of death,*" characteristic of the drug.

Rectum and Anus: "*Burning* after stool; tenesmus; painful spasmodic protrusion of rectum; also hemorrhoids with the intense burning, relieved by heat."

Bladder and Urethra: Burning, urging, desire which cannot be satisfied.

Uterus and Vagina: "Leucorrhea; menorhagia and metrorrhagia; granulations and ulcerations, aphthæ. The discharges are usually thin, acrid and offensive."

Respiratory Organs: "*Asthma at night making him spring out of bed,*" "*short difficult, anxious, distressed, painful* *breathing*," "dryness of the air passages, spasmodic cough, threatening suffocation, spitting of blood."

The modalities are agg. after midnight and from cold air with exception, viz., fresh cool air relieves the asthmatic attacks.

Skin.

"White and pasty looking; white, later turning yellow; scaly; producing irritating eruption all over the body; blue spots on abdomen and genitals, sometimes on the neck and back; dark and livid spots on hands and forearms; dry, rough, scaly, sore, red, moist; painful petechiæ which burn after scratching; burning, painful eruption around the mouth; miliary eruption; swelling about the orbit, especially beneath the eyes; edema about face and neck; desquamation from hand to foot; *pimples* burning, itching worse by scratching; vesicles; ulcers."

We find our *white, pasty, waxy* skin in the *chronic* forms of *nephritis;* the *red, puffed, swollen* in the *acute*. In simple dermatitis and *psoriasis* we have the fine, *dry, scaly* skin with the intense *itching* which changes to burning after scratching. With the Arsenicum *herpes* we have the *blue vesicles* which dry into *brown* and even *black scales* or *scabs*. With *erysipelas* and *carbuncles* of the drug the *discharges* are *serum* and *blood* which also dry into *black crusts*. I have more confidence in the use of Arsenicum paste and the administration of Arsenicum internally, for epithelioma, than any other method.

Urinary Organs

Urethra: "*Burning* in the urethra on voiding; *frequent desire* which he cannot satisfy; *involuntary* micturition; urine *scanty;* urine retained; urine scanty, burning, passed with difficulty; urine *bloody;* urine copious; glycosuria and hematuria."

In *acute nephritis* we have the following symptoms: "convulsions, intense *thirst* followed by *vomiting*, and *flushed* face with the puffiness beneath the eyes," and in most cases the characteristic *diarrhea.*

Kidneys: In *chronic* nephritis we find the "sallow, *waxy, cachectic* face" instead of the flushed *blood* casts and *pus* in the scanty urine.

Acute nephritis following the exanthemata is the form I find most frequently calling for *Arsenicum.* I have found and cured with it a few cases of "*glycosuria*" and *diabetes* when we had high specific gravity, low per cent. of sugar, great dryness of the mouth, thirst with the irritable stomach, emaciation, mental depression and rapid prostration. Fatty degeneration of the kidneys is the final result of Arsenicum.

Thermic Centers.

"*Chilliness* with shuddering, stretching, and drawing of the limbs;" "shivering when in open air after drinking."

"*Coldness* with chattering of teeth; coldness of body and dryness of skin alternating with cold sweat;" internal coldness in the P.M. with external heat and flushed face; "coldness of legs with diarrhea."

Heat with thirst; internal heat with inclination to uncover, with thirst and vomiting; feeling as if blood in the arteries were boiling hot; "sensation as if blood coursed through the veins too rapidly and were too hot."

Sweat in bed causing faintness; sweat, copious, offensive, over whole body; cold, clammy sweat on forehead, on face also over whole body. In our intermittent fevers the different stages of the paroxysms are all mixed up, *i. e.*, any one of the three may be missing, the chill and fever may be at the same time or the fever may come with the sweat. But with these fevers you always get the restlessness, the thirst, the irritable stomach and bowels and the great prostration. The sensation of the blood burning as it courses through the blood vessels has often been verified.

Blood.

"Sensation as if the *blood* coursed through the veins too rapidly or were too *hot;* feeling as if blood of arteries were *boiling* hot".

Arsenicum produces *changes* in the blood *simulating* those produced by *typhoid fever,* erysipelas, *carbuncles, intermittent fevers, yellow fever,* remittent, *diphtheria* and general *Sepsis.* The Arsenicum alb., also its compound of Chininum and Iodium, are among the five remedies most frequently called for in general sepsis.

ARSENICUM IODATUM.

Make-up: *Catarrhal;* debilitated.

Loc.: *Mucous membrane;* skin; lungs; blood.

Sen.: *Weakness,* sharp pain, itching, *thirst for cold water; burning.*

Mod.: *Agg. from cold wind;* dry weather; exertion.
Amel. from warmth.

Leaders: *Profuse,* acrid, burning corrosive *discharges with* profound *prostrations.*

Mucous Membrane.

Nose: "*Excoriating gluey discharges,* like yellow honey; chronic nasal discharge."

It has been most useful for nasal discharge of the above character in *patients of* a *tubercular diathesis.* Also for corysas and *hay fever.* With these conditions the yellow, thick discharge alternates with or follows a thin watery discharge. Both are always acrid and corroding.

Eyes: "Weak, burning, smarting; secretions greatly increased."

It has cured *parenchymatous keratitis,* also *scrofulous* ophthalmia with the acrid secretions and tendency to *ulceration* of the lower lids.

Ears: "Very sharp pains in ears when riding in a cold wind."

This is about all we have from the provers but clinically we have found it useful for the following according to Allen: "*Otitis,* with *fetid, corrosive discharge;* catarrhal inflammation of the throat, nose and middle ear; swelling of the tissues within the nose; *hypertrophied* condition of the opening of the Eustachian tube and increasing deafness; chronic irritability of the middle ear following scarlet fever; thickening of the tympanum."

I have found it the only remedy when the eye, ear, nose and throat symptoms combined produce the condition known as *influenza, grippe, flu* and sometimes "*epizootic.*" There is no condition for which hydrogen peroxide, one part to four of water, used as a douche, gargle or spray, will assist the action of the indicated remedy as in the above. Use the 3x two grains every three hours; the hydrogen every six hours before taking the medicine or food.

Genital Organs: All we have from the provers are "lumps in mamma, sensitive to touch and painful; nipple retracted." But many times have I used it successfully for the above condition when there was in addition a *bloody, yellow leucorrhea.* Also for *indurated labia* with an excoriating discharge. In one case a woman with a t. b. c. diathesis had abscess of the labia. The abscess had been drained three times and had again returned. I lanced it again and gave Arsenicum iod. 6x two grains night and morning. The woman claims it also cured her of an acrid leucorrhea and an annual attack of hay fever.

Stools: "Diarrhea five to ten stools each day, not at night, but the urging began on moving about in the morning; stool mushy, almost black."

Respiratory Organs: "*Frequent cough* with *muco-purulent* and occasionally stringy expectoration; *greenish-yellow, pus-like* expectoration; *expectoration* heavy at night and morning: asthmatic sensations; must sit up to breathe."

"Arsenicum iod. has demonstrated its usefulness in many cases of pulmonary disease, both subacute and chronic, and various forms of phthisis pulmonaris have been cured. It seems probable that in the Iodide of Arsenic we have found a remedy most closely allied to manifestations of *tuberculosis.*"

Allen wrote the above in 1889. Experience has demonstrated the accuracy of the statement not only for the conditions he mentioned but also for acute and chronic bronchitis, acute catarrhal pneumonia with the "caseous degeneration and fibrosis."

In addition to the symptoms enumerated under the heading of respiratory organs the patient suffers from rapid and profound prostration; night sweats; *emaciation;* weak irritable pulse; the exhausting diarrhea and very frequently the nose and throat symptoms of the drug. It has *relieved* the *"shortness of breath"* (genuine *air hunger*) of patients whose lung conditions had *passed* beyond the curative stage.

Skin.

"Dryness; itching; stinging."

Very little, you note, from the provers but the clinical results give it a very wide field in this location. I have cured a few cases of *psoriasis* with it, depending upon the t. b. c. diathesis and the general symptoms. However, I have found it most useful for cases called "moist desquamative eczema." Let me cite an illustrative case: Mr. C., age 57, came to the hospital with body covered with *thick scales* and a great deal of *moisture* (an ordinary tea cupful of scales was found in the sheets the first night); intense *itching; burning* after scratching; stools dark, watery and frequent; great thirst; marked restlessness; irritable stomach; weak and prostrated. The latter condition he attributed to loss of sleep. Not only was the Wassermann positive but also the test for t. b. c. Aided by a fruit and cereal diet and arsenated baths, Arsenicum iod. 3x, 6x and 30x cured him in four months. The baths were

Iodide of Arsenic, 1 to 5000, at first twice daily, then once daily and finally once a week.

Blood.

Besides the scrofulous and t. b. c. diathesis already mentioned, Arsenicum iod. has been used for general sepsis, the symptoms being those of Arsenicum alb. plus the catarrhal symptoms. Allen says: "*Blood poisoning with debilitating night sweats* but for that condition you will find China ars. better.

CHININUM ARSENICOSUM.

Make-up: The weak; debilitated; septic.

Loc.: *Blood;* skin; alimentary canal.

Sen.: *Weakness;* soreness; *urging;* nausea; vomiting; chilly."

Mod.: Agg. stimulants and open air.

Blood.

Sepsis: "*PROFUSE SWEAT;* great prostration; *rapid,* weak *pulse;* watery, *fetid,* pappy *stools.*"

Illustrative case: Mrs. B., aged 28, whose mother and one aunt had died of t. b. c., gave birth to a child. On the third day a *severe chill* was followed by a *rapid rise in temperature,* restlessness and cessation of the lochia. About 24 hours afterwards the temperature fell to 97 and was followed by a very *profuse sweat.* There were the *high and low temperature,* alternating for two days more, while the sweat continued all the time and was so profuse as to necessitate changing her clothing every few hours. The patient had become very weak and delirious. At this stage Chin. ars., 3x, three grains every two hours, was given. The disease was checked after about 24 hours and the patient made a full, though slow recovery. I have frequently observed good results in such cases, since that time, which was in the fall of 1899. In this case the woman was infected during delivery. It has acted just as favorably in *malignant diphtheria, malaria fever, scarlet fever* and in a few cases of influenza. The *profuse sweat* is the *characteristic* symptom of the *group*. Use it low and repeat often.

BAPTISIA.

Make-up: Weak; depressed; low vitality.

Loc.: *Blood.*

Sen.: *Confusion; bruised;* aching; rumbling; distention.

Mod.: *Agg. hot weather;* on waking; walking.

Leaders: *Very foul discharge;* confusion; rapid prostration; *dusky, besotted countenance.*

Blood.

Typhoid: "Chilliness with *bruised* pains and *soreness* over entire body; heat of *face* with *dark* redness; tongue coated white at first, then yellow, then brown with red edges; tongue dry on waking and feeling burnt; excited feeling; *mind cannot be confined,* a wild, wondering feeling; indisposition and inability to think; sore feeling in brain, worse from stooping; appetite lost; *distention* and *rumbling* in *abdomen;* pain in region of the gall bladder; diarrhea in the morning; *papescent* painless *stools.*"

When Baptisia was first introduced into medicine it was proclaimed a specific for typhoid fever and was tried by all schools of medicine. It was soon rejected by the old school; but verification of so many of the above symptoms gave it a place in our school for a certain form of typhoid fever, also for many *typhoid conditions.*

The *mental confusion;* the inability to think; the low delirium during which the patient is *trying to get himself* or his tools *together;* the *horrible odor* of the *discharges* and *rapid prostration* are the symptoms which have been verified again and again.

Diphtheria: The *mental confusion,* delirium, even unconsciousness; *inability to swallow* solids; the besotted face with the *horrible odor* from the mouth have led to its successful use in this dreaded disease.

You should take special pains to *guard* your Baptisia *patients against bed sores,* as I know of no remedy except Arnica which has such a tendency to develop them. .Use the tincture and 3x internally and a solution of 20 minims to the ounce locally for the bed sores and for a mouth wash. I have found that beef, mutton or chicken broth agrees better than milk for the diet of the Baptisia patients.

GELSEMIUM.

Make-up: Nervous, weak, debilitated.

Loc.: *Nerves;* muscles; blood; membranes and sexual organs.

Sen.: Weakness; *trembling;* heaviness; vertigo; *fullness.*

Mod.: Agg. motion for most symptoms; damp weather; summer heat; 4 to 8 P.M.

Amel. stimulants; cool, open air; heat for the headache; voiding large amounts of clear, watery urine.

Characteristics: Hot; flushed; besotted appearance of the face; chilliness; blunted sensibility; partial paralysis.

Nerves.

Paralysis: "Drooping of the eyelids; eyelids closed in spite of him on looking steadily at object; apparent inability to move the eyelids, to open them or to keep them open. Numbness and thickness of the tongue so that he could not articulate. Spasmodic, cramp-like pains in the gullet; difficult swallowing: complete inability to swallow due to paralysis of the muscles of the throat. Partial *paralysis* of the *sphincter ani;* prolapsus ani; constant dribbling of the urine. Difficult respiration; struggling for breath: stertorous, irregular, imperfect breathing. Feeling as if the heart would stop beating if she did not move about; palpitation and irregular beating of the heart. *Trembling* of the *extremities; weakness* of hands and feet with indisposition to move; gradual *loss* of *control* of the *extremities;* staggering; fatigue after slight exertion."

The stage of irritation of Gelsemium is not marked. We have a little neuralgia and some headache which may be called nervous. On the other hand the paralysis of the drug is frequent. You will find it useful for patients suffering from vertigo due to paralysis of the recti muscles, causing first diplopia and then vertigo; for ptosis; for asthenopia; for strabismus; for aphomia due to emotions or diphtheria; for paralysis of the *tongue, throat* and organs of respiration due to emotion or diphtheria. For paralysis of any organ or tissue, caused by diphtheria, Gelsemium shares the honors with Lachesis. The cause of the paralysis of the bladder and rectum I have found to be fear, joy and excitement more often than diphtheria.

Membranes.

Eyes: "Eyes suffused, bloodshot; vision dim with vertigo; vision smoky with pain above the eye; blindness."

Gelsemium is probably the most frequently called for of our remedies for serous inflammation within the eyeball. With it T. F. Allen saved what eyesight there was left in a man's eye. The sight of one eye and part of the other had been destroyed by serous inflammation of the retina which had become detached. It is also useful for iritis with the serous exudate.

Nose: "Watery discharge from the nose; sneezing with tingling and full sensation in nose."

Although we have but a few symptoms from the provers under nose, these few are found so frequently in practice that they become first rank symptoms. With the head, face and nose symptoms we get what we call the hay fever group.

With the great prostration, the chill up and down the back,

the aching in every muscle, etc., we have the grippe or "flu" symptoms. Also for acute nasal catarrh with sore throat, pain extending into the ear and some deafness with the weakness and trembling it is often called for and responds at once. The action of Gelsemium upon the membranes of the intestinal canal is due in great part to impression upon the nervous system. The result is *emotional diarrhea.* An illustration: An officer was leading his men in a charge upon the enemy. A bullet struck him in the chest. His men led his horse to the rear, supporting the man on the way. All the time the officer could feel the *blood* running down his legs into his boots. But when he was undressed it was found that his order book had stopped the bullet and the boots were full of feces, not blood.

Blood and Thermic Centers.

We have in the blood changes which correspond to those which take place in the eruptive fevers: *yellow, typhoid, remittent fever* and *influenza.*

The most striking case of remittent fever which Gelsemium cured presented the following symptoms: Temperature for three days was between 106 and 106.5 from 4 to 6 P.M.; between 100 and 100.6 from 6 to 8 A.M.; severe, shaking chill from 1 to 3 P.M.; the patient was stupid from 3 to 5 P.M., and unconscious from 5 to 8 P.M.; the face was almost purple; the eyes suffused; the skin yellow; the stool thin yellow and involuntary; thirst just before the chill for only three days. Gelsemium 3x was given. The man made a good recovery and returned to Alabama. Several cases of measles with marked prostration; a livid eruption; profuse, watery discharge from nose and eyes; mental stupor and diarrhea, were helped by Gelsemium. In typhoid the early and great prostration; the mental confusion, soft feeble pulse; trembling and great weakness with lack of thirst call for Gelsemium. In our epidemic of "Spanish influenza" of 1918 and 1919 Gelsemium lessened the severity of the symptoms and hastened convalescence.

The chills up and down the back, the aching of all the muscles; the great prostration, the loose stools, the suffused face were the prominent symptoms. Fear of the disease and its results was a symptom of high rank in this Gelsemium group.

Muscles.

"Weakness and trembling through whole system; relaxed muscles and motor paralysis; easily fatigued, especially the lower limbs; drooping of lids; paralysis of muscles of the eyes, throat, and sphincters; fatigue after slight exertion; pains, sharp, drawing, cramping, aching, sore in any and all muscles."

The above symptoms are usually combined with the nervous symptoms in the "Flu" group.

Sexual Organs.

"Sharp, labor-like pains in uterine region, extending to back and hips; emission at night without erection, irritation of right testicle in P.M. and evening; dragging pain, extending into groin and hypogastrium, genitals cold and relaxed; sexual powers exhausted; inefficient labor pains or none at all; sensation as if the uterus were squeezed by a band; almost continuous flow of blood from the uterus from 4 to 6 P.M."

Gelsemium has relieved the following conditions: Suppressed menses with congestion of the brain and the sensation of fulness or expansion of the head so characteristic of the drug, and pain extending from the uterus upward and downward. During labor when the pains are too weak or have ceased, or do not force down but fly upward. *Congestive dysmenorrhea* with vertigo, headache, faintness and when the pains shoot up the back and down into the legs. This condition is usually accompanied by ovaritis. Threatening *puerperal convulsions* with the flushed face, twitching of muscles, albuminuria and stupor.

Gelsemium is one of the greatest of our polychrests. There

is not another remedy with so few symptoms which covers so large a field. It might well be called an every day remedy. This is easily explained by the cause of the symptoms which it simulates. They are every day incidents like: *fright; anger; self-abuse; alcoholic excesses;* bad news; exposure to the sun; changes of weather. And in addition such communicable diseases as tpyhoid; remittent; intermittent; and the eruptive fevers, diphtheria, etc. It has responded successfully in the tincture, the 3rd, 30th, 200th, and 1000th.

CHINA OFFICINALIS.

Make-up: Anemic; hemorrhagic, debilitated.

Loc.: *Blood;* circulation; liver; spleen, nerves; M.M.

Sen.: *Weakness;* vertigo; suffocative; *roaring.*

Mod.: Agg. loss of fluids; touch; drafts; *periodicity.*
Amel. hard pressure.

Leaders: Profuse, exhausting discharge, intermittency; exhausting sweat at night. The action of China on the blood is the foundation of most of the conditions for which we use the remedy. This result may be summed up in a few words, viz., *anemia* and *devitalization* of blood and tissue. It *poisons* the *protoplasm,* retards the elimination of nitrogenous *wastes* and *retains* the *effete products* (Mercurius) in the system. By this action it *causes congestion* of the *brain,* irritates the serous membranes and skin, and from lack of proper nourishment produces all sorts of *disturbances* in the *digestive* tract.

Blood.

The most pronounced effect is a condition simulating that of *malarial poisoning* but it is seldom an antidote for it. Another condition it simulates is that of *leucocythemia* and finally as stated above *anemia* with its long train of ills, a few of which we will study by groups.

Brain and Nerves.

Mind: "Sudden screaming and tossing about during a cheerful mood; excitability with intolerance of noise; solicitude about trifles: discouraged; discontented; disinclined to mental labor. Slow flow of ideas."

For a confused *delirium,* rarely with the *intermittent fevers.* more frequently *from* loss of fluids. For *melancholia* of pregnant women or chronic malaria, with which we may have an extreme apathy alternating with marked irritation.

Head: "*Aching* as if the skull would burst (Bryonia, Ferrum), brain *beats* in *waves* against the skull, as if brain were pressing together from both sides and out at forehead, agg. walking in the open air; confusion with tensive pain in forehead and orbits; in the morning as after intoxication, Nux; *vertigo* at night on waking so that he is afraid to sit up; agg. motion; amel. lying down; scalp extremely sensitive to touch."

The *headache* of China is a violent one. You will find it hard to differentiate it from Ferrum, Belladonna or even Bryonia unless you take the make-up of the patient and the cause into account. There is intense, throbbing (Belladonna) pain; the scalp is so sensitive that the patient cannot have her hair combed. The pains are worse in the temples. The agg. are by noise, odors, bright light, and the touch; amel. *binding the head tight* (Silica, Gelsemium).

Ears: "*Deafness as* if something were before the ear internally; *ringing,* with pain in the temples; *roaring;* ticking as from a distant clock."

China produces all sorts of effects upon the auditory nerve, *e. g.,* from a *slight irritation to atrophy,* with total deafness. It stands in the same relation to this nerve that Strychnine does to the optic.

Eyes: "*Pain* on motion, with sensation of mechanical hindrance; *biting* as from salt; pressure; weakness."

Hemeralopia; *ciliary* and *supraorbital neuralgia* (Cedron, Spigelia), agg. slightest touch. These neuralgias are often associated with extreme soreness of the spine which comes up to the occiput and even into the eyes.

Nose: "Pain in root; sneezing; *bleeding.*"

The only symptom in this section is the acuteness of smell with the anemic headache.

Respiratory Organs: "Whistling and wheezing in trachea when breathing; *cough caused by laughing* (Phosphorus, Stannum); *irritation as from sulphur fumes* but nothing loosened; *suffocation* as if larynx were full of mucus, agg. towards evening and at night."

The only one of the above symptoms I have verified is found *in idiopathic asthma.*

Back and Spine: "*Sticking tensive* pain in *sacrum as from a heavy load* or long stooping; in small of back as from cramp or as if bruised and crushed, *with sudden crying out on motion.*"

Very often useful in *spinal irritation* of anemic persons. The spine is very sensitive to touch and the symptoms shoot into the head (Actea, Nux, Lycopodium, Gelsemium). *Tabes* has been amel. by China where in addition to the above you had: "*Sensation as if garters were too tight and leg would go to sleep and be numb.*" Also as if cob-webs or cords were tied about the legs.

Thermic Centers.

"*Intermittent chill* all day agg. forehead, where there is cold sweat, with thirst after the first chill; *cold hands and feet; general coldness with sticking in skin* (Mercurius), *agg.* neck with thirst for cold water, *from 5 to 7 P.M.*, also agg. walking; *internal* and *external heat* with thirst for cold water; *SWEAT* in sleep *general, as soon as he is covered.*"

Without doubt our greatest remedy for intermittent fever, *i. e.*, for the pure marsh malarial variety *not dependent* upon some diathesis, unless you call anemia a diathesis. *The paroxysms are fully developed, i. e., A CHILL, A FEVER, A SWEAT.* There is a distinct interval between each stage.

Note also that ***preceding*** the ***chill*** there is a ***violent*** temporal ***headache, marked thirst. During*** the ***heat*** there is also marked ***thirst*** and usually great hunger; there is also thirst with sweat which is profuse and very debilitating. Between the paroxysms and after the attacks there is soreness of the liver and spleen, general weakness, disturbances of the stomach, etc.

Mucous Membranes.

Stomach: "***Appetite*** variable, ***increased for*** various ***things*** but *does* not ***know what; indifference*** to eating and drinking, only while eating appetite and natural taste for food returns; *empty eructations; soreness* in pit of stomach."

Dyspepsia is the most frequent condition produced by China. The *cause* as stated above is ***vitiated gastric juice.*** The digestion is very slow. The patient feels distended and drowsy after eating (Lycopodium), ***craves sour, pungent*** spicy *things,* also stimulants. With the *acid* dyspepsia we have heartburn, even from milk, satiety with no relief from belching gas. Sometimes this distention from gas causes ***distention*** of ***stomach, palpitation*** and ***dyspnea.*** You will also note in this group ***weakness,*** causing inability to work. China is occasionally useful for ***hemorrhages*** of the stomach, but more frequently for the *effects* of ***hemorrhages.*** It is ***after hemorrhages*** and ***intermittent fever*** that we have the ***tenderness*** and ***soreness*** of ***stomach, liver*** and ***spleen.***

Abdomen: "*Distention* after eating (Lycopodium), with griping and here and there sharp pain. *Fermentation from fruit* (Arsenicum, Bryonia, Pulsatilla); rumbling between 6 and 10 P.M., with emission of offensive flatus; swelling of liver (Chelidonium, Mercurius, Lycopodium); intermittent pressure in region of liver while standing, amel. bending forward with pain on touch as from suppuration: fullness after eating."

Useful for *gastro-duodenal catarrh* (Hydrastis, Kali bich., Pulsatilla) with canine hunger yet loathing of food (Ignatia);

yellow scaled tongue, often profuse vitiated saliva, oppressive headache agg. night; ***enlarged spleen*** after intermittents (Ceanothus, Cedron), when you have sharp sticking pains. Also the painless stools. Finally for gall stone colic? and the ***jaundice of babes*** (Podophyllum), when the abdomen is much distended, the spleen and liver enlarged.

Stool: "*Diarrhea after eating;* of *undigested* food in feces (Ferrum), stools white with dark urine; frequent, ineffectual urging with biting, burning pains in rectum; painless stools."

The *diarrhoea* of China is usually painless. With it bloated abdomen, *great fermentation in bowels;* general desire for acid spiced things. The stools are *cadaverous,* at times involuntary, *painless,* contains undigested food. This diarrhoea is caused by too much fruit (Arsenicum), too great loss of fluids and following the intermittent fever of the drug.

Female Generative Organs: "*During* the *catamenia, starting* with *cramp* in the *chest* and *abdomen,* or *congestion in head,* with pulsations in the carotids, face puffed, eyes prominent and watery, *convulsive movements* of the eyelids and *loss of consciousness; metrorrhagia,* with discharge of black blood, with fainting and convulsion; *leuchorrhoea* even before the menses with cramp-like contractions of the uterus and painful bearing down towards the groins and the anus; *watery* and *bloody flux* from the *vagina* with clots of blood or fetid pus."

Many times have I had the *best* of *results from China* in uterine hemorrhages due to atony of the uterus. There were large quantities of blood, *fainting spells,* cold, clammy skin, convulsive jerks and frequently unconsciousness. I have found this condition just after labor, sometimes during the menses. If the flow is very severe I give five drops of the tincture in water every fifteen or twenty minutes till the flow lessens and then lengthen the interval. China will not only control the hemorrhage in such cases, but will prevent the violent headache which follows such a condition.

For leucorrhoea which comes at the times of the menses, a

bloody, fetid, purulent, profuse discharge which produces marked prostration. Both the *leucorrhoea* and the *profuse menses* are frequently the *result* of *prolonged lactation.* Another cause is *sexual excesses.*

Respiratory Organs: "Suffocative attacks as if the larynx were full of mucous, agg. towards evening and at night on waking; sensation of soreness in larynx and trachea; expectoration of purulent matter on coughing; expectoration of blood."

I have used it with success for *bronchorrhoea* with *loud rales* in chest (Tartar emet., Ammonium carb.), great prostration, muco-purulent expectoration and *profuse night sweat.* For *hemoptysis,* also *phthisis* of the lung when you had marked general *weakness,* night sweat and the stomach irregularity and profuse, painless, undigested stools. Use it from the tincture to 200th, according to the conditions.

CHININUM SULPHURICUM.

This is the commercial quinine of the market, the active principle of China. Many consider the action of the two identical, saying that they consider the quinine more reliable and scientific for accurate prescribing. There is, however, some marked differences between the two both in degree of action and in variety of symptoms. The melancholia is intensified in the Chininum sulph., and there is added the symptom "feeling of impending evil." With the vertigo we find "Whirling in heal like a mill-wheel. There are no cases of China having produced atrophy of the auditory nerve and deafness but there are many Chininum sulph. China has never helped pneumonia but Chininum sulph. has. In the intermittents there is more regularity of the paroxysms and its prophylactic powers are greater than those of China. I have seen marked delirium followed by complete unconsciousness from 25 grains of Chininum sulph. The patient "took it to break up a cold."

ECHINACEA PURPUREA.

Make-up: Tendency to suppuration.
Loc.: Blood.
Sen.: Biting; tingling; *tired;* confused.
Mod.: Agg. evening; stooping.
Amel. rest in bed; pressure; bending double.
Leaders: *Tired,* drowsy, listless feeling, agg. evening.

Blood.

Echinacea presents changes in the blood simulating typhoid, pyemia, diphtheria, scarlatina, septicemia, also the effects of vaccination (Thuja). The following is the group: "*I feel so tired, so tired;* temperature from 97 to 105, up and down; *flushed face* (Baptisia), marked chilliness; offensive discharges (Arnica, Baptisia), mental confusion."

I have used it for *FURUNCLES* with a dry skin. The boils were small ("cat-boils"), *very sensitive* and seemed to come *in crops,* more about the neck and shoulders. For *carbuncles* with profuse sanguino-purulent discharge, marked prostration (the *tired* feeling), some rise in temperature and large sloughing. They also come in crops and mostly about the neck, sometimes on perineum. I usually give such patients five drops of the 1st every three hours and apply, hot, a solution of 1 part of the tincture to 9 of water; change the application often.

In a similar manner, treat bruised, lacerated wounds. In a case of a strumous, young bricklayer whose hand and fingers were so injured that he was advised to have the fingers amputated because of symptoms of sepsis (*i. e.*, enlargement of the glands under the arms and temperature), Echinacea 1st internally and tincture locally checked the sepsis and saved the fingers. In this case the skin and muscles were brought as nearly as possible to normal position and the Echinacea applied and changed every hour for 48 hours.

I never have used it with success but once for suppurative appendicitis, *i. e.*, after pus had formed and evacuated into the intestines. Mercurius sol. and Hepar had both failed to heal but Echinacea 1st, five drops every night and morning for three weeks, cured. It has been used with success in oft recurring attacks of chronic inflammation about the cecum and in a few cases of typhoid when the *tired feeling* was the ranking symptom.

LACHESIS.

Make-up: Anemic, nervous, sensitive.

Loc.: Blood, brain and nerves.

Sen.: Tearing; constriction; weakness; restlessness; soreness; rawness; beating; throbbing; sensitiveness.

Mod.: Agg. after sleeping; morning; heat of sun; summer heat; hot drink and hot room; empty deglutition; alcohol; at climacteric; retarded discharges.

Amel. open air.

Leaders: Nervous excitability; aimless raving; great loquacity; hemorrhages; blue, mottled, livid skin; suffocation on falling asleep; extreme sensitiveness; can't bear anything about throat; excessive fetor.

Blood.

Typhoid Fever: "Tearing, sticking headache extending into the eyes, always worse in the morning; thick, dark blood from the nose; distention of the abdomen with extreme sensitiveness to all pressure; low muttering delirium; putrid, offensive, yellow, watery stools which are often involuntary; tongue red, dry and tremulous."

Lachesis is not frequently called for in typhoid but for those rapid, prostrating cases with the extreme sensitiveness of the abdomen and the loquacity it will save the patient when no other remedy will. In the few patients I have had calling for Lachesis swollen glands was a complication in all of them. I generally use the 30x for typhoid.

Infected Wounds: "Sore spots become fungoid, dark red to brownish; blueness; swelling; old wounds reopen; great sensitiveness of the affected part; dry red tongue; tendency to gangrene."

Carbuncles: "Excruciatingly sore; bluish-black areola; discharge of thick black blood which soon becomes sanguino-purulent." The ranking symptom of this group is *the tendency of the areola tissue to become bluish black.*

Scarlet Fever: "Red spots on various parts of body; inflamed spots with sticking and burning; vesicles which suppurate and break; ulceration of the throat with soreness and difficult swallowing more so for liquids than solids; extreme sensitiveness of the left side of neck to external impression; urine dark red, at times black, *i. e.*, containing particles like charred straw; trickling of thick, dark blood from the nostrils; face swollen and livid; pulse rapid and small; stools loose, putrid and in severe cases involuntary."

Erysipelas: "Erysipelatous eruption beneath left eye, itching at night, in the morning the skin begins to redden and swell, worse after the midday nap, next morning very thick and red with itching; sore spots become fungoid, dark red to brownish."

With the erysipelas of the face, especially if it goes into the scalp, you have the muttering delirium with great loquacity. The face is greatly swollen and of a purplish color.

Purpura Hemorrhagica: With this condition you will find the "*dark red* almost *purple spots* which have a tendency to ulcerate or become gangrenous." The characteristics of the condition however are the *marked soreness* and *sensitiveness.* The entire body is badly swollen.

Indolent Ulcers: Lachesis is frequently indicated for indolent ulcers, especially varicose ulcers, which are very sensitive, of bluish purple color and exude a thick, dark blood which is offensive.

Smallpox: I used it with much benefit in one case of smallpox during the suppurative stage, when there was a great deal of pus and some blood. The spots became blue at first and then black but did not form scales.

Congenital Cyanosis: I have used it a few times for the "*blue baby*" when the color became *worse after sleep.* This modality was so marked in one case that the mother would wake the child. The baby cried a good deal when dandled.

Brain and Nervous System.

Mind: "*Lively* and *wide awake* for a long time in the *evening; loquacity* worse in evening; excitement with physical exhaustion; sadness; confusion; delirium."

Lachesis has a great deal of delirium with its fevers. Also useful for delirium tremens. The patient is continually talking. It has also been used with success in cases of religious melancholia when the patient was continually bemoaning the fact that he was lost.

Neuralgia: You find the peculiar pains of the drug with the extreme sensitiveness to all impressions in all parts of the body, *e. g., neuralgic headaches* which extend to the nose, face, eyes and even shoulders, always worse after sleep; *odontalgia* with swollen, dark, purplish, bleeding gums; *orbital* neuralgia when the *eye* feels as if it had been *squeezed.* The *sharp pains of throat extend* into the *ear.* The *cardalgias have great soreness* of the pit of stomach *to touch* and the intolerance of clothing which is such a marked symptom of the drug.

Heart: In nervous affections of the heart you find severe pains, palpitation, intolerance of pressure about the heart; very irregular action and a feeling as if the heart turned over (Angina pect.).

Back and Extremities: "Sticking, drawing pains in the spine extending into hips and legs, especially the ischia; sticking, tearing in arms and legs."

The most frequent use has been for neuralgia of the coccyx worse from getting up, so must sit still, and for sciatica.

Paralysis: The best remedy in our materia medica for paralysis following diphtheria, especially paralysis of the vocal cords and heart. In most cases there is an increase of sensibility with a loss of motion. I do not remember ever having a case of post-diphtheritic paralysis when Lachesis had been indicated and used during the attack of the disease. So I consider it a prophylactic in many cases.

Reflexes: "Hot flushes; hot vertex; pain in ovaries with marked intolerance to weight of clothes."

With Sepia and Sanguinaria, Lachesis forms a trio which will relieve most of the annoying symptoms of the climacteric.

CONIUM MACULATUM.

Make-up: Lively; quick, sanguine disposition.

Loc.: Brain and *nerves;* glands; sexual organs.

Sen.: *DIZZY;* weak, listless, erratic.

Mod.: Agg.: *Alcohol;* seeing moving objects; lying down, *excesses,* continence.

Leaders: *Reeling vertigo;* hardening, swelling and soreness of the glands; *tremulous weakness.*

Brain and Nerves.

Mind: "Inability to sustain mental effort (Phosphoric ac.), stupefaction, difficulty in understanding what he is reading; loss of memory; aversion to being near people and to talk to those passing him, with inclination to seize hold of and *abuse them;* disinclination to business; anxiety, as if great guilt weighed upon them."

There are various conditions represented by the above symptoms for which reason it is difficult both to group them and to determine their rank. Take the symptoms "aversion to being near people," for an example. What is the cause which produces it? What is the general condition which would lead a person to such a state of mind? The reply off hand would be sexual organs. The experienced observer would in turn reply: "Oh, yes;" but be more definite, for we may have "desire with erections or without," also "enlarged or atrophied testicles." We may also have pruritus vulva, uterine polypi, or cancer of the uterus, either of which conditions may produce a host of symptoms. The experienced man will tell you that the symptom in question will be presented by masturbators and those who, though having fiery passions, are too conscientious to either masturbate or gratify their desire in any other way. The fact that the symptom is found in the great majority with such habits makes it of the highest rank. What are the other symptoms of this group and how do we select them? Again, by experience, by knowledge of the effects of the habits. So we explain "*Mental weakness,*" "Inability to sustain mental work," "Loss of memory, mental *confusion and worry,*" "as if a great guilt weighed upon him." There is one more mental symptom I have met in nearly every such patient for which I will use the word "*sheepish*" (Staphisagria); their face, speech and action are hard to describe. The stomach symptoms are "*variable appetite* usually *lost.*" The remainder of the group are: "*frequent micturition* sometimes *involuntary, urine flows by fits and starts,*" "*weakness* on walking even to *trembling,*" in fact *general tremulousness.* Staphisagria and Conium are the two remedies which have served me best for the above group of symptoms.

Head: The other mental conditions are *melancholia, hypochondriasis* from excessive venery, and *brain fag.*

"*Aching* on waking in morning, as if brain were too full and would burst (Bryonia), *intoxication* from slight amount of spiritous drink; vertigo in morning on rising (Lycopodium, Phosphorus); on walking; *sensation* in right half of brain as *of a large foreign* body; one side of head numb and cold; pain in occiput as if pierced with a knife."

Vertigo is the symptom of this group which needs studying. It is not caused by disturbances of stomach (Nux) nor by paralysis of the recti muscles (Gelsemium) nor by atrophy of the optic nerves (Strychnia), neither by middle-ear trouble as in Menier's disease (China), but *vertigo due to* exhaustion of brain force (*functional* not *structural changes*) caused by a blow either *physical* or *nervous* (shock); *sexual excesses or abstinence.* With the vertigo the patient reels, staggers, agg. on turning the head; also on lying down. When he lies down the couch seems to move back and forth, especially is this true if the patient turns in bed. Our well known superintendent of education sent for me once because he was suffering from excessive vertigo. It seemed to him as if his bed was moving up to the ceiling and that he would be suffocated. So real was this to him that he reached up to show me he could touch the ceiling. The cause of this particular attack was that he had attended a meeting of the Amherst Alumni the night before and had made a long address. He was 82 years of age. *Another cause of* this *vertigo* is the use of tobacco. I have demonstrated this by prescribing it to *boys after their "first smoke"* and to *adults who smoked* to *excess.* Finally Conium has cured headaches from a variety of causes when the brain felt too large (Gelsemium, Argentum nit.) and was very sensitive. A feeling of coldness and numbness in or on the side of the head remained for hours after the headaches ceased (Aconite, Veratrum alb.).

Eyes: "Pupils dilated; lids seemed pressed down, and sleepiness; *vision weak with dizziness, vertigo, and general debility* worse in arms and legs, so that he staggered; sluggishness of adaptation; vision double."

Often useful for *partial or complete paralysis* of *muscles.* It is an *effort sometimes painful* to focus upon any object and you have *vertigo,* running together of letters; dimness or vanishing of vision. For scrofulous ophthalmia with *marked* photophobia. *Cataract* has been *arrested* by the use of Conium.

Stomach: "Pressure in pit of stomach as if a ball rose from it to the throat (Ignatia)."

This symptom belongs in the hysterical group.

Sexual Organs.

Male: "*Desire without erections*, emission even when frolicking with a woman (Phosphorus); *e. g.*, without dreams at night; discharge of prostatic fluid at every excitement, without voluptuous thoughts, with itching in prepuce."

Female: "Itching deep in vagina (Kreosote); leucorrhea ten days before menses, with colic before the discharge, with weakness and paralyzed sensation in the small of the back before the discharge; l. of *white* acrid *burning* mucus (Phosphorus, Kreosote); l. thick milky with contractive, labor-like pains coming from both sides; menses suppressed."

I will simply emphasize two or three of the conditions of this location. Useful for *sexual nervousness* of strong, healthy men who are unable to have an erection, *e. g.*, a strong, healthy business man came to me about four months after his wedding with the statement that although the erectile power had been perfect all his life he had not been able to have intercourse because of lack of erection. Conium 12th cured the defect within two weeks. He took five drops before each meal and at bedtime.

The next condition is for *hard, indurated enlargement of* the *testicles following injury* (Arnica). Third, in boys, old maids and old bachelors, for symptoms caused by having the mind dwell on sexual subjects and then suppressing the desires which the thoughts create. The symptoms of this group are almost identical with those of masturbation.

Conium is one of our best remedies for *scirrhous tumors* of the *female genitals;* for *hard, smooth, large, induration of* the *mammary glands;* with the sharp knife-like pains, also for hard nodular tumors in the mammary glands which appear just before menses and disappear with the menses. These tumors are very sensitive and the patient knows she is going to have cancer. Conium and Kreosote have saved many women from the knife.

The *nervous night cough* of *old people* is the only other condition I have used the remedy for. This condition combines "a dry hacking cough," "spurting of the urine," and "sleeplessness." The cause is a dry spot in the larynx which is agg. at night.

CICUTA VIROSA.

Make-up: Old people and children, prostrated; neurotic.

Loc.: Medulla oblongata, the gastro-intestinal tract, and skin.

Sen.: Stiff, tearing, jerking, trembling.

Mod.: Agg. cold; touch; concussion; jarring.
Amel. warmth and quiet.

Leaders: The violence of the attacks. The frightful distortions during convulsions.

Nerves.

"Convulsion with wonderful distortions of the limbs, head turned backwards, back bent as in opisthotonos, with unconsciousness; spasms of all the muscles, with dark redness of the face, blue lips and bloody froth from the mouth."

It has been used for *convulsions of all forms,* chorea-like, epileptiform, tetanic, puerperal, from worms, from indigestion, from injuries, from the use of opium, with the violent contortions and distortions mentioned above and with the modalities agg. touch, noise, cold, wet (Nux vom.).

I have found it successful after eating, for worms, and after using morphine. The latter patient had been an addict for years. Her usual dose was 2½ grs. Morphine daily. She had had a good deal of excitement one day when convulsions followed. Her daughter did not dare give her more Morphine so sent for me. Cicuta 3rd, 10 drops every 15 minutes, quieted her in about an hour and the convulsions ceased in about two hours. She then went to sleep and rested 11 hours. I continued the remedy for two weeks to see if it would have any affect on the drug habit but it did not, neither did she have any more convulsions.

Head: "Jerking; vertigo and reeling; falling to the ground; stupefying pain in forehead externally, agg. rest, tearing pain in occiput followed by a feeling of exhaustion."

It has cured many cases of *cerebro-spinal meningitis with convulsions* as mentioned above. For *concussion* of the brain *with* the same *convulsions*. With both there were the violent shocks through the head and body and the agg. of the drug. In one case the *child would scream* from the pain *before* the *convulsions* came on.

Eyes: "Staring; pupils dilated and insensible; objects seem to approach and recede when attempting to stand; all objects double."

The only use I can vouch for here is for strabismus following convulsions (Apis).

Throat: Rarely you will need it for *spasms of the esophagus from worms* when the child strangles so as to make deglution impossible. The action then will only be palliative. Cicuta will not destroy the worms, so you will use some other remedy like Cina after the spasms have been controlled by Cicuta.

For *violent hiccough* with screaming; red face; trismus; distortion of the limbs and unconsciousness (Tabacum). Sometimes you will find with the hiccough group such tightness of the muscles of the chest that the patient can breathe only with the greatest difficulty.

Back: "*Bent backward like an arch* (Nux vom., Cuprum ars.); tearing, jerking in coccyx."

In addition to the terrible spasms it has cured *neuralgia* of the coccyx with the tearing, jerking during the first few hours of the menses especially when the menses have been delayed.

Extremities: I have already given you the character of the symptoms for this section. They all belong to the general convulsion group, the causes and modalities being the same.

Skin.

"Elevations over the face and hands with burning pain on touch; red on scapula, painful to touch."

Cicuta has cured *eczema capitis* when the entire *scalp* was *covered* with a *solid mass.* Also for epithelioma when the growth is covered by a thick yellow scab. The growths were about the corners of the lip (Arsenicum iod.). The field of Cicuta is a narrow one. The 3rd is the only potency I ever used.

SPIGELIA.

Make-up: Neurotic.

Loc.: Nerves.

Sen.: Shooting; *tearing;* burrowing; sticking.

Mod.: Agg.: *Touch; motion;* jar.

Leaders: *Violence of pains;* left side.

Nerves.

Head: *Burrowing; tearing pains in head.*

Agg.: Left side; *towards evening.*

Agg. by motion, on *walking; a jar;* pain in brain; shaking the *head;* dull pain with pressure outwards so that reflection was difficult; *shooting through forehead* behind and above eminence; *tearing, tensive* pain *beneath left eminence* extending towards orbit; burning pain in forehead extending to the eyes so that he could not move them without pain; *deep seated* pain in right side in evening, in eye in the morning agg. motion, especially by suddenly turning head, when brain seems loose.

Useful only for *purely neuralgic headache, i. e.,* no *structural changes,* with *tearing,* burning, jerking pains usually beginning at one point and radiating over and through the entire head. Sometimes they cease suddenly in the head and go to the heart and nerves of the left arm. Occasionally there is the sensation as if the head were opening. Often the pains begin in the morning and cease when the sun goes down. This is called the "*sun headache.*" A jar causes the greatest agg.

Eye: "Pain *on turning the eyes;* feeling as if eyes were too large for their orbits; *pain* in balls of eyes *in turning them* and *vertigo* on attempting to look with eyes turned *forcing* him to turn the whole head."

Face: We have three conditions indicated by these symptoms, viz., *ptosis, ciliary neuralgia* and *rheumatic iritis.* The symptoms of facial neuralgia have already been given under head. They are shooting, burning, tearing.

Ear: The toothache is agg. by cold water (Arnica, Chamomilla).

Chest: "*Cutting, tearing beneath* left *nipple, extending* into region of *upper arm* agg. *deep breath;* cutting constriction, with anxiety; tearing constriction above the pit of the stomach, with oppression, then below throat pit, with palpitation."

Useful for intercostal neuralgia generally associated with rheumatism; sometimes for an aggravation of pain in the muscle of a hypertrophied heart.

Heart: "*Palpitation* (Arsenicum, Pulsatilla, China, Natrum mur., Cactus). P. *with anxious oppression and trembling of heart, agg. siting down and bending forward, the palpitation was felt by the hand at pit of stomach; violent beating in the morning as soon as he sat down; after rising, with weight upon the chest above the point where the beating was felt, with cutting and digging in the hypogastrium as from incarcerated flatus, which lasted longer than the palpitation;* irregular action of heart, with suffocation; heart beats audibly and visibly through the clothes with pain causing desire for fresh air (Cactus)."

Spigelia is most frequently called for in *neuralgia* about the heart when the pain extends up over the shoulder and down the nerve of the left arm, often accompanied by pale face and profuse sweat about the face and head. For pericarditis and endocarditis with the severe irregular tumultuous action of the heart, severe pain, dyspnea from lying on the back and a dry hacking cough. Sometimes useful when the inflammation of the heart extends to the aorta with pain under the sternum, numbness of the arm, violent irregular pulsations also irregular pulse. I use it from the 3rd to the 200th.

CACTUS GRANDIFLORUS.

Make-up: Emotional, neurotic.

Loc.: Circulation; *heart;* blood.

Sen.: Pulsations; chilliness; *constriction;* suffocation; sharp, shooting.

Mod.: Agg. when walking or lying on the left side; from missing a meal or fasting; at night; at 11 A.M. and 11 P.M.

Characteristics: *Sensation as if the heart were alternately clutched and released by an iron hand.*

Heart.

"*Constriction as by an iron band;* acute pain, with stitching, causing loud cries, with obstruction of breath; rapid, short, irregular beats on rapid motion; violent, irregular beats with pressure and heaviness; *palpitation worse* at night; *walking* and lying on left side; palpitation in small irregular beats *from* slight *excitement* or deep thought, with necessity for deep inspiration."

Cactus has won success in the treatment of patients suffering from acute myo- endo- and pericarditis; hypertrophy of the heart; angina pectoris; cardiac dropsy and palpitation. With the dropsy you have *labored breathing* causing the patient to sit up, edematous extremity and cold sweat. With all the conditions the characteristic feeling as if the heart were alternately clutched and released by an iron hand. If that symptom which has been verified be not present better look up some other remedy for your patient.

Circulation.

Head: "Pain like a *weight on vertex, better from pressure, worse* from sound of talking and from any *noise;* feeling as if head were compressed in a vice and would burst from the severity of the pain; vertigo; *pulsations* in *head.*"

Has cured congestive headaches and neuralgic headaches, the latter being *periodical. Pulsations in the* pit of *stomach* and *hemorrhages from* various organs, *e. g., uterus, nose, rectum* and *lung* plainly *show* its *use* for *equalizing* and tranquilizing the *circulation.*

Blood.

"*Chilliness* with chattering of the teeth not relieved by covering, at 11 A.M. and 11 P.M.; burning heat with shortness of breath; scorching heat at night with headache following a chill and terminating in perspiration."

Cactus has cured patients of intermittent fever with the regularity of paroxysms. The cold predominates. Hemorrhage from different organs occurs during some stage of the paroxysms. The paroxysms are often incomplete. Intermittent neuralgias frequently precede or follow attacks of intermittent fever. The attacks of neuralgia are also periodic.

Notwithstanding the fact that many insist that Cactus has no remedial virtue I can testify to its efficacy in many cases. I use the 1st, 2d and 3rd x.

DIGITALIS.

Make-up: ————

Loc.: *Heart;* kidneys; circulation of *liver* and lungs; genito-urinary organs.

Sen.: Palpitation of heart; weakness; drowsiness.

Mod.: Agg.: Rising from a reclining or sitting position; lying on left side (Phosphorus).

Amel. lying flat on back.

Leaders: The *slow,* weak, *irregular, INTERMITTENT* pulse; the attacks of great weakness, with the sensation as if the heart would stop.

Heart.

"*Sudden sensation as if it stood still.* In P.M. with anxiety and necessity to hold the breath; action feeble, frequent, *intermittent,* irregular (Apocynum, Cratægus) action of heart and pulse feeble and small with palpitation."

The *intermittent pulse* is the ranking symptom of this group. The *intermittence* is *irregular.* The *second ranking* symptom of the group is the rapid and *violent change* from *slow to rapid* on the least excitement or emotion. This change shows the feebleness of the heart muscle. Anxiety and oppression are very prominent. Dyspnea and cyanosis occur in many cases.

Digitalis is useful for pericarditis with effusion; in fact cardiac dropsies from any cause with the above symptoms.

I have found it the most frequently indicated remedy for acute dilation of the heart. Given for a long period of time it regulates the heart's action and hastens compensating hypertrophy. I give it in the 2d or 3rd, five drops three times daily. It has also helped clear up many cases of "Blue babies," when given in drop doses of the 3x twice daily.

For *cardiac dropsies* or *edemas* or *dropsies* elsewhere, when you have the above group of symptoms, *use* an *infusion representing three* or *five grains* of the leaves. Give it every four hours till you get relief. Always see to it that the bowels are acting freely before you begin this treatment.

Liver.

We can say that *all conditions* of the *liver* are *secondary* to some *affection* of the *heart.* Here is the group as I have found it; *liver enlarged, tender, sore; stools light-colored;* skin jaundiced; pulse irregularly intermittent; acites; dropsy; nausea and vomiting; the patient is drowsy, dull, sluggish in all his actions.

I want to speak of Myrica in this connection. It is a remedy which has most of the liver symptoms of Digitalis, but it acts primarily upon the liver. In two cases when Digitalis failed to act Myrica the 3rd cleared up the case. This is the only mention I will make of Myrica as I have never used it for any other condition.

Lungs.

"*Respiration irregular and performed by frequent, deep sighs;* respiration difficult, deep, slow; constant desire to breathe deeply but it seemed as if the chest could be only half filled because of some impediment deep in the chest with a cough agg. by deep inspiration; edema of lungs; suffocative constriction of the chest as if the parts were grown together."

The above symptoms are usually found in edema of the lungs and effusion into the pleura in patients who have weak hearts. Occasionally in pneumonia of old people when in addition to the pathognomonic symptoms of pneumonia you have the feeble *intermitting* pulse, the cyanotic lips and fingers and cold, clammy extremities.

Kidneys.

"Function of the kidneys suspended; urine scanty, dark, of high sp. grav.; urine red, depositing a sediment."

It has helped me in a few cases of *post-scarlatinal nephritis* with the scanty albuminous urine and weak pulse, also tendency to dropsy. This is the only curative action I have found in this section but I have had it act as a palliative in chronic nephritis when the heart threatened to stop and when there was edema of the lungs and dropsy. For this condition use the effusion as directed above.

As a *result* of the *effusion* it will cause, Digitalis has been used for *detachment* of the *retina* (Gelsemium).

Although our authorities speak highly of it for gonorrhea, hydrocele and sexual weakness, I have never verified the statements except a symptom of minor importance in patients suffering from heart trouble.

ALUMINA.

Make-up: Thin; anemic; nervous; lacking normal vital force.

Loc.: Mucous membranes; spinal nervous system.

Sen.: Faint; weak; tremulous; drawn tight.

Mod.: Agg. from starch, salt, wines, cold air, in the morning on awakening.

Amel. from *cold bathing,* but warm food or drinks and by *warmth* generally.

Characteristics: Paralytic loss of power; inactivity of rectum and bladder; dryness of the mucous membranes.

Mucous Membranes.

Eyes: "Agglutination in the morning on waking, with *burning* when opened, and dread of light; dim vision, obliging her to wipe her eyes constantly with sensation as if lids would adhere in corners; *dryness.*"

For subacute and catarrhal *conjunctivitis* with smarting, marked *dryness* and *burning,* very little discharge and no destruction of tissue. Also useful for granular lids, chronic blepharitis.

Throat: "Dryness with burning in the evening, at night inducing *frequent clearing;* shooting here and there and sticking in the throat; soreness on swallowing; scraping and rawness; roughness with accumulation of mucus; pain as if part of the esophagus were contracted or compressed."

Alumina has been quite extensively used for the sore throat

of public speakers when there is great irritability and dryness. The sticking pains and inclination to clear the throat are marked. General relaxation of the uvula is also marked.

Rectum and Anus: "Rectum seems paralyzed; pressure and sense of excoriation after a small, hard stool; dried and constricted feeling during stool; excoriated feeling in anus after stool attended with contraction of anus and rectum; bleeding after stools; stools hard, scanty, difficult; stools dry like laurel berries."

Nose: Alumina 30th is the best remedy for constipation of children with the above symptoms. Such children are anemic. In seven cases out of ten the children will suffer from a dry, chronic catarrh of the nose. The mother will say: "*Baby* has *snuffles* and is constipated." The mucous membrane is so dry that the stool causes fissures and bleeding. Alumina 30th will cure such patients.

Vagina: "Leucorrhea, acrid, worse after the menses with burning in the genitals and rectum which parts seemed inflamed and corroded so that walking was difficult, better from washing with cold water; profuse leucorrhea which flowed almost to her feet, excoriating the skin."

This condition is usually gonorrheal, accompanied by bubo, burning and itching along urethra, more at the meatus.

Respiratory Organs: "A *continual, dry, hacking cough* at night, *with vomiting* and arrest of breathing; irritation of the larynx inducing cough; fatiguing cough with much expectoration."

Useful in *catarrhal laryngitis,* the result of talking in the open air.

Spinal Nervous System.

Back: "Bruised feeling; *pain* in the lower vertebræ *as if* a *hot iron were thrust through,* shooting pains in back."

Extremities: "Tearing in thighs and legs; tension almost like a cramp in thighs and legs, intermittent, extending downwards; tearing in patella; *heaviness* and *staggering* in evening;

weariness when sitting; tension on face as if the white of an egg had dried on it; lightning-like pains; inactivity of rectum."

Alumina has cured a few cases of locomotor ataxia and relieved the sharp pains of many other cases. Its most frequent use is for constipation. Use the 12th and higher.

GLONOINE.

Make-up: Florid; plethoric; sensitive; nervous; sanguine.

Loc.: Brain and nerves; heart.

Sen.: Throbbing; *fulness;* weakness; aching.

Mod.: Agg. heat generally, heat of sun especially; damp weather; wine; jarring.

Amel. cold applications and cold air; pressure.

Leaders: The *throbbing* and *fulness* in head; *the suddenness* and *rapidity* of the *attack*, and *agg. by heat.* The use made of it by epileptics.

Brain and Nerves.

Mind: "Familiar things seemed strange; confusion of ideas so that he could not tell where he was; scarcely knew what he was about; unconsciousness."

For acute *mania* or insanity when the *head* is *hot, full, throbbing,* the face either flushed or very pale; eyes staring; pulse very rapid and full; pulsations in carotids; for *mental confusion* when the patient *loses all sense* of *location;* for insanity caused by the long continued heat of the sun, when the patient has exalted ideas (Platinum), thinks she is the Almighty and every one her inferior.

Head: "*Fulness with full quick pulse and red face;* throbbing without pain at base of brain with throbbing of all the arteries of head and nape of neck; *shocks synchronous* with every *pulsation* of the *arteries; undulating sensation; sensation* as if *hanging with* the *head downward and all the blood were rushing into the head;* throbbing in arteries which felt like whip cords; skull feels too small."

Our best remedy for *violent* congestive headache from shock, excitement, etc. (Aconite, Belladonna, Ferrum phos.). The pains are as stated above and are felt with every heart beat. The lips and face are sometimes pale but usually bluish and swollen. The patient speaks of the brain surging in waves.

Glonoine is a valuable *remedy* for the effects of *sunstroke.* For *threatening apoplexy* of excitable, full-blooded persons. Occasionally useful for the characteristic headache caused from traumatism when the pains run up and down from head to spine, especially for concussion of the brain (Belladonna, Hypericum, Arnica). Glonoine has cured some cases of *cerebro-spinal meningitis* when the pains come from the spine up through the neck into the occiput with the same throbbing, pulsating pains as in the head.

Eyes: "Staring, wild, protruding; vision dim; dancing of objects; he thinks he sees with every beat of the pulse blood-globules passing before the eyes; black, floating spots on stooping."

Useful for only two conditions in this section, viz., *supra-orbital neuralgia* and congestion of the retina after exposure to bright light. With the neuralgia you have the pulsating, throbbing sensation.

It is a good remedy for those who are obliged to work with a bright light, men and women who work nights on delicate machinery or fine sewing.

Female Genital Organs: "*Menses suppressed;* instead of menses congestion to head."

The most successful use of Glonoine I have made was for *cerebral congestion during pregnancy.* There was congestion of the chest as well as head and in one case facial neuralgia with the headache.

At the *climaxis,* the drug will help the flushes of heat, the pressure in head, vertigo and unconsciousness. For *eclampsia* with the flushed face, staring eyes, full hard pulse, urine copious and loaded with albumin, and unconsciousness. I also saw a case of *dysmenorrhea with unconsciousness,* in which both Cocculus and Nux mosch. had failed completely, cured by Glonoine.

Heart.

"Violent action of the heart; distinct pulsations over the whole body; excessive perceptible palpitation of the heart with *sensation* of *fulness,* heaviness and *heat;* sharp pains in heart."

For *Angina pectoris* with any or all of the above symptoms. In this group I have seen the face alternately a blue, pale and purple, at one time pale and covered with cold sweat, at another flushed, hot and dry. Sometimes there are severe pains radiating in all directions from the heart; again no pains but the terrible dyspnea.

If you will bear in mind that the action of Glonoine is identical with Amyl-nitrite, you will get a better idea of its use.

One word in closing about the repetition of the dose. If you recall the rule I gave you, you would expect Glonoine to need repeating every few minutes for it has sent the pulse of a prover from 72 to 140 in less than a minute. In all cases for which I have used the remedy the interval between the doses has been minutes instead of hours, except for chronic headaches caused by exposure to heat. Give from 30th up.

CHIONANTHUS.

Make-up: Sallow; jaundiced; plethoric.

Loc.: *Liver,* diabetic diathesis center?

Sen.: Rumbling; sore; shooting; griping; weak; trembling; drowsy.

Mod.: Agg.: From stooping; from motion; after eating; especially from a jar.

Amel. in open air and rest.

Head: "Dull frontal headache, better in the open air."

Eye: "*Conjunctiva* and *sclera yellow;* burning and smarting when reading; sensation of dryness relieved by cold water; *eyelids heavy.*"

Face: "A drowsy, *listless appearance;* flushed, hot face; *sallow, yellow complexion.*"

Mouth: "Profuse, sticky, saliva; sensation of dryness even with the profuse saliva; yellow coating of the tongue."

Stomach: "Eructations, some sour, some tasteless; variable appetite; nausea; dull pains; feels as if full of undigested food."

Abdomen: "Dull, sore pain in region of liver; shooting, sharp, griping pains in lower abdomen; all abdominal pains relieved passing flatus."

Rectum: "Filled with flatus."

Stools: "Variable, yellow and watery; yellow and pasty; soft; lumpy; brown; dark."

Urinary Organs: "Urine increased in quantity; increased in urea; traces of sugar; traces of bile.

The grouping of the above symptoms shows the use of the remedy as applicable to patient suffering from liver troubles, either catarrhal or functional. The *dull frontal headache* is the most prominent of the concomitant symptoms. *Bile in* the *urine* the second rank. The headache, *increased quantity* of urine, *sugar in urine* and *dryness* of the *mouth* are a group of symptoms which have been the indication for the drug for *diabetes* of which many cases have been relieved and some cured by the use of the tincture and 1x. For the liver conditions use the tincture 3x, five drops, four times daily.

ALOE.

Make-up: Indolent; plethoric; "liver."

Loc.: Veins; liver; intestines and rectum; female generative organs.

Sen.: *Heavy;* dragging; urging; *insecurity* of anus; cutting: sensation as of a *plug.*"

Mod.: Agg.: Heat of summer and early morning.
Amel.: Cool, open air.

Portal Circulation.

Abdomen: "Distended; gurgling with motion of flatus; weak feeling as if diarrhea would occur; sensation of a plug between symphysis pubis and os coccygis with urging to stool."

Rectum: "Heaviness; fear lest stool should escape with flatus; feeling as if thin stool would escape on passing urine; with the stool always a feeling as if more were at hand; urging to stool with passage of urine or flatus; urging to stool worse after eating and in early morning."

Anus: "Hemorrhoids swollen and sore; weakness of sphincter."

Stool.

"Liquid, yellow, copious, involuntary with passing of flatus or urine, falling out without exertion."

The field of action of Aloe is not large but it is unique in its field. There is engorgement of the liver and the organs supplied by portal circulation.

The desire for stool is very urgent but the patient cannot say whether it is caused by flatus or feces. The *hemorrhoids* are large, very angry and painful. The pain is relieved by the application of *cold water*.

Female Generative Organs.

"Menses too early and copious; cramp in uterus; determination of blood to uterus."

Aloe has been used successfully for uterine hemorrhage due to congestion. The sensations of a "*plug*" and *heaviness* are most always present with this condition.

Potency 3rd and 6th.

PODOPHYLLUM.

Make-up: Dark; bilious; sluggish.

Loc.: *Rectum;* liver; female sexual organs.

Sen.: Gurgling; heaviness; nausea; soreness; faintness.

Mod.: Agg.: in *early morning; hot weather;* during dentition; eating.

Amel.: massaging liver; lying on abdomen.

Leaders: Gurgling; profuse, fetid morning diarrhea; prolapsus.

Liver.

Abdomen: "Fullness, burning and twisting in right hypochondrium with flatulence, pain and soreness; pain in region of liver with tendency to rub the part with the hand; flatulence, with abdomen swollen almost to bursting; abdominal plethora with soreness, bloated feeling and uneasiness better after stool; pain with coldness then heat with warm sweat; heat with inclination to stool; excessive secretion of bile with irritability of liver."

Rectum and Anus: "*Protrusion* of *rectum* after stool or motion; sometimes protruding for days owing to the swelling and congestion; hemorrhoids."

Stools: "*Diarrhea* in *morning* and through the forenoon, then natural stool in the evening; *diarrhea* alternating with constipation; liquid, yellow, offensive stool every hour."

Stomach: "Desire for something sour; indifference to food, appetite lost; thirst; gagging; nausea; *vomiting* of hot, frothy *mucus,* of *contents* of the *stomach,* then of bile, of thick, dark-green bile mixed with dark coagulated blood; griping, sticking in stomach about 4 P.M.; an offensive, yellow, undigested stool mixed with mucus; empty, hollow sensation in the epigastrium."

Mouth: "Tongue coated white in morning with much viscid mucus in mouth; smell of food causes loathing (Colchicum); bad taste."

For *chronic hepatitis* with the fullness, soreness and dull pain in hepatic region. Associated with this condition you may have one or more of the following, viz., prolapsed rectum and uterus, acute and chronic indigestion, catarrhal inflammation of the bowels, especially the duodenum, jaundiced skin, diarrhea and dysentery.

For *diarrhea of infants* in hot weather, not even Arsenicum excels Podophyllum. The most frequent cause of this diarrhea is dentition. Here is the picture: several stools in the morning so thin that the greater part passes through the diaper, leaving some feces which resembles yellow corn meal. Preceding the stools marked *nausea*, the "*everlasting gagging*" of the drug. You can tell this in babies by watching the expression of the *face*, which is deathly *pale* just before the stool, also *puckered mouth* as if something sour or bitter came up. In severe cases the child rolls the head which is covered with sweat.

For a *general diarrheic condition*, the result of sluggish liver. This group comprises most of the symptoms found under infantile diarrhea except the rolling of the head and the convulsions which occasionally occur in the other form.

Constipation. Podophyllum also has a large gray or white, well formed stool. You usually find this condition when the flow of bile is obstructed, usually by hepatic calculi. For the constipation I use 3rd, for the diarrhea the 30th.

Podophyllum has cured more cases of *prolapsus ani* in children than all other remedies combined. I use three doses of the 30th daily. I leave the following directions: first cleanse the protruding part with a solution of calendula, then apply calendula cerate and push the rectum into place. After which put on a perineal bandage to keep the organ in place. As the gut protrudes after each stool the above process should be repeated. If the M.M. of the rectum has become ulcerated, as it sometimes does, substitute hydrastis or glyco-thymoline for calendula.

Next to children, women are most subject to prolapsus ani and in half the cases it is associated with *prolapsus uteri*. I find the great majority of such cases *in parturient women*. In addition to the care of the rectum mentioned above, use a douche of hot calendula or normal salt solution and have the woman take the "knee and chest position" three times daily.

For *catarrh* of the *duodenum* (Kali bich., Hydrastis) and *dysentery*. I never have met an acute dysentery calling for Podophyllum but occasionally a *chronic*. I can testify to all the symptoms given by Allen, viz., "discharges like meat washings, burning pain in rectum, severe tenesmus, sinking feeling in abdomen, nausea, efforts to vomit and prolapsus ani", except the severe tenesmus.

Female Generative Organs.

"*Sensation* in female *genitals* as if they *would fall out* when at stool; ***pain in uterus and right ovary;*** symptoms of prolapsus of uterus with pain in sacrum, flatulence, infrequent, muco-gelatinous stools."

The prolapsus group contains heaviness, backache, feeling as if genitals would fall out and the occipital headache, endometritis, flabby vaginal walls and a thick, transparent leucorrhea. I have already given you the treatment.

Let me in closing give you a case to illustrate its use in *vomiting* of *pregnancy*. A graduate of our college of nervo-bilious temperament, usually constipated, eighth week of gestation, found the following: the *constipation worse, stools large,* almost *white;* aversion to food, craved cold drinks; both food and drinks vomited soon after eating; *constant gagging* between meals, but seldom vomited except after eating, bad taste in mouth which was filled with offensive saliva. She was emaciated and weak. Her physician, having tried everything without success, had insisted on emptying the uterus. Guided by the stool and the gagging we prescribed Podophyllum 3x, two grains every three hours. She began to improve after 36 hours, was up and about in a week and went to full time without any further trouble.

CHELIDONIUM MAJUS.

Make-up: Sluggish, bilious, lazy.

Loc.: *Liver;* mucous membranes and lungs.

Sen.: Weariness; weakness; heaviness; nausea; constriction; sticking.

Mod.: Agg. from motion; change of weather; 4 A.M. and 4 P.M.

Amel. from *hot food.*

Leaders: *Pain under lower angle of right scapula;* sallow, jaundiced face.

Liver.

There is probably no remedy in the materia medica whose manifestation of a disordered liver appears in so many different locations as do those of Chelidonium. Let us trace a few of them. "*Pains through liver* and *in right scapula;* pains in region of liver and spleen; pain in hepatic region extending downward and across the umbilical region as if constricted by a string; soreness in region of liver worse from pressure of clothes; enlargement of liver."

Stools: "*Bright yellow,* copious stools with much mucus; *pasty; watery;* slimy; also stools *hard,* light gray."

Chelidonium, like Podophyllum and Aloe, has both the constipated, hard and diarrheic, loose stools. *For* the *diarrhea* give Chelidonium 30th or higher; for the *constipation* give the remedy in the 3rd.

Urinary Organs: "Urine *dark yellow;* turbid when boiled; dark *brown* like brown beer; urine stains diaper reddish-brown; red sediment in urine."

Eyes: "*Dirty yellow* color of whites; sore sensation on looking up."

Face: "*Yellow,* worse about nose and cheeks; the usual redness of the cheeks has a mixture of *dark yellow.*"

Mouth: "*Tongue yellow* with red margin showing imprint of teeth; salivation; collection of bitter water obliging constant expectoration; *bitter* taste when eating and drinking."

Back: "*Sticking* pains *beneath right scapula;* pain extending from right scapula through chest to sternum; with oppression."

Skin: "*Yellow, jaundiced; itching* of whole body; painful pimples and pustules in various parts of the body."

With the *acute* and *chronic hepatitis* and *hepatic calculi* we often have migraine, pains extending down the neck and shoulders to the angle of the right scapula; vertigo and violent prosopalgias. We also find *gastric disturbances* relieved by hot drinks and hot food. The characteristic stools are also found. With the hepatic calculi you find the yellow sclera and the yellow, itching skin.

Lungs.

Respiratory Organs: "Cough; after waking and on rising with sensation of dust under the sternum; cough as in incipient whooping cough; racking cough as in consumption, worse in the morning with much expectoration from deep in the lung, difficult to loosen the rattling in the chest, worse changing position after waking."

Has been successful in *bronchitis* of children but I have most frequently succeeded with it in cases of chronic *catarrhal pneumonia* with the above chest symptoms and in addition a fluctuating temperature.

CINA.

Make-up: *Ill-humored;* restless; over-sensitive; *sickly.*

Loc.: *Nerves* of *spine,* brain and abdomen; stomach; thermic centers.

Sen.: *Ravenous* hunger; tearing; sticking; restless.

Mod.: Agg. *Worms; during sleep; touch;* vexation; yawning.

Amel. Lying on abdomen.

Leaders: *Grinding of teeth;* cross, *touchy* disposition; picking and burning of nose; paleness about the mouth; *milky brine.*

Brain and Nerves.

Stomach: "*Great hunger soon after meal* (China, Calcarea carb., and Nux vom.); *desires many and different* things; thirst; *vomiting* of mucus only, of food, then general chill, then heat with great thirst."

I give you this group of symptoms first because it seems to be the center of all the others, of which it seems to be both cause and effect.

Mind: "*Cannot be quieted by any persuasions; proof against all caresses* (Nux vom.); piteous cries if one attempted to touch or lead him; weeping and complaining; *unconscious* and *frothing* at the *mouth.*"

There is *no child more contemptible* than the *Cina.* He is easily excited; weak; screams, strikes and bites; is cross and obstinate.

Head: "Internal, stupefying headache on walking in the open air more in sinciput than in occiput; drawing pain from left eminence to root of nose, causing confusion of head; stitching above orbital margin extending deep into the brain; intermitting weight in middle of vertex as if brain were pressed down, amel. by pressure."

These symptoms are found with the others, especially the gastric, and constitute a group we may call "*cerebral irritation.*" I recall only one case of inflammation, *cerebral meningitis, which called* for *Cina.* It was that of a nervous, sickly, pampered girl of 3 years, following what her physician called acute gastritis with a high temperature, a hot, swollen belly, diarrhea and spasmodic twitching of muscles. The treatment had been "calomel and starvation" which cured? the child. About three weeks afterwards a maiden aunt gave the child a large dose of some "*vermifuge,*" *which* brought several worms. This was followed by a rapid rise in temperature and convulsions. The physician was recalled and advised consultation. When I first saw the child the face was pale, the head hot and retracted, some rigidity of the muscles of the neck, was vomiting mucus and voiding a whitish, copious urine. She had had several convulsions, was just coming out of one when I arrived. There was a little frothing of the mouth and slight strabismus. There was no question as to the diagnosis, *cerebral* meningitis with a tendency to *spinal*. Her physician suggested a dose of castor-oil, flushing the bowels with normal salt solutions and following that with calomel and soda, and starvation. I agreed to the flushing of the bowels, objected to the oil and starvation and suggested Cina 3rd, in place of soda and calomel. The child got the Cina, five drops every hour for three doses, then every three hours for 48 hours. After that, as the child was convalescing, we changed to the 30th. night and morning. The convulsions continued for about 12 hours, the child passed many large worms for a week. Her appetite began to improve after three weeks and she was a normal child in six months.

Eyes: *"Sickly look about the eyes, with pallor of face;* pupils dilated; pulsations of superciliary muscles, a kind of convulsion."

I never knew Cina to help any kind of eye trouble.

The *above symptoms and* the *strabismus* mentioned in the case above *are* all *reflex* symptoms.

Nose: *"The child bores into the nose until the blood comes;* sneezing."

Face: "Twitching of muscles; sticking, cramp-like pains; *pale and cold; white and bluish about* the *mouth;* red; alternate pale and cold and red and hot."

There is *something* about the *face* which *indicates* that the *troubles* for which Cina is useful are *deep-seated.*

Abdomen and Stools: "Pinching or cramp-like pressure transversely across in the region of stomach, after eating; twisting about navel; loose, involuntary white evacuations."

The few symptoms quoted above are all we have from the provers but from patients we have in addition: "Abdomen hot, swollen, sore about the navel, with a great deal of colic", also

"Stools with maw-worms; loose evacuations with the consistence of pap; discharge of ascarides and of other worms from the anus; itching of the anus; diarrhea of bile and of stercoraceous matter."

All of these symptoms confirm the presence of worms.

Respiratory Organs: "*Hoarse, hacking cough* in the morning *after rising,* caused by a sensation of dust in trachea; cough and in paroxysms in the evening; *gurgling* is heard going downward during which the *patient* is anxious, pale and *clutches* at her *throat;* cough, then patient cries 'ah! ah!'; mucus hangs in larynx in morning after rising, soon collecting again after expectoration."

Aside from the cough which is reflex we have a cough group of *capillary bronchitis* and pertussis calling for *Cina.* In both of these groups we have the symptoms: "*swallows after coughing,* screams when any one approaches the bed (Arn.), also screams and talks in sleep."

Thermic Centers.

The thermic symptoms of Cina are peculiar. They are the unexpected and as changeable as the general symptoms of Pulsatilla. Here are a few. "Chill daily at the same hour, then heat witout thirst (Ignatia), shivering over the whole body, then heat without thirst; shivering creeping over trunk so that he trembles; heat mostly in head during fever, with yellow color of face and blue rings around the eyes; rising heat and redness of cheeks, sometimes one cheek hot and red and the other cold and pale (Chamomilla)."

I have never seen Cina do any good in such fevers as typhoid, malarial or septic. On the other hand I have never seen a marked, clear, Cina group without some thermic symptoms in it.

Cina is without question the best remedy, in fact, the only remedy for the above groups of symptoms representing, with possibly one or two exceptions, conditions caused by worms.

What causes the worms? The condition of the alimentary canal. What is the cause of the condition of the alimentary canal? Mal-nutrition. What is the cause of mal-nutrition? In my opinion the causes are two, viz., some inherited weakness (diathesis) and improper diet. Let me make clearer my meaning by illustration. Take three *old* apple orchards, the trees infested with worms (grubs) and three *young* apple orchards with no grubs, adjoining each other. You say the difference is in the age of the trees or the care given them. All are in the same soil, get the same rain, sunshine, heat and cold. The cause is not in the elements. The young orchard has been well cared for so you say it is all in the care. But you examine the old orchard and find that certain rows of trees are as free from grubs as are those in the young orchard. You further learn that the trees free from grubs are of a different variety, more sturdy, longer lived. You ask the farmer why one variety is more hardy than another. He does not know. I do not know. Another illustration: The owner of one of the old orchards takes a grub hook, digs out the grubs and scrapes the bark of the tree. The grubs increase and his trees die. The second owner plows up his soil and digs about the roots and then fertilizes with some substance which has proven to be specially adapted to apple trees in orchards where the soil is poor or not suitable. Get your dietician to indicate the proper diet for your Cina patients and put a copy of his directions in with to-day's notes.

IRIS VERSICOLOR.

Make-up: Nervo-bilious.

Loc.: Liver; kidneys; stomach.

Sen.: Nausea; raw; brassy taste; griping; sore.

Mod.: Agg.: *Periodically*, spring, fall, *weekly; mental exhaustion;* hot weather.

Amel.: Vomiting; good night's sleep.

Leaders: Headaches when relaxing after severe mental

strain; *bilious,* acrid, brassy tasting, *vomit* with burning, acrid, watery stools which burn like fire.

Iris seems to have an "elective affinity" for organs as a whole rather than for the individual tissues which make up the organs.

Liver.

Abdomen: "Pain in the region of the liver agg. motion; sharp, griping pains in the bowels; pain in abdomen amel. discharge of flatus; pain, heat and soreness in hepatic region."

Rectum and Anus: "*Burning in anus after stool* (Aloe, Sulphur), distress in anus as if prolapsed; *anus sore* in the morning as if there were points sticking in it (Ignatia, Æsculus)."

Stools: "*Frequent; watery* with *burning* in anus with disposition to strain (Mercurius) and bear down (Sulphur, Podophyllum); *mushy;* copious; yellow; also *constipated.*"

Stomach: "*Burning distress* in the *epigastric* region (Sanguinaria); empty eructations; nausea; vomiting of a watery, very acid substance; contents of stomach "turn to vinegar;" *great, burning distress in* mouth and *stomach;* vomiting of food; of sour, bilious, watery substance."

Mouth: "*Mouth and tongue feel scalded;* profuse, *ropy saliva* drops from the mouth during conversation; *acrid, peppery* taste."

There are only two conditions for which I have used Iris. The first for want of a better name I will call "*bilious attack*" (Bryonia); the second, *nervo-bilious sick headaches.* I will give for you a case from my records illustrating each. A banker, age 32; dark, sallow complexion; who took no exercise; was habitually constipated; used meat and milk freely; felt dull and drowsy after noon and evening meal; tongue coated; bad taste in mouth which was full of saliva. Whenever the man took cold, or sometimes without any apparent cause, he became more nauseated than usual, then vomited and purged. The stools were, at first, very offensive but became odorless by the time the attacks were over. They were thin, burning rectum and anus and leaving the latter sore. The *vomited material* was a green, *watery liquid,* tasting *hot* and as he expressed it, *brassy,* puckering the mucous membrane. The attacks would last from 24 to 72 hours, leaving him weak and exhausted for a week or ten days after which he felt better for three or four months, when the same symptoms would recur.

The second was a dark, olive-colored woman of 28, a school teacher. She was of a nervo-bilious temperament and worked very hard. By Friday P.M. she was exhausted. Saturday she usually relaxed ("rested" she said). Sunday A.M. she would awake with a fearful *ache* all *through* the *head, blurred vision, vertigo* and marked *nausea.* All the above were agg. motion. The aching would increase till towards noon and then continue till evening when she would vomit an acrid, hot, peppery liquid. The vomiting was accompanied by much retching. *After* the *vomiting* she rapidly *improved;* usually slept well Sunday night and returned to her schoolroom Monday morning in fair shape. This had been going on for several years. Iris 3x, five drops morning and evening, cleared up the case in three months. A case similar in regard to cause was a railway mail man with long, hard run and then a rest. I have had many such cases and all were of constipated habit.

IPECACUANHA.

Make-up: Morose, disdainful; scrawny; spare.

Loc.: M.M. of stomach, intestines and respiratory organs; blood; sexual organs.

Sen.: *Nausea;* sinking; crushing.

Mod.: Agg.: *Warmth;* damp; overeating; periodically.
Amel.: Open air.

Leaders: *Persistent nausea;* profuse, bright-red hemorrhage; *loose whistling in chest* without expectoration.

Mucous Membrane.

Respiratory Organs: "*Rattling* in *bronchi during respiration, suffocative cough* whereby the *child becomes* stiff and *blue in the face;* cough causing inclination to vomit without nausea; cough from constrictive tickling extending from the upper part of larynx to the lowest end of bronchi; dry cough from tickling on the upper part of larynx. Expectoration of blood (Ferrum, Phosphorus, Aconite); spasmodic asthma with constriction of throat and chest *with peculiar wheezing; dyspnea* in evening *with wheezing, and weight and anxiety about precordia.*"

Before taking up our grouping I want to explain the two words "rattling" and "wheezing." I prefer the word *whistling*. You will note that in the first symptom the rattling was heard "during respiration." That is the key to our explanation. The mucous membrane excretes a substance which is sticky enough to adhere to the walls of the tubes in shreds, so that as the air passes in and out it moves the shreds and produces the whistling. This indicates a different stage of the disease than does the "bubbling" and "rattling" of Tartar emet. caused by the air passing through the debris, pus and mucus, which lies loose in, not adherent to, the walls of the air tubes.

Ipecac is most frequently used for *capillary bronchitis* with great accumulation of mucus in the larger tubes, violent paroxysms of coughing, retching and vomiting, also expectoration of a good deal of mucus. The usually pale, sunken face becomes flushed; the temperature rises; there is hot and cold sweat in alternation. The child is nauseated and frequently vomits greenish mucus, or mucus and blood. I have helped many cases like the above with Ipecac 6th or 12th when the whistling (mucous rolls) was the ranking symptom.

Pertussis comes next to bronchitis for frequency of use. The *spasms* of cough are *so violent* that the *child* almost *loses* his *breath,* his *face becomes blue,* the *blood flows* from *nose* and *lungs;* much nausea and some vomiting which relieves the nausea and cough.

I remember one case, the child of a physician, who was drowsy all the time. He would wake, cough, vomit, nurse and go to sleep while nursing (Aethusa). The father, doctor, stated that he could not get the child to hold the medicine down long enough to do any good. If he gave it when the child first waked up he vomited; if he waked him after nursing the child would repeat the paroxysms and so loose the medicine. We decided upon Ipecac 12th to be given just after the vomiting, before nursing. It worked.

For *false* or spasmodic croup (Cuprum) *coming* on *about 10 P. M.* with inability to lie down *because* of some *irritation* as from sulphur fumes causing dyspnea. *Blueness of the face* is nearly always *present* in this group.

I have often met this group. Many physicians of the old school claim brilliant results in such cases from giving wine of Ipecac to produce vomiting. I have seen palliation of croup symptoms by such large doses; but the potency not only palliates more quickly but cures. My experience in these cases is that more or less bronchitis follows the spasmodic attack (croup?) or in other words that the cough is the premonitory symptom of bronchitis. I wish you would also bear in mind that both pertussis and genuine laryngismus stridulus are nervous affections and that I am combining two localities in these two groups.

Eyes: "Hardened mucus in the external canthi; eyes red and inflamed; eyelids closed, painful expression of the face; *the pillow* was soaked with tears and tears flowed freely on opening the eye; conjunctiva rose-colored; cornea opaque."

It has cured *subacute inflammation of* the *cornea* with intense *pain,* marked *photophobia* and profuse *lachrymation.*

Ipecac has been found extremely helpful in *pustular conjunctivitis* of *children with* some *ulceration.* The inflammation is general, the pains are tearing and sticking and you have the gushing of tears in this group also.

Nose: "Violent paroxysmal sneezing with thin mucus, sneezing with cough and expectoration; bleeding."

Occasionally useful for acute *coryza* or *catarrh with loss* of *smell* and nausea. However, the above symptoms belong with the bronchitis and pertussis groups.

Mouth and Stomach: "*Salivation, obliged to swallow constantly;* saliva runs from the mouth when lying down (Mercurius); eructations with rumbling in abdomen; *nausea,* with *empty eructations* and *salivation* (Pulsatilla, Cuprum); distress; *vomiting* of everything swallowed (Eupatorium perf.): of food (Nux vom., Ferrum), agg. stooping.

To understand the symptoms of this section you must bear in mind that they represent disturbances of two locations, viz., the M.M. and nerves. This is why the nausea is so persistent and violent and yet with little or no inflammation of the mucosa; also why the *vomiting* of bright red *blood* is *followed* by *cold extremities, hippocratic face,* feeble pulse, etc., and that you may even have the vomited blood black, tar-like but *no burning, sticking* pains *indicating* marked inflammation or ulceration. Again we find the stomach group in the fever (malarial) group, the respiratory group, the group of female generative organs. However, we do find Ipecac curative for *gastric catarrh* the result of injudicious partaking of fruits and cold drinks (Arsenicum). You have the nausea, vomiting of mucus, green mucous diarrhea, often frothy (Magnesia carb., Lithium carb.), the tongue coated white or sometimes perfectly clean.

Abdomen and Stools: "Griping, clawing as if grasped by a hand so that each outstretched finger pressed sharply on the intestines, amel. rest, agg. motion; cutting about umbilicus, with shivering; pinching in hypogastrium, pit of stomach; diarrhea; as if fermented; soft, *frequent, of green mucus* (Argentum nit., Pulsatilla, Magnesia carb.), *bloody,* covered with bloody mucus."

The most frequent use I have made of Ipecac in this group

is for what we call *cholera infantum.* With the peculiar stools, colic, nausea and vomiting we find the hot head, còld feet and clean tongue and red, scanty urine.

Sexual Organs.

Female: "Dragging towards uterus and anus; menses fourteen days too soon."

For *all forms* of *uterine hemorrhages* I place *Ipecac third* (China, Phosphorus). It has *helped* me in *metrorrhagia, menorrhagia;* two cases of *placenta previa;* threatening abortion; *following abortion and parturition.* The *blood* has *always* been *bright red* and *liquid;* the nausea has always been *present* but it was *neither* the *nausea or* the character of the *blood* which *led to* the *selection* of the *remedy* but the *face.* In all cases there was the dark, heavy, bluish ring beneath the eyes, most marked in menorrhagia; the anxious, pleading look of the eyes most marked in the miscarriages; the faintness and gasping for breath out of all proportion to the loss of blood. Use the 3x five drop doses repeated as often as 15 minutes.

Blood.

Anemia and *intermittent fever.* The Ipecac patient is always anemic. The red blood cells, less than half what they should be. The blood is so thin that it oozes from every orifice. The patient is small, scrawny (Ergot).

Thermic Centers: The intermittent fever picture is an incomplete one. The *persistent nausea* is the *center of* the *group.* There is *great thirst* but while *drinking* does not quench the thirst, it does *increase* the *nausea* and cause *vomiting.* The "bruised feeling in brain and skull, piercing through skull into root of tongue," which is the most prominent head symptom is usually present with nausea.

PHOSPHORUS.

Make-up: Tall; stoop-shouldered; hollow chested.

Loc.: Mucous membranes; circulation; brain and nerves; bones; *blood*.

Sen.: *Burning;* heaviness, *oppression;* nausea; vomiting.

Mod.: Agg.: *Lying on left side,* on back; mental exertion; emotions; cold water; warm food and drinks; evening.

Amel.: Eating; sleeping; *resting*.

Leaders: *Hemorrhagic diathesis;* heaviness of the chest, craving cold drinks which are vomited after becoming warm; *burning;* special affinity for bones.

Phosphorus enjoys the *highest rank* as a *tissue remedy*. It is also a most virulent poison and many of the symptoms have been taken from the record of cases of poisoning. It is a *powerful irritant* and produces *violent inflammation,* and *marked functional* and *structural changes*. Marked tendency to fatty degeneration; the mucous membranes are pale (anemia); the muscles are lax; emaciation great (Iodium).

Mucous Membranes.

Nose: "Swelling painful to touch; nose *swollen* and *dry,* cannot draw air through it; internal inflammation, with dry sensation and *slow bleeding,* soreness in nostril, even to touch, with bloody scabs on margins of nostrils; fullness, stoppage; sneezing; blowing out of blood."

One of our best remedies for nasal polypus (Sanguinaria) which bleeds profusely and interferes with the breathing; for chronic catarrh with a bloody mucous discharge sometimes yellow or green. With this condition there is frequently *ulceration* of the *membrane* and *caries* of the *bones* which cause pain and soreness. The swelling and discharges cause marked obstruction shown by the "fan-like motion of the wings of the nose" (Lycopodium).

Mouth: "*Gums* inflamed, *bleed easily* and are separated from the teeth; gums ulcerated and so sensitive cannot eat;

tongue chalky white with red in middle, also dry, red and even black along median line (Veratrum alb.); saliva runs from mouth during sleep."

Useful for inflamed, ulcerated gums; for *toothache caused by working with hands in cold water;* for the persistent bleeding after extraction of teeth (Mercurius viv.).

Throat: "Sore, painful on swallowing; *burning,* raw, scraping feeling in throat; *tonsils* and *soft palate dark red;* small ulcers with yellow centers in pharynx; constriction of throat and dysphasia; swallowing saliva very painful."

For simple and ulcerative pharyngitis when the nervous symptoms combine with those of the M.M.

Stomach: "*Ravenous appetite* at night; longing for acids and spicy things; *unquenchable* thirst for cold water; empty *eructation* while eating; of food; gas tasting of food (Pulsatilla) ineffectual, with pressure in chest; *nausea* at night with eructation of food; *nausea* relieved by drinking cold water but is increased after the water becomes warm and the nausea is associated with *vomiting;* vomiting of food, of blood, of *pure blood* or mixed with dark acid matter, bile or mucus; V, like coffee grounds; *distention* and *pain* in pit; sensitiveness to pressure *in region of pylorus; pressure as* from a *hard substance* above pit; *burning* in pit; *drawing* in pit extending into chest, heaviness after eating worse form pressure."

Very useful in *gastritis, gastralgia, ulceration, vomiting of pregnancy,* atonic *dyspepsia.* Note that the chief modalities are: *Worse* during *hot weather;* hot ingesta or after cold becomes hot, *better temporarily* from *cold drinks;* that the coffee grounds and bloody vomit and the *sharp, excruciating pains running through to the back* mean ulceration, while the empty, faint feeling is usually found in the dyspepsia, and the great thirst with those conditions having marked inflammation.

Abdomen: "*Empty and weak feeling;* tense, distended; tympanitic; coldness; weakness in ab. and back so she must lie down; emission of flatus."

Rectum: "Sticking; smarting during stool that was not hard; *burning* in rectum and anus after stool, with exhaustion; *urging* on rising; urging before a stool, which shot out as from a gun."

Stool: "*Gray, whitish gray, long, hard; hard,* small, *dark,* difficult; *soft* with *lumps* of white mucus; involuntary, of slimy mucus and mucus mixed with blood like scrapings of intestines (Colchicum); involuntary the moment anything entered the rectum; semi-fluid, pasty, hard."

With these symptoms of the four sections of the M.M., viz., stomach, abodmen, rectum and stools you should include those of the liver, especially those of fatty degeneration of the liver and of the pancreas.

Bearing these in mind you will understand the significance of "small lump of white mucus" like cooked sago, also greasy stools. These from the pancreas. Again the *white,* hard stools show absence of bile. The yellow skin is a prominent symptom of this group.

Phosphorus is useful for chronic *enteritis* with *diarrhea* as the *ranking symptom* of the group. The stools are often painless (China) *worse* in *hot weather,* cold drink and urging whenever the feces enter the rectum. For bleeding *hemorrhoids* from which blood streams after every stool.

Respiratory Organs and Chest: "Rawness in larynx and trachea with hacking cough and hawking; *burning; soreness* of lungs, difficult to take a full breath; *tighness* of the upper part of chest worse lying on left side; *suffocative pressure* in upper part of chest; *hoarseness* in the morning, and larynx seemed coated; voice husky, rough; inability to speak aloud, could not speak above a whisper; *cough,* dry, hollow, hacking, spasmodic tickling; cough with *expectoration* of blood, mucus, pus, viscid, muco-purulent; expectoration tasting salty, sweet and of blood; expectoration red, white, green or yellow; *respiration* oppressed, anxious, panting, impeded, short, difficult, suffocative, fatiguing."

Here again many *symptoms differing in rank* according to their use in many conditions, which conditions may vary from a simple irritation of the brain to complete destruction of the lungs and be complicated with many other conditions, *e. g.*, *fatty degeneration of the heart.* The conditions are *laryngitis, bronchitis, pneumonia, pleuritis,* any of which may be acute or chronic. The causes, anything from excitement to t. b. c. The hoarseness is worse from using the vocal cords. The cough and expectorations are worse evening and morning. The heaviness is the most marked in the pneumonia, of which profuse, bloody expectoration is the characteristic symptom. *All conditions* of this section are *agg.* by *lying* on *left side. Anxiety* at first *followed* by *delirium* usually present.

Brain and Nerves.

As in other locations so in this, Phosphorus is capable of causing any and all of the four conditions: irritation, etc. This fact will account for the apparently contradictory symptoms in the same section of the location, *e. g.*, mind lively and stupid, pain sharp and dull, appetite increased and lost. As you know, the *first step* of *fatty degeneration is irritation.* So we have neuralgia, neuritis, paralysis, hypertrophy, atrophy and the changing of nerve and muscular fibers to oil cells. Let us now run through the different sections and see what symptoms are found under each.

Mind: "Ill humor; excitement; delirium; *worried* anxious; disinclination to work; inability to think; *forgetful, apathetic;* stupor, complete dementia."

Head: "Aching all day with vertigo; *dullness;* weakness; vertigo with heaviness and pain in the head as if he had been lying with the head too low; *vertigo* on rising from a seat or from lying down, worse looking up or turning around quickly; rush of blood to head."

The Phosphorus patient feels as if the brain were tired and could not be rested, especially is this true of the brain fag of those "who think on their feet," *e. g.*, public speakers, lawyers, ministers. With these cases you have pressure on vertex, coldness in cerebellum and the sensation of stiffness in the brain as of impending paralysis. It is in these cases as well as the neuralgias of the brain that you have the "rush of blood" to and shocks in the brain.

Phosphorus can cure neuralgias, and brain fag, will *restore* the function, *check* and *retard* the process of fatty degeneration but it *cannot* change the oil cell back to fiber. *Rest* and *foods containing Phosphorus* are great adjuvants.

Eyes: "Eyes give out when reading, *vision* dim for distant objects, sees better by shading eyes with the hand, sees more distinctly in morning, in twilight than in middle of day, sees a green halo about candle light; black floating points."

Our oculists have used it for *blindness* which comes in paroxysms, caused by sexual excess with a sensation as if everything were covered with a mist or veil, either gray or black; for *retinitis* simple and albuminurious, also for *detachment* of retina; for *neuritis;* for retinal apoplexy; and muscular asthenopia.

Ears: "*Hearing difficult; re-echoing of* his own and other's *words;* of every tone that is spoken distinctly in the same pitch; ringing; roaring."

Clearly a condition of functional and structural changes combined.

We have already discussed the *gastralgias, enteralgias* and *proctalgias*. Under *anus* there is one condition I wish to call your attention to, viz., *paralyzed sphincter*. The symptom is "*anus always open*" (Secale, Apis).

Sexual Organs: "*Irritation;* erections day and night; *desire marked,* when feeble erections afterwards disappeared and erectile power left him."

For *sexual excitement* also for *impotency*. With the impotency you always have a history of the excitement with weakness, erotic dreams and seminal emissions. For nymphomania (Hyoscyamus) which condition is usually accompanied by sterility.

Back and Extremities: "*Weakness* of muscles as if crushed, then weakness in limbs and *trembling on* least *exertion;* spinal *processes* of dorsal vertebræ *sensitive* to *pressure; burning* pain between the *shoulders.*"

Useful for *spinal irritation,* with heat and sensitiveness; *for locomotor ataxia* with burning in the spine, *lightning-like pains,* formication and exhaustion; for general, *subacute neuritis* followed by numbness, the "girdle" sensation and feeling of constriction in the extremities; for *paralysis* due to exposure and excesses. Among the symptoms of this group the clinical one, "sensation as if quicksilver moved up and down the spine" is one of high rank.

Bones.

It destroys bones, having a special affinity for the tibia and jaw bones. It begins with irritation and ends with caries. *Bleeding and sensitiveness, prominent* symptoms of this location. It helps in the union of fractured bones but Calc. Phos. and Symphytum are more frequently indicated for that purpose.

Blood.

It *disorganizes* the *blood* causing hemorrhages from every pore and a jaundiced skin. Its action simulates that of *typhus* and *typhoid fever,* also of *anemia, simple* and *pernicious.*

Skin.

Useful for fungous *hematodes* and *excrescences.* Occasionally for psoriasis of palms and soles.

The diathesis for which it is most useful is the t. b. c.

Use the 30th and higher.

SANGUINARIA.

Make-up: Irritable, florid; bilious.

Loc.: Brain; *nerves;* M.M.

Sen.: Flushes of heat; *burning,* aching.

Mod: Agg. with the sun; walking; odors; climaxis.
Amel.: *SLEEP*, vomiting.

Leaders: Pains shoot from occiput and settle over eyes. Pains increase and decrease with the sun.

Brain and Nerves.

Head: "*Aching beginning* in the *morning;* agg. stooping and moving about, *with nausea* and *chilliness,* then *flushes* of heat extending *from head* to *stomach; paroxysmal* pains, as if the head would burst (Bryonia) in the P.M., worse in the temple; amel. walking in open air; throbbing pain agg. stooping (Bryonia) with *bilious vomiting;* rush of blood to the head, with *whizzing* in *ears* and transitory heat, then *water-brash as* if *vomiting would occur; vertigo* in morning on rising quickly from stooping; on turning the head quickly (Bryonia); with faintness; pain over the eyes in the morning agg. exercise, sympathizing with stomach, like sick headache; lasting all day; pain in the occiput and nape in P.M."

Sanguinaria is one of the four great remedies for nervous (American) sick headache. The pain usually begins in the morning and lasts all day. The pain is severe, agg. by motion, amel. by sleep, also by voiding a large amount of urine (Gelsemium).

For *climacteric* headache *with* the *rush* of *blood to* the *head,* hot flushes; noises in the ears, nausea and vomiting, burning, empty, faint, feverish feeling in the stomach; shivering, amel. in open air. As a rule we have menorrhagia with this headache, but it may not come till after menstruation has ceased. Finally for a *neuralgic headache.* The pains commence in the *occiput radiating* all over the head, finally settling down over the *eyes. With* these pains you have *redness of conjunctiva,* marked *photophobia; humming* and roaring in ears, the same as you have at the climacteric. I once knew an anemic headache relieved by letting the head hang over the side of the bed.

Mucous Membrane.

Throat: "Dryness of throat with dry, tearing, hacking, cough, *dryness* with tickling cough not amel. by drinking (Belladonna)."

Often helpful for *ulcerated sore throat* which is red, dry, hot. Associated with the *sore throat* you often find a sore mouth, with the sensation as if it had been burned or scalded. The tearing, burning pains of throat extend into the ear and stomach.

Stomach: "Longing for spiced things, for indefinite things: *nausea not relieved* by *vomiting;* nausea with profuse saliva; with headache, chill and heat; emptiness with faint, feverish feeling."

About the only condition I have verified is *ulceration* of the stomach. The ranking symptom of the group is *rising of heat from stomach to head.* The other symptoms of the group are: *burning* pain with nausea which is not relieved by vomiting, tenderness of abdomen; diarrhea with undigested stools.

Sexual Organs: "*Uterine hemorrhage;* menses profuse, with pain in the right side of forehead and sensation as if eyes would be forced out of head (Spigelia, Cedron, Natrum mur.); sticking in right nipple; pain beneath the sternum and in the right breast; burning, sharp, myalgic pains midway between sternum and right nipple, with tenderness of surface to pressure."

This is the second most important section of Sanguinaria. In fact this and the head section are so closely related that we might call them one.

I will first mention the *HEMORRHAGE.* You recall that I mentioned this symptom in the *climacteric group* under head.

In addition to that you may also find it a ranking symptom in the *polypus group*. In the former group it was meno- in the latter metrorrhagia. The hemorrhage is profuse in both, is offensive and usually bright red, but it is much more profuse in the menorrhagia. With the polypi you usually find pieces of mucous membrane, with both the florid face, the dry hacking cough and often burrowing pain and soreness of the mammary glands. Also useful for *delayed menstruation* (Pulsatilla, Phosphorus), in the florid person, with all the heart, stomach and lung symptoms of the other uterine groups.

Respiratory Organs: "*Hacking cough, evenings after lying down,* from tickling in throat (Rumex, Arsenicum, Hyoscyamus); agg. eating; *dry cough* with *tickling in throat-pit* and *crawling* extending beneath sternum; *dry cough* waking him; *amel.* sitting up in bed and *discharging flatus upward* and *downward;* dyspnea and desire to breathe deeply; cough with the expectoration of thick blood-streaked mucus."

Useful for eight conditions; 1. *Croup* with the whistling cough, hot throat, redness and burning of the fauces with marked dyspnea. 2. *Aphonia* from congestion and dryness of the parts. 3. *Laryngitis* with soreness, a *sensation* of dryness and heat but with some expectoration of thick mucus sometimes streaked with blood. 4. Pertussis when the *cough* is dry, *agg. on lying down* at night. The stools are usually loose and there is some vomiting with pain in stomach after the paroxysms. 5. *Edema of the glottis* when the *mucosa* is *red* (Belladonna) *not pale* (Apis). 6. *Bronchitis* with much heat in the larynx, sharp pains beneath the sternum, dry cough agg. lying down and a scanty, glairy expectoration with just a little blood. 7. *Subacute, typhoid* and especially *hypostatic PNEUMONIA* (Chelidonium, Veratrum vir.), *cough agg. lying on back,* face livid, dark red; pulse rapid; very *little* blood streaked *expectoration.* 8. *Ulceration* of the lung and phthisis. With which condition you get the *burning* in chest with congestion, the *hectic flush,* circumscribed *redness* of the *cheeks,* hemoptysis.

Note that red and redness and flushing often appear in the different groups. It is a picture in red. Belladonna is the acute, Sanguinaria is the chronic.

RUMEX CRISPUS.

Make-up: ————————.

Loc.: M.M. of *trachea,* larynx and bowels; nerves, skin.

Sen.: Restless; aching; bruised.

Mod.: Agg. *inhaling* cold air, rapid changes of air; uncovering.

Amel. covering mouth; wrapping up.

Leaders: Every breath of air causes tickling in the throat pit and coughing. Covering of the mouth to prevent coughing.

Mucous Membrane.

Throat and Respiratory Organs: "Tough mucus removed from larynx by hawking; tough mucus agg. night with a constant desire to raise it; cough on breathing cold air (Phosphorus) in the evening, on lying down, from tickling in pit of and behind sternum; a dry, spasmodic cough, like the beginning of whooping cough."

The modalities *agg. from cold air* and *amel. from covering the mouth* are the two ranking symptoms of the cough groups. Rumex has been successful in relieving the annoying night-cough *of phthisis* when the tickling was caused by a little adhesive mucus (Kali carb.), of *asthma* when the violent attacks with a sense of suffocation come at 2 A.M. For those *incessant paroxysmal coughs* of *incipient t. b. c.* which recur on the least provocation or exposure, and produce soreness of the chest. Finally for what people call a *"stomach cough,"* which is *accompanied* by an early morning diarrhea, driving the patient out of bed (Sulphur). The stools are brown and watery, the time is from 4 to 9 A.M. and there may be a normal stool in the P.M. (Podophyllum).

Stomach and Stools: "Feeling of repletion (Lycopodium),

weight in pit, and epigastrium after eating, sensation with upward pressure to throat-pit, every empty swallowing carried it down but the pressure immediately returned; watery, brown stool in the morning."

We have a combination of M.M. and nerve symptoms of the stomach, first a *flatulent dyspepsia* often *due* to excessive *tea* drinking (Thuja). There is distention of the stomach with much flatulence and *severe* pains shooting from pit of stomach into chest and throat. Second *gastralgia* with an aching extending from pit through to the back causing patient to take a long breath. Sometimes these pains extend into the chest and throat. In all conditions we find marked *agg.* from *motion* and *relief* from *rest* especially rest for the stomach, *i. e.,* fasting.

I have already spoken of the *chronic morning* diarrhea in connection with the cough. The *stools* are *brown* and watery.

Skin.

"Severe itching on any part of the body but most often on legs and thighs with a nettle rash, agg. by exposure to air, such as undressing at night or getting out from under the covers in the morning" (Rhus tox., Causticum), *chronic urticaria* with the above symptoms and the dyspepsia; *prurigo* agg. cold, amel. warmth. *Prairie itch.* We have a condition in the middle west called prairie itch which has every modality of Rumex itch for which they give the remedy in the 3rd, and bathe the parts with a solution of 1 part of the tincture to 20 parts water. Use the solution hot. The 3rd, 6th and 12th for internal use.

ANTIMONIUM TARTARICUM.

Make-up: Lacking in reaction; weak; listless.

Loc.: Respiratory organs; skin; mucous membrane.

Sen.: Weakness; nausea; *suffocation.*

Mod.: Agg. *Warm room,* wraps or weather; anger; lying down; morning.

Amel. Expectoration; motion.

Leaders: *Loose, coarse, rattling cough;* lungs seem full, yet little is expectorated or absorbed; cold sweat; ***suffocative shortness*** of ***breath.***

Respiratory Organs: "Suffocation at 3 A.M. with necessity to sit up; agg. cough and expectoration: S. in the evening in bed with necessity to sit up all night; short breath; heavy, anxious rapid breathing; rattling of mucus in lungs; oppression; constriction of chest."

These are conditions which Antimonium tart. has relieved many times. I have repeatedly used it with success for patients suffering with *Asthma* with the "Suffocation in the eve. in bed and ***necessity to sit up*** all night;" the "***rattling*** of ***mucus,***" audible through the entire bedroom; "cold sweat;" and "rapid, weak, trembling pulse." Give it in five or ten grains of the 2x or 3x every fifteen minutes till the patient relaxes and goes to sleep. *Bronchitis* of children or old people with the same "rattling in chest," caused by the accumulation of free mucus in the tubes. There is marked dyspnea and the child gets angry with the cough; some nausea and occasionally the patient vomits; often cyanosis. *Pneumonia,* the last stage when resolution takes place so much more rapidly than absorption and expectoration that the lungs fill with mucus and pus. There is the "*loose, rattling cough,*" but little or no expectoration. The face is hippocartic and covered with beads of cold sweat. The pulse is very rapid and *weak.* The above is the only condition of patients suffering from pneumonia for which I have ever used stimulants. I use some such preparation as Arlington Co.'s liquid beef peptonoids freely and give Antimonium tart. 3x, two grains every hour, till improvement begins; then every two hours.

Skin.

Smallpox: Guided by the symptoms, "Poxlike eruption, often pustular, as in smallpox, forming painful crusts with itching on genitals, scrotum, arms and back," I have used the remedy for smallpox of a low type in the pustular stage. In such cases the tongue is dry and red in streaks, the stools thin and offensive and there is marked prostration, sometimes nausea and vomiting.

Mucous Membrane.

Stomach: Appetite *variable,* sometimes great for apples, with thirst for cool water; again lost, with no thirst; anxious *nausea* after eating; *vomiting* difficult, with trembling of hands, frequent stools and weakness."

The vomited matter is usually tough mucus and the vomiting is frequently accompanied by watery stools. The tongue with the gastric symptoms is coated thick, white and pasty. Antimonium seems to act best in the low potencies.

AMMONIUM CARBONICUM.

Make-up: Weak; low vitality.

Loc.: Heart and circulation; *respiratory* organs and blood.

Sen.: *Weak;* fullness; *oppression.*

Mod.: Agg. cold; wet; raw, open air; washing; during menses.

Leaders: *Wanting* in *reaction; weak heart;* dyspnea.

Heart and Circulation.

Head: "Light feeling in; fullness as if the head would burst. Palpitation after every effort with blood rising to the neck and dyspnea; weakness in the precordial region; pulse rapid."

Face: "Pale as a rule but flushed and besotted with heart and lung troubles."

Extremities: "Swollen veins and bluish color of the extremities."

Ammonium carb. is used for patients having a *weak heart*, with frequent fainting attacks; also for the effects of charcoal fumes. For the latter open windows so as to give plenty of fresh air and give Ammonium carb. 3x five grains every fifteen minutes. The impeded circulation of brain and extremities is also noticed in the pneumonia, cerebro-spinal meningitis, and scarlet fever calling for the drug. There is a tendency to heart clot in the pneumonia.

Respiratory Organs.

"Heaviness; accumulation of mucus in the larynx; cough at night; cough with bloody mucous expectoration; *rattling* of mucus in the lungs; *wheezing*, oppressed breathing; heaviness of the chest."

There is no remedy as good as Ammonium carb. for the last stage of *pneumonia* when resolution is taking place more rapidly than expectoration and absorption. The patient presents the following picture: "*puffed, besotted, hot face;* coarse rattling râles; weak, feeble pulse; unconsciousness; and general cyanosis."

Tartar emetic for similar condition differs only in that the *face is pale* and covered with cold sweat.

Blood.

Hemorrhages: "Bleeding from the intestines; discharge of blood during and after stools; menses too early and copious; hemorrhages under the skin."

Next to China I consider Ammonium carb. the best remedy for *anemia* caused by loss of blood.

Scarlet Fever and Measles: "Redness like scarlet fever over the whole upper part of the body; desquamation of hands and feet; painful swelling of the glands of the neck and axilla;

throat dark red and swollen; involuntary stool and micturition; child stupid; pulse weak and rapid."

Prof. W. H. Dickinson, who had a large experience in two epidemics of scarlet fever, gives the following group of symptoms as calling for Ammonium carb.: "Great prostration with gangrenous ulceration of the throat; tonsils dark red; hemorrhage of dark blood from mouth and throat; drowsiness; coma; involuntary stools; pulse small and thready."

For its physiological effects use 5 grains of the crude drug; for its homeopathic effects use 5 grains of the 2x or 3x. In either case repeat often.

IGNATIA.

Make-up: Dark, firm-fibered, emotional.

Loc.: Brain, especially sensorium; nerves.

Sen.: Sharp; sticking; sad.

Mod.: Agg. emotions, *e. g.*, worry; fright, mortification, reprimand; cold, open air; coffee.

Amel.: When alone; change of position; profuse urination.

Leaders: *Constant sighing;* erratic; the *unexpected, unreasonable,* by which we mean *fever without thirst, cold* but *wants to be uncovered,* congestive headache, relieved by stooping, cough agg. by coughing, etc. Be prepared to find "contrariness" in every condition and group of symptoms.

Brain and Nerves.

Mind: "*Sensitiveness, delicate, conscientiousness; changeable mood,* inconstant, impatient, irresolute; anger at slight blame or contradiction and then angry at herself; howls, cries, and beside herself on account of trifles; anxiety as if he had committed a crime; cries if one hesitates to obey her or tries to persuade her."

A great remedy for grief. I made that statement to one of the professors of this University once and he asked, "What is grief? There is no such condition, is there?" I asked him if he had ever met a patient with the following symptoms, the result of some great trouble: "Weeping, *sighing,* chilliness, frequent micturition, loose stools, difficult deglutition, lost appetite and sleeplessness." He replied, "Often." I told him, and I tell you, that the above group means grief to me and Ignatia is the best, the only, drug for it.

Hysteria is the *other condition.* In a few instances the cause may be the same. To any or all of the grief group you may add globus hystericus, syncope, unconsciousness and even paralysis.

Head: "Inclined forward; aching with every beat of the arteries agg. stooping, talking, aching in forehead, sensation as if a ball would be pressed out; *sticking* pains; sharp pains."

Nervous headaches usually confined to one spot, a foramen or ganglion of nerves, *e. g.,* supra-orbital foramen. The sensation is as if a *sharp nail were being driven into* the *brain.* For a *congestive* menstrual headache amel. by having the head low (Sanguinaria). I have met one case in which were marked symptoms of *hydrocephalus.* It was a case resulting from giving laudanum and checking stools of entero-colitis of a teething baby. There were spasms of the throat, eyes and mouth, one cheek red, one pale, both hot. Chamomilla had failed but Ignatia cured. *Sighing* was the ranking symptom.

Stomach: I will give you but one symptom here, viz., "hiccough." I found this once in a case of a smoker, who for some reason he could not give me, suddenly became aversed to his cigars. However, when his desire for the quieting effect overcame his aversion and he smoked, attacks of hiccough would follow, accompanied by nausea. Ignatia 30 cured.

Stools: "Stools thin, *involuntary,* small and frequent."

The only remedy which will more often be called for in *emotional diarrhea* is Gelsemium. As has already been stated grief is the cause of the diarrheic stool of Ignatia. The patient *fears something* terrible *will happen* to *some one else,* or it may have happened; while with Gelsemium it is *for oneself* that there is fear or that something has happened. With the diarrhea caused by fright or other emotion, there is usually much flatus in the abdomen which causes an ineffectual desire for stool (Cantharis). Like Nux, Ignatia may have *constipation alternating with diarrhea.*

Urinary Organs: "*Frequent voiding of watery urine;*

The most notable condition I have noticed in this section is the "watery" urine. As stated above I find it present in hysteria. The most marked case I ever saw in which the symptom was one of the group was a dark-haired, nervous girl of ten. The amount of urine passed in 24 hours was 11 pints, the sp. grav. was only 1001–2, constant sighing was the only other symptom. Ingatia 30th checked the condition at once. As the parents would or could assign no cause, I assumed it was a case of discipline.

Retention of *urine* (Belladonna) *after confinement* and during the menses has often yielded to the remedy.

Rectum: "*Prolapsus ani from moderate exertion at stool* (Podophyllum), *frequent, sharp, cutting pains* in anus (Silica, Sulphur), contraction and soreness (Lycopodium, Silica), ineffectual urging, in evening from middle of abdomen with protrusion of rectum."

Anus: "Blind piles, with pressure in anus and rectum, *painful when sitting* and *standing* (Æsculus), less when walking, *agg. after taking fresh air;* occasionally for *fissures with constipated* stool (Silica)."

For *bleeding hemorrhoids.* Rarely for prolapsus following confinement (Podophyllum). Violent itching of anus caused by swelling due to acrid stools. This itching causes many of the nervous symptoms, even hysteria.

Sexual Organs: "Erections on going to stool; menses late; lasciviousness with prominence of clitoris."

The most prominent symptom here is *suppression of menses,* prominent *because* with it are *associated* many of the *mental symptoms* also because it is *of frequent occurrence* in Ignatia women.

It has often quieted *labor-like pains during gestation,* caused by emotions, and by so doing *prevented miscarriage* (Actea rac.). Finally if you have the *weak, sinking* sensation in stomach *amel. by eating* in *morning,* sickness of pregnancy, Ignatia will cure.

Respiratory Organs: "*Provocation* in larynx *to hacking cough* in evening on lying down, *not amel. by suppressing* the *cough;* inability to talk; *inspiration impeded* as from a load on the chest, *expiration* just so much *easier.*"

Let us combine these with the symptoms of the throat section for a better understanding of both.

Throat: "*Sticking when not swallowing, the more he swallows, the more it disappears, entirely relieved by swallowing* anything *solid;* choking *constriction in* middle of the *esophagus,* in the evening, *from a plug agg.* when not swallowing; crawling."

The symptoms of these two sections enter into groups representing: *nervous spasms of the glands, globus hystericus, hysterical aphonia,* sympathetic cough *reflex from* the *stomach,* rectum (worms), *ovaries, uterus, etc.*

Many cases of *diphtheria* have been *cured by Ignatia.* In all throat and respiratory organ affections the unexpected, contrary symptoms should be the *ranking,* guiding ones.

Extremities: "*Jerking on falling asleep* (Chamomilla), crawling, asleep sensation; twitching of deltoid; *jerking* in forearm *as if a mouse were crawling under the skin;* sticking, jerking, bruised pain in posterior muscles of the thigh; tearing in back of legs; worse in tendo-achilles and its muscles as if the parts would be cut off, agg. by standing."

For *sciatica* generally *occurring* in the *fall.* The pains are violent, burning in character; always preceded by coldness and accompanied by coldness and shivering. It generally comes at night and is worse from warmth and quiet. The patient is forced to get up and walk to get relief.

If you *noticed* the sensation of "*mouse crawling under skin,*" you *thought* of *aura* and *epilepsy*. Ignatia will cure some cases caused by fright.

Chorea has very often been cured by Ignatia. I think the ranking symptom of this group is *amel. motion*. I had one case of a nervous, anemic girl of nine years, who would begin to twitch about the face, arms and legs if she could not have her own way. All choreic motions ceased if the mother took her by the hand and went for a walk. It was necessary to walk till the patient was tired.

Thermic Centers.

The above are a part of the nervous symptoms and conditions of Ignatia. I must not bore you with more but I cannot close without saying a word about the intermittent fever which the drug will cure because it shows the characteristic modalities, viz., *thirst during chill,* no thirst during fever, *heat relieved* by *covering* up warm, one ear red and hot, the other pale and cold; one day heat first, the next chill first, the third sweat, or all mixed up (Arsenicum). Ignatia seldom cures a case of intermittent but clears up the case so that the indicated remedy may be selected and cure.

NUX MOSCHATA.

Make-up: Neurotic: changeable; dark.

Loc.: Sensorium; nerves; female generative organs.

Sen.: Faint; sleepy; cold; dryness.

Mod.: Agg. emotions, menstruation, pregnancy, cold, damp wind or drafts.

Amel. dry weather; warm room.

Leaders: *Extreme dryness* of *mouth* and *throat without thirst,* marked distention of abdomen.

Brain and Nerves.

Mind: "Confusion, coma, *unconsciousness; inability to think;* indifference to everything; a senseless, intoxicated condition when reading which passed into sleepiness; incoherent; faint (Moschus, Sepia, Digitalis, Cocculus)."

For *general tendency* to syncope from many causes, I cured with the 30th a case of dysmenorrhea, the patient becoming completely unconscious with the severe pain which came in paroxysms. The menstrual flow was at times bright red and free, at others dark, scanty, clotted. Just before the dark clots were expelled came the severe cramping pain and the syncope.

We also have *hysterical* coma or *unconsciousness.* I had a patient who had these attacks when her husband came home drunk. One day the man came and found her stretched out on her bed. A note on the table stated she had taken poison. Powder papers by the side of bed were supposed to confirm the fact of suicide. I found the pulse regular at 60, breathing 16, temperature normal. As I had seen her in this condition before, I told the husband to let her sleep. Twelve hours after, no change having taken place, I tried the reflex, to find them all abolished. I told the husband it was hysterical catalepsy but put a trained nurse in charge. Twelve hours more and the nurse's statement was no change, no stool, no urine, no movement of the muscles. Had Dr. W. H. Dickinson see her with me. In his examination he broke her finger nail without her flinching. No change till after 75 hours, when she gave up and said she made up her mind to frighten her husband into a total abstainer. But she failed. I had just seen a case in consultation with Dr. H. S. Aldrich of a young girl—19—who was very fond of nutmegs, and while making pies one Saturday A.M. she grated and ate a whole nutmeg. About 4 P.M. Dr. A. was called because the maid was unconscious. Pulse and respiration normal, perfectly quiet. Sunday A.M. there had been no change. The use of catheter showed bladder was empty. Expectant treatment. Monday A.M. no change. Monday P.M. I saw her. Strong aqua ammonia caused a little turning of the head when it was held to the nose. Strong vinegar on a cloth over the nose caused her to regain consciousness, when she told us about eating the nutmeg.

When case 1 had another hysterical attack some six months after the one recorded she was given Nux mosch. 30th and never had a return although the husband kept getting drunk.

In some cases of *hysteria* there has been *profuse urination;* in others *urine scanty* or *suppressed;* some cases have been extremely hilarious but with most there has been unconsciousness.

Head: "Head dropped forward with the chin resting on the breast, could be raised with difficulty; was obliged to support it with hands, it seemed so bulky and rolled about; pain in spots; agg. hot weather."

This congestive headache comes from overloading stomach or at times of menses. There is always drowsiness.

Eyes: For ptosis there is one symptom in regard to vision that goes in the hysterical group, viz., "*everything looked large.*"

Heart: "Awful feeling, feeling as if blood rushed to it, thence to head, then over whole body; again to heart and repeat."

This condition is found in persons whose heart muscles and valves seem perfectly sound. The attack often ends in syncope.

Female Generative Organs.

We do not get anything from the provers which is marked, but clinically we find in addition to the dysmenorrhea and syncope frequent *suppression of menses* with all the symptoms mentioned above. It is hard to tell which is cause and which is effect. The suppressed menses have been caused from emotion, *i. e.*, followed it; again the syncope, mental excitement and emotion have followed the suppression of the menses from going bathing in cold water. The 30th seems to act best.

COFFEA CRUDA.

Make-up: Irritable, restless; lean; tall; dark.

Loc.: Nerves; *circulation;* sexual organs.

Sen.: *Sleeplessness,* trembling; weary.

Mod.: Agg. Noise; touch; mental exertion.
Amel. Lying down; rest.

Leaders: *Sleeplessness;* can't bear pain or noise; *acutely sensitive.*

Brain and Nerves.

Mind: "*Unusual activity* of *mind* and body *till midnight;* lively fancies; great anguish; cannot be composed; *power to think increased;* excessive *weeping* and lamentation at trifles."

For *delirium tremens* when the *hands* and even the body *tremble;* extreme *restlessness,* full of fear; thinks he is not at home. Such patients are in the habit of using *champagne,* not beer nor whisky.

For *sleeplessness* when the patient is of *nervous temperament;* easily affected. She cannot sleep because the *brain* is so *active.* Everything is running through her mind. Sometimes the *thoughts* are unusually *pleasant,* again extremely *sad.* There is no pain *if* the thoughts are *pleasant,* she *lies quiet* and revels in them. *If sad* she is *restless* and tries to get away from them. She may lie awake all night because of some remark made to her, either of praise or condemnation.

For *hysteria* with *repeated attacks* of *weeping and laughing,* tremulousness, excitability, *sleeplessness.* May be the *result* of *pleasurable emotions.* I recall a case of an extremely excitable, well educated, ambitious little woman, who went into hysterical attacks of weeping and laughing with all sorts of silly action and talk, on hearing over the phone that her husband had been elected to a position for which he was running. Coffea 30th in all such cases.

Teeth: "Sticking, jerking pains from above downwards into the nerves of the roots of teeth, amel. cold."

Coffea is even better than Pulsatilla for toothache which is intolerable and can only be endured by holding ice water in mouth.

Female Generative Organs: We have no symptoms here from the provers but clinically we find Coffea a most valuable remedy for the *"after pains" of nervous, excitable women.* The patient says the pains are unbearable, that she *must* have morphine or *something* to relieve her from such *terrible suffering.* You will find that such women have suffered from uterine hemorrhages, the menses having been dark and clotted, especially the first day, also that there is extreme sensitiveness of the genitals (Platinum). Also that they have been subject to hysteria.

The woman I referred to above kept the nurses and myself busy for sometimes after her confinements even with the use of Coffea. This is all there is to the drug. It should be classed with Platinum, Scutellaria, Zinz. phos. and Chamomilla.

COCCULUS.

Make-up: *Neurotic;* overworked; *sleepless.*

Loc: *Brain and nerves;* blood.

Sen.: *Vertigo;* restlessness; *weakness;* griping; distention.

Mod.: Agg. from *motion* of *car,* boat or *carriage;* anxiety; night watching; emotion.

Leaders: Vertigo; occiput seems to open and shut; empty, hollow feeling.

Brain and Nerves.

Mind: "*Mania* with irresistable inclination to sing; *sad,* as if he suffered an insult; *sensitive,* everything offends; absorbed in self; sudden anxiety as if she had committed a crime; sits in deep thought; stupefied."

The Cocculus mind seems *benumbed.* The patient cannot think; cannot express himself, *has lost control of himself.* The causes which bring about this condition are: severe prolonged mental exertion and prolonged loss of sleep, sometimes also suppression of the menses.

Head: "Confusion and stupefaction worse from drinking and eating; dullness and confusion, must read a passage over several times in order to understand it; vertigo, on rising up in bed compelling him to lie down; vertigo as from intoxication, with dullness in forehead as if a board were across forehead (Rhus tox.); headache as if the eyes would be torn out; aching as if something forcibly closed the eyes."

For *sick headaches* caused by worry, loss of sleep, overwork; *riding* in all kinds of *motors*. Whatever the cause *vertigo* is a *constant symptom* of the *group*. With the headaches you have the extreme *sensitiveness* of the drug, the *nausea* and vomiting; also marked insomnia especially when loss of sleep is the cause. It seems as though the patient had lost the habit of sleeping, or rather formed the habit of not sleeping.

Stomach: "*Aversion to food;* even the smell of food causes aversion (Colchicum); nausea when riding in a wagon; griping; pinching; sensation as if a worm were moving in stomach."

All the *stomach symptoms* are of *nervous* origin and are usually associated with the head symptoms. You never find ulceration, very rarely inflammation. The desires and aversions are marked; eating and drinking agg. all the symptoms. Weakness and faintness are usually present.

Abdomen: "*Distention by flatulency,* waking about midnight, causing oppressive pains here and there, some flatus passed without much relief, new *fltus collected for hours,* relived by lying on one side or the other; *griping in epigastrium* taking away the breath; *painful inclination* to inguinal *hernia;* internal feeling in groins as if stuffed."

Useful mainly for two conditions, viz., *flatulent colic* and *hernia.* The flatulent colic may come during pregnancy. The hernias are the result of loss of nervous tone of the abdominal muscles plus the enormous distention. It acts like Lycopodium in causing hernia.

Female Generative Organs: "*Cutting, contractive pains* in pelvis and abdomen."

Cocculus cured a patient who, in addition to the above sensation, would become unconscious when the pains reached their height. Nux moschata is the only other remedy I have successfully used for menstrual colic producing unconsciousness. With the menstrual colic of Cocculus the patient complains of a sensation in lower abdomen as if the parts were being rubbed or squeezed between some sharp, rough bodies.

Extremities and Back: "*Trembling of hands* when eating, worse the higher the hand is raised; now one *hand,* now the other *insensible and asleep; knees threaten* to *sink* from weakness, he *totters when walking* and threatens to fall to one side; feet and hands alternately asleep; paralytic pains in small of back, with drawing across the hips preventing walking."

The trembling and weakness are a part of the general nervous group. The paralysis usually follows the convulsions of the muscles in various parts of the body and is usually transient. The case in which paralysis of the extremities was most prolonged was purely hysterical. Spinal irritation is a prominent and frequent condition. Some cases of cerebro-spinal meningitis have been reported cured by Cocculus.

Blood.

In the clinical of Allen Handbook under the heading of fever you find some of its uses in intermittent and typhoid fever, but I have never met any such cases. Use the low and medium potencies.

MOSCHUS.

Make-up: Neurotic; excitable, *hysterical.*

Loc.: *Sensory nerves;* genitals, respiration.

Sen.: Twitching; cramping; trembling; cold.

Mod.: Agg. excitement; suppressions.

Amel. fresh, open air.

Leaders: Frequently recurring, easy fainting in attacks of hysteria. "Patient faints completely away from the least excitement."

Brain and Nerves.

Mind: "*Anxious;* fretful; easily excited."

Melancholia of hysterical patients when the pulse becomes rapid, soft, and tremulous, followed by complete syncope.

Head: "Aching deep in the brain on violent motion, agg. in evening with coldness as from cold application."

Moschus cures violent *neuralgic headache* with the sensation of coldness, amel. in fresh air, agg. warmth of room. The cause is usually suppression.

Menses: "Menses irregular; dragging towards genitals as if menses would appear."

Useful for suppression of menses (Sulphur, Pulsatilla, Platinum) with globus hystericus, choking sensation, general spasms and *fainting.*

Respiratory Organs: "Sudden sensation in upper part of larynx as if it closed upon the breath; breathing oppressed and she must take a deep breath; short respiration amel. during rest."

Many of the cases calling for Moschus have in the group of symptoms the *spasmodic constriction* of *larynx and chest,* causing a sense of impending suffocation. They are the ranking symptoms in *asthma, angina pectoris, hysteria, whooping-cough* and *laryngismus stridulus.* Many of these attacks are brought on by excitement, laughing and eating. It seems to work better in the 30th and upward.

COLCHICUM AUTUMNALE.

Make-up: Gouty and rheumatic diathesis.

Loc.: Heart; muscles; digestive tract; kidneys; skin.

Sen.: Tingling; nausea; icy coldness; *tenesmus;* weakness.

Mod.: Agg. from mental or physical exertion; night and evening; from *cold* or *damp;* lying on left side."

Amel. from warmth and bending forward.

Leaders: *Acute sense of smell;* nausea; *loathing* the sight or *smell of food; cold, weak* but *restless,* with tendency to collapse.

Heart.

"Trembling in the precordial region with sticking; anxiety in the precordial region provoking sighing; oppression obliging deep inspiration; dull, irregular, suppressed beats; with indescribable sensation in chest; fullness as from stagnation of blood; impulse not felt, even heard with difficulty, a blowing sound like a heart heard at a distance; pulse small, weak, irregular, at times rapid, at times slow, intermittent, scarcely perceptible."

Very useful in chronic or subacute *bronchitis* with water in the pericardium, marked dyspnea, contraction as from a tight band around the chest. In these cases you will find the heart's action weak and indistinct, the pulse often thread-like. It is also with these cases that you get the icy-cold feeling at pit of stomach. In the personal history of your patient you will find the record of attacks of gout or rheumatism.

Muscles.

Extremities: "Drawing, sticking, jerking pains in joints of fingers, toes, wrists and ankles; also in shoulder and knee. worse during rest; rheumatic pains in hands and feet so that she could not bear to have her finger joints pressed or extended from their semi-flexed position; joints stiff, red and feverish: *paralytic pain so that he cannot hold the lightest thing firmly.*"

With *both* the *gouty and rheumatic diathesis* you have the *mental irritability* of the drug. With both you also have the extreme soreness so that the patient cannot have the part touched or any one come near him. With the *gouty diathesis* you *have* the *gastric irritability;* with the *rheumatic* more of the *cardiac* complications and sequellæ.

Urinary Organs.

Kidneys: "Urine scanty, dark, dark brown, bloody, with strangury."

For *acute and chronic nephritis.* In both conditions you have in addition to the above, pain in back and sacrum, worse from pressure, from stretching out the legs; also the *icy coldness* of the *extremities* and in *stomach.* The kidney conditions usually follow attacks of rheumatism and precede or accompany the heart conditions.

Digestive Tract.

Stomach: "Great appetite for different things but *as soon as he sees them,* or, worse, *smells them,* he shudders from nausea and *cannot eat;* appetite lost; unquenchable thirst for cold water, violent vomiting with watery diarrhea relieved by bending himself up and lying still; burning in epigastrium; coldness in pit of stomach."

For *gastritis* accompanied by violent attacks of gastralgia with the above symptoms. The causes are: repression of gout; grief; getting wet; checked perspiration; and inherited rheumatic diathesis.

Abdomen: "Distended as if she had eaten too much; spasmodic contraction before vomiting; tenderness."

Rectum: "Tenesmus; with only a little fecal matter at first then transparent, bilious, membranous mucus with relief of colic; tenesmus relieved by frequent passage of flatus."

Anus: "Spasm of sphincter, with chilliness running up the back, then urging to stool and insufficient stool."

Stools: "*Contained many white shreds;* slimy and bloody with tenesmus; copious; offensive."

One word as to the "*white shreds*" and "*membranous mu-*

cus." They are the ***product*** of an ***organized exudate.*** In a few cases this exudate was exhibited by the patients and in one case by the doctor, with the expression, "See! the lining of the intestines!" In all of these cases careful examination proved the substance to be the vitiated product of the mucous membrane and not the membrane itself. We do not get the intense inflammation and destruction of the mucous membrane in Colchicum that we do in Mercurius cor. but we get more exudation. Most *frequently useful in dysentery.*

Skin.

We have no symptoms of either first or second rank from the provers. Allen, however, taught us that "tingling in finger nails" was found in no other remedy and hence was characteristic of Colchicum. I have never found the symptom but have used Colchicum in a few cases for prolonged desquamation and following enormous distention of the skin of the lower extremities in a case of dropsy. Apis had removed the swelling but the skin remained livid, dry and rough. I was led to its use by the stool which was clearly that of Colchicum. The abuse of the use of Colchicum in its various forms by the old school, given in large doses, shows the benefit of our method of preparing and administering drugs. The 3rd, 6th and 12th are the potencies most frequently used.

BORAX.

Make-up: Pale; flabby; irritable; sickly.

Loc.: Mucous membrane; nerves; urinary organs.

Sen.: Sticking; dryness; fretful; irritable.

Mod.: Agg.: Warm weather; after menses.

Amel. *downward motion.*

Leaders: The peculiar aphthous group; viz., *white patches* with *red areolæ, hot mouth, hot urine* making the child cry when urinating.

Mucous Membrane.

Eyes: "Eye lashes turn inward toward the eye and inflame it, especially at the outer canthus, where the margin of lids are very sore."

For *blepharitis* with much soreness of the lids and agglutination after sleep. The margin of lids is very red (Sulphur).

Mouth: "*Mouth of infant very hot* (Kali chlor., Silica); mucous membrane of fore part of palate shrivelled, as if burnt, with pain agg. by chewing; aphthæ on the inside of the cheek, bleeding when eating; taste bitter, if patient eats anything or swallows saliva everything tastes bitter (Bryonia)."

A frequently indicated remedy for *aphthous sore mouth,* the *ulcers bleed easily,* the white of the center is surrounded by little red points, the mouth is hot and dry; the patients are irritable; the *children scream before* and during *micturition* because the urine is hot *and contains red sediment;* the stools are soft, light-yellow, offensive with this mouth group.

Urinary Organs: "Frequent urination, often with cries before the urine passes (Nux vom.); urging to urinate, often ineffectual; *smarting, in the urethra, after urinating;* pain in the orifice as if sore after urinating; *urine hot* (Cantharis); pungent odor (Benzoic ac.)."

For a *urethritis,* usually of children suffering from stomatitis, when there are little red particles left in the diapers.

Female Generative Organs: "*Leucorrhea like the white of an egg,* with sensation as if warm water were flowing, as thick as paste and white; menses irregular, too soon, too late; menses profuse with griping in abdomen, nausea and pain in stomach extending into small of back."

For *dysmenorrhea, often membranous.* It is one of the few remedies with which I have cured *membranous* dysmenorrhea. The others are Sepia, Sulphur, Natrum mur. The two patients which Borax cured of membranous dysmenorrhea had an unhealthy, itching skin, the mucous membrane of the vagina was inflamed before and after the menses, and there was a profuse, acrid, albuminous leucorrhea. The pains during the menses were like labor pains and the membranous shreds were large and numerous. The uterus had been curetted on several occasions. Both women were barren before taking the Borax but both had children after taking it. I used the 6th in one case and the 30th in the other.

Sleep.

The sleep of Borax is worth special attention as it often leads to the discovery of the urinary condition and aphthæ. From the provers we have: "Wakes at 3 A.M. and cannot sleep again for two hours on account of general heat, especially in the head with sweat on the thighs." From patients cured by the remedy we have: "*An infant cries out, wakes from sleep and anxiously grasps its mother, as if* he had been *frightened by a dream;* the child tosses about, cries till 4 A.M., frequently cries out while sleeping, and in the morning is in a whining mood."

These symptoms are caused by the condition of the urinary organ as stated above. Examine the urine also the diaper and urinary organs. Use 6th and 30th.

KREOSOTUM.

Make-up: Dark; lean; leucophlegmatic; sad; irritable.

Loc.: Female generative organs; digestive tract; gums; teeth; *blood.*

Sen.: *Burning;* itching; soreness.

Mod.: Agg.: *Dentition;* rest; after eating.
Amel.: Warmth; motion.

Leaders: Profuse, acrid, foul discharges; early decay of teeth; vomiting; burning.

Teeth and Gums.

"*Jerking, throbbing,* drawing *pain* in hollow *teeth* and teeth which are beginning to decay; drawing pain in upper gum with inflammation; gums bluish red, soft, spongy, bleed easily; bad odor from decayed teeth."

I give you this location first because I have used Kreosotum more frequently for it than the others. The symptom which ranks the highest is a clinical one, viz., "*early decay of teeth.*" Before giving the other symptom of the group let me say a word about this. The *teeth begin* to decay *in* the *enamel* and transversely, next to and parallel to the gums. A little black stub is left in the unhealthy gum. In addition to the decayed teeth and unhealthy gums the child has a *white, coated tongue,* a *foul breath;* nausea and *vomiting* which is persistent, *of undigested food* even hours after eating; profuse saliva of bad odor and *cadaverous* smelling *stools* which *contain undigested food.* These symptoms you will not usually get from the mother without quizzing her. She will come to you to see what you can do for baby's teeth. Seven tenths of my Kreosotum patients with the above group of symptoms are babies and half of them will add one more symptom, viz., "*bedwetting,*" which comes during the first sleep. If old enough they will tell you that they dream they are urinating during the act (Pulsatilla). For this condition use the 12th and 30th.

Female Generative Organs.

The second location in regard to frequency is the female generative organs. From the provers we have: "*Burning between pudenda on urinating; soreness between labiæ* and *thighs* with *burning* (like fire), biting pain, *corrosive itching* between labiæ and in vagina, then burning and swelling in labiæ; vagina itching in the evening, then smarting; external genitals swollen, hot and hard, and on urinating sore pains in vagina; *discharge from vagina* white (Graphites), and of the *odor of green corn;* yellow leucorrhea, staining linen yellow, causing itching and biting on external genitals with weakness in the legs."

A very valuable remedy for *leucorrhea* following inflammation, also ulceration of cervix and vagina. The characteristic symptom of the group being the peculiar sickening odor of green corn; for *cauliflower excrescences* of the *uterus* with profuse ichorous discharge burning like red hot coals; frequently palliative in scirrhus of the *uterus* and *epithelioma* of the pudenda, also with the burning pains and offensive discharge. The menses of the Kreosote woman are too profuse and usually followed by the peculiar leucorrhea of the drug. With the menstrual irregularity I have occasionally found *swellings in* the *mammary glands,* a little hard, very sensitive lump *just before the menses which disappears when* the *flow begins.* For these conditions use the 3rd and 6th and in addition a 1 to 2000 solution of the 1x locally.

Digestive Tract.

We have already spoken about the mouth and teeth and included a few stomach symptoms in that group. The remaining stomach symptoms are: "Nausea with burning in the mouth; spitting of saliva and general chill, without heat or thirst; urging to vomit, nothing but saliva results; vomiting of sweetish water, of food, in the morning when fasting."

For the *vomiting* of *pregnancy* when the food which was eaten the night before is undigested, and the stools are diarrheic, offensive and also contain undigested food. There is also soreness at the pit of stomach, often vomiting.

Blood.

Changes in the blood simulate those which take place in the blood in only two conditions, viz., *diphtheria* and *tuberculosis.* The group for diphtheria is: *Burning* in the *throat,* much bloody, slimy saliva with the horrible odor and marked swelling of the glands of the neck. Its place in tuberculosis has not been definitely determined as yet. We have "*burning spots and soreness* in the *chest;* both dry and moist cough," the latter accompanied by "*expectoration sweet* in taste, mucous, bloody, and *very offensive* in odor." We also know that there is "*marked emaciation*" and "*loss of weight,*" all symptoms of tuberculosis. We further know that inhalation of Kreosotum vapors and the internal use have relieved many of the above symptoms. We further know that Kreosotum in malt and other media in the large doses usually given has done more harm than good. I feel, however, that I have checked the progress of t. b. c. of the lung and pharynx by the use of the 6th and proper diet. I also feel that the results accredited to kreosote on workers in smoke shops or from too much smoked meat are as much from the action upon the mucous membranes of the respiratory and digestive tracts as upon the blood. I hope we may make a thorough proving on our animals with the object of deciding this point, viz., its relation to tuberculosis.

MURIATIC ACID.

Make-up: Black hair; dark eyes.

Loc.: *Blood;* mucous membranes; skin; muscles.

Sen.: Weakness.

Mod.: Agg.: Touch; wet weather.
Amel.: Warmth.

Leaders: *Tendency to low typhoid condition; intense, burning heat* with aversion to coverings.

Mucous Membranes.

Mouth: "*Mucous lining of lips red,* inflamed *and painful,* stripped of epithelium to a considerable extent and *dotted with whitish points; tongue* thick, dark and with most of the *mouth fauces covered with* a *grayish-white membrane;* bluish and sore; painful blisters with burning on tongue; redness of the inside of cheek and arch of the palate; raw spot on palate with soreness; *fetid breath.*"

Aphthous sore mouth of ***nursing children or occurring in*** the *last stages of wasting diseases* are the two conditions most frequently calling for the drug. The other conditions are ***inflammation*** and ***ulceration of the tongue*** also ***epithelioma.*** The stomatitis of children presents the following symptoms: aphthous patches over entire surface, including the tongue; *fetid odor of breath;* diarrheic stools, also offensive; loss of appetite. For this condition use the 6th and a solution of 10 drops of the acid to four ounces of water. Have the mother or nurse wrap the finger with gauze, dip it into the solution and swab the entire mucous membrane, taking special care to get into the buccal cavity. If the child is old enough, have him wash out the mouth with the solution. Cleanse the mouth before feeding or giving medicine.

For the stomatitis of wasting diseases use the 3rd instead of the 6th but the solution the same as in the other variety.

For the *epithelioma* of the *tongue with* the *bluish-red edges* use a stronger solution, 10 drops to two ounces of water, locally, and use the 6th internally. It is with this condition that you have the "*burning*" and "soreness in spots" of the provers.

Throat: "Swelling of uvula, tonsils, of mucous lining of fauces with inability to swallow, the attempt causing spasm and choking; mucus that he must swallow; grayish-white deposits, then ulcers; dead white patches over velum and pillars of palate, tonsils and posterior part of pharynx like the false membrane of diphtheritic angina."

We use Muriatic ac. in this section for ***non-diphtheritic angina*** when besides the above we find the *lips sore, cracked, scabby;* redness, rawness and soreness of the fauces and larynx. Treat this condition as you did infantile stomatitis.

Most of the above symptoms are present in the diphtheritic

form and in addition you have the "*putrid breath*" and the *diphtheritic baccilli* which appear early in this form; irritable stomach with vomiting; albuminous urine; drowsiness and sometimes stupor. Here use the swab, the gargle when you can and the 3x.

Anus: "Swollen *hemorrhoids* with burning sore pain (Nitric ac.), blue swollen hemorrhoids with pain and pressure; itching before, cutting during and burning after stools."

The *hemorrhoids* are *agg.* by *cold water,* amel. by warmth. They are found in three conditions: first with the *stomatitis of infants,* bluish in color and very sensitive, second of *pregnancy,* bluish-red and very sore, third *after child-birth,* when you have excruciating pains with the prolapsus ani. Here *use* your weaker *solution hot* for an application and bathing the parts.

Blood.

Changes simulating those which take place in *diphtheria; carbuncles; scarlet fever, typhoid* and *remittent.*

Carbuncles with red, *angry, bleeding* ulcers especially with the *scorbutic gums* and ulcers on other parts of the body. Malignant scarlet fever when the rash is rough and irregular, when you have great prostration, rapid, weak pulse but especially when the *mouth* is *filled with ulcers.*

The typhoid picture of Muriatic ac. is a gloomy one. The *patient* lies in a *stupid,* often *unconscious,* condition and yet he is restless, rarely quiet; the *mouth* is *open, covered* with *aphthous patches,* usually with a horribly foul discharge; the *tongue* is dark and *dry;* the discharges are involuntary, stools offensive, marked tendency to hemorrhage (Nitric ac., China); the patient is *constantly sliding down in bed; bed sores* come *easily* and are *difficult* to manage, with bad odor. Give the 3x five drops in an ounce of water; always have the nurse cleanse the mouth and teeth before giving medicine or food.

PETROLEUM.

Make-up: Persons with an unhealthy skin.

Loc.: *Skin;* M.M.; nerves.

Sen.: Sticking; burning; *sore;* cutting.

Mod.: Agg.: *Motion,* cars or boats; *cold. Winter weather;* eating; worry.

Amel.: Warm air.

Leaders: Vertigo; nausea; rough, thick, *cracked skin,* with *deep fissures* which are excruciatingly sore and bleed easily, agg. by cold.

Skin.

"Finger-tips rough, cracked, with cutting, sticking pains in them (Graphites); hands cracked and rough; redness behind the ears with rawness, soreness and moisture; skin unhealthy suppurates readily and spreads; boils on nape of neck with moist eruption, great soreness preventing motion of the head."

Petroleum has been used for *herpes zoster, eczema, psoriasis* of hands, *intertrigo,* ulceration and *fissures.*

The only success I have had with the drug has been for *fissures* usually of the fingers. Many farmers have come to me during husking time with deep fissures of the fingers, and tips which become so sore they cannot use them. They bleed easily and are greatly agg. by the cold weather. I give five drops of the 6th, four times daily and have them stick the fingers into cots lubricated with crude petroleum at night.

I have also used it for *eczema* or *herpes* of the *perineum.* There is a great deal of *moisture* and often fissures with much *burning* and *smarting.*

It has also been used with success for the *eruption* of *secondary syphilis,* especially of the scrotum which is fiery red almost raw, with burning, smarting and much oozing of a thick, glossy, acrid fluid (Staphisagria).

Mucous Membranes.

Eyes: "Stitches and itching; burning and pressure; inflammation of conjunctiva and lids."

Useful for *conjunctivitis* and *blepharitis*, usually accompanied by lachrymal fistulæ.

Ears: "Swelling of meatus; inflamed and painful; diminished hearing, with roaring as of wind; ringing; cracking at times."

It has helped *catarrh* of the *Eustachian* tube with the noises and hardness of hearing also for otorrhea when the discharge leaves rawness and soreness of the skin (Tellurium).

Nose: "Ulcerated nostrils and stopped catarrh; with necessity to blow out small masses at night."

An excellent remedy for *post-natal catarrh*, discharge is purulent and obstructs the nasal passages. The odor is offensive. The *nostrils* are *full* of *cracks* which *bleed readily*. Use the petroleum ointment in connection with the internal remedy.

Throat: "Throat covered with mucus; rawness of pharynx on swallowing; dryness and burning; tickling on swallowing extending to ear."

Catarrh of the *pharynx* with a *sense* of *dryness* and *burning* notwithstanding the fact that there is *much mucus present*. The pains extend into the Eustachian tube.

Stomach: "Ravenous hunger often making her sick; hot, sharp, sour eructations; *nausea all day with accumulation of water in mouth; incessant* nausea; violent vomiting; empty feeling."

For acid dyspepsia with temporary amel. from eating (Pulsatilla, Anacardium). The pains are violent and extend into the chest with nausea and vomiting. Next to Cocc. it is our best remedy for nausea from riding in cars or boats (Seasickness). For *nausea* and *vomiting* of *pregnancy* due to gastric catarrh often accompanied by leucorrhea, like white of an egg."

Anus: "Burning pain in region of anus; itching, burning and weakness in anus."

For hemorrhoids and *fissures* of the *anus,* use the remedy locally as well as per mouth.

Stools: "Diarrhea of profuse bloody mucus, violent, often involuntary with weakness."

We find that the diarrhea is agg. during the day and is accompanied with *soreness along* the *colon.*

Brain and Nerves.

Mind: "*Imagined some one was lying near him* (Graphites); irritable; quarrelsome; violent; offended at trifles."

This peculiar symptom of the Petroleum patient that some one is lying in bed with him is marked. It has been verified many times in both typhoid and puerperal fever.

Head: "*Pressure in occiput* in the morning, also pinching, throbbing; *leaden heaviness in the occiput* (Picric ac., Chelidonium).

Petroleum is useful for *neuralgic headaches* which begin in occiput and go up into and over the head (Actea, Gelsemium, Agaricus). The pains are accompanied by stiffness of the neck and *vertigo,* sometimes nausea and numbness. The feeling of *numbness* is *general* and is *amel.* by *motion,* especially of the hands and arms.

Abdomen: "Distention; *cutting* with diarrhea; colic with retching."

For *gastralgia* and *enteralgia* amel. bending forward (Colocynth, Colchicum, Tabacum). With both conditions you have a sensation of coldness and faintness.

PHYTOLACCA.

Make-up: Muscular, rheumatic.

Loc.: Glands, mammary, tonsils and of the throat; fibrous tissues of neck, back and joints; bones; brain and nerves.

Sen.: Burning; sore; faint; stiff.

Mod.: Agg.: Hot drinks (Lachesis); heat of bed (Mercurius); swallowing; motion; cold damp.

Leaders: Stony hardness of the mammæ (Conium) with tendency to suppurate (Hep.).

Glands.

Throat: "*Tonsils* and *palate dark purple; tonsils swollen* and red; with soreness and dryness; fullness so that it felt choked; hawking, to rid throat and posterior nose of mucus; swallowing impossible with shooting through ears on attempting to."

For *follicular tonsilitis* with the *peculiar color* mentioned above, with *backache* and stiffness; *urine dark* and *scanty*, sometimes *albuminous;* tongue heavily coated; temperature from 101–104, *agg. warm drinks;* great prostration. For a *general sore throat* with the above symptoms minus the follicles in place of which you get ulceration. For *diphtheria* for the above group only substituting the *diphtheritic* exudate for the follicles. Next to the baccilli the *purple color of* the *membrane* and *high temperature* are the ranking symptoms of the diphtheria group. In my experience high temperature is not as bad a symptom in diphtheria as a subnormal temperature such as you get under Lachesis or Mercurius cyn.

"Mammary glands swollen, hard, painful; breasts full of painful hard nodosities."

It is for diseases of the mammæ that Phytolacca has won its reputation. Before it was proven and incorporated into our Materia Medica, the dairy maids used it for caked udders.

We use it for *mastitis* occurring during the first few days after child birth. The breasts have been enlarged, hard, painful. Now comes a slight chill, a rise in temperature, a slight line of demarcation which indicates that suppuration is about to take place. At this point Phytolacca 3rd, five drops every two hours, given internally and the tincture of Poke root, 1 part to 4 parts water, hot, applied to the breast, will prevent suppuration.

The second condition is for inflammation of the mammæ after the acute symptoms given above have subsided, but whenever the breasts fill with milk or the babe begins to nurse, violent pains begin at the nipple and radiate over the whole body, especially up and down the back bone.

Sometimes for *mastitis during pregnancy* with pains from nipples to all parts of body.

Finally for *tumors* of the *breasts* when the *axillary glands* are *enlarged,* the skin over the tumors red or purplish and the radiating pains. These tumors are apt to appear and disappear at the menstrual period (Kreosote).

Muscles and Joints.

Neck and Back: "Stiffness in the morning on waking, also at night; shooting in sacrum, extending down the outside of hips to the feet; sticking from within outward in various parts, always near the surface; rheumatic pains in arms and legs below elbows and knees."

Extremities: "*Sub-acute rheumatism* of the long bones or tendinous attachment of muscles. The pains are shooting, burning always agg. at night and during stormy weather (Mercurius, Rhus, Rhododendron). The pains fly from one part to another." There is a ranking symptom of this group, viz., "*very severe and obstinate pain in the heel* only amel. by keeping the heels higher than the body. Another symptom of high rank with the rheumatic group is "*patient pale* and *puffy.*" This is a *heart symptom showing* that we have a *complication,* of either gouty heart, fatty degeneration or endocarditis (Colchicum). The last condition of this section is syphilitic or gonorrheal *rheumatism* with swollen joints, also red and swollen; rheumatism with swollen joints, red swollen glands agg. by damp weather. Use 3rd, 6th, and 30th, also tincture locally.

RHODODENDRON.

Make-up: Sensitive to storms and changes of weather.

Loc.: Periosteum; brain and nerves; fibrous tissue.

Sen.: Tearing; drawing.

Mod.: Agg. *approach of stormy weather;* rough, cold, windy weather; rest.

Amel. heat, especially dry.

Leaders: The agg. of all symptoms on the approach of storms; rheumatic pains agg. cold, rough weather and amel. moving (Rhus tox.).

Fibrous Tissues.

Head: "Tearing, boring in the forehead spreading to the temples, agg. wine; as if everything would fall out."

For *rheumatic headaches* involving the *forehead* and temples with tearing of the bones of the skull. These pains are always *agg.* by *cold, wet weather* (Kali carb.) and *wine.* Amel. by wrapping the head up warm (Silica).

Neck: "Stiffness of the nape in the morning in bed and after rising, with rheumatic pains."

It has often relieved rheumatism of the tendons of the neck and periosteum with the modalities of the drug.

Back and Extremities: "A drawing, tearing, sprained pain in the bones of the lumbar region agg. rest and in rainy weather; pain as if one had been bent too long, amel. motion, agg. stooping; pain in bones or periosteum of the extremities, bruised, cramp-like on every change of weather."

For *rheumatism* not only when an attack is agg. by change of weather but when the condition which was apparently cured reappears before changes of weather.

There is one point of difference between this modality and a similar one of Rhus tox., namely, that the Rhododendron patient's pains are relieved when the storm breaks, while Rhus pains continue till the storm or rain is over.

Rhododendron has relieved many cases of rheumatoid arthritis.

Nerves.

Eye: "Burning *pain, and* on reading or writing *heat* in eyes."

For *ciliary neuralgia* accompanying muscular asthenopia threatening glaucoma in rheumatic or neuralgia patients. With the asthenopia the *pains dart through the eye.* Both have the *agg. before the storm* and *amel. after the storm breaks.*

Ears: "Pain in outer ear nearly all day; humming, buzzing, ringing; *sensation as if* water were rushing into them; loud sounds re-echo for a long time."

Very useful for otalgia of rheumatic patients who have the above symptoms and the modalities of the drug.

Teeth: "Drawing, cutting pain in teeth before a thunder-storm or cloudy, windy weather."

For *odontalgia* caused by cold *accompanied* by *tearing, jerking pains* in the *face* agg. by change of weather, amel. by eating and warmth.

Stools: "Diarrhea in damp weather; food passed undigested."

For *diarrhea* caused by eating green or over-ripe fruit *accompanied* by neuralgic *colic* in various parts of the abdomen, especially under the short ribs, *amel. eating.* Use the 6th and 30th.

RANUNCULUS BULBOSUS.

Make-up: Prone to vesicular eruptions.

Loc.: Brain and nerves; skin; mucous membranes.

Sen.: Stitching; burning; biting; sticking and smarting.

Mod: Agg. *Drafts* of damp; open, cold *air* (Hepar); alcohol; *motion of arms;* evening; change of weather.

Leaders: The bluish vesicles in herpes and the stitching, shooting pains, especially in the chest.

Brain and Nerves.

Mind: "Fear in the evening, does not want to be alone; fear of ghosts; thoughts vanish."

Head: "Distended feeling; confusion; vertigo making it difficult to think; pain in forehead and into eyes; pressure outward."

Neuralgic headaches in *forehead* and *vertex* as if forced asunder, agg. in evening, also on coming into a warm room. This headache usually *accompanies herpes frontalis.* The pain is very very violent *agg.* by *change* of weather (Rhododendron, Rhus tox.).

Eyes: "Pain in balls pressing out; pressing downward as with a dull point; vision misty."

For intense *ciliary neuralgia* and *iritis* usually following herpetic eruptions with the modalities of the drug.

Chest: *"Sticking pains above the nipples, agg. touch and motion;* sticking, *bruised pain* about the ribs, with *sensitiveness* of that spot to touch, the pain arresting breath, with stitches and pressure on top of shoulder; burning pain agg. moving, whether stooping or breathing, with pressure and tightness across the lower part of chest; bruised pain in region of short-ribs, with pain in the back, lassitude and ill humor."

The above are only a few of the many symptoms given by the provers. They represent five conditions; *inflammation* of the *diaphragm,* pleurodynia, *intercostal neuralgia, herpes zoster* and *muscular rheumatism.*

Besides these nervous manifestations one may have pleurisy or peritonitis.

Skin.

"Ulcers and vesicles on the fingers, dark blue elevated blisters the size of a pin's head with red skin underneath; burning and itching; itching, herpetic, horny scurf; groups of openings emitting yellow lymph-like drops of sweat, these openings changing into flat, spreading ulcers."

For *vesicular eruptions* and *ulcers* with the above symptoms especially the burning and itching.

One of our best remedies for *herpes zoster,* usually of the chest with the blue discharge and the burning and itching.

The pain is very severe just before the eruption and prostration is equally marked. This form of herpes seems to be found in older people. The seat of these herpetic eruptions may be about the eyes, lips, forehead and occasionally the genitals, but usually it is the trunk.

Mucous Membranes.

Nose: "Tingling pressing upward from tip to root and from root to brow and temple; frequent necessity to blow the nose, during which blood is discharged therefrom; stoppage in evening with painful soreness extending deep into the nose; discharge of tenacious mucus."

One of our leading remedies for *hay fever* (Arsenicum, Gelsemium, Euphrasia). There is smarting and burning in the eyes, the nose is stopped up, agg. evening, pressure at the root of nose. The *crawling, tingling sensation* in the *nostril* is the most annoying and obstinate of the group. The patient hawks, blows the nose and does everything to get rid of the sensation but without result, unless as is sometimes the case, blowing of the nose causes epistaxis.

CARBO VEGETABILIS.

Make-up: Loss of vitality; failing reaction.

Loc.: M.M. of the digestive tract especially of stomach; heart; blood; skin.

Sen.: *Weak; cold;* sharp; numb.

Mod.: Agg. *warmth* (Secale), *exhausting diseases; dissipation, especially eating;* extreme temperatures.

Leaders: *The pinched, blue or dusky face;* air hunger; cold, short breath; excessive flatulency with *rancid* belching and tendency to hemorrhage in low types of diseases (Lachesis (Muriatic ac.).

Mucous Membranes.

Ears: "Discharge of thick, flesh-colored, offensive moisture; ears seemed to be stopped up, something heavy seemed to lie in front of them; roaring, ringing."

For *otorrhea,* offensive, accompanied by deafness, with an excess of unhealthy cerumen and exfoliation of epidermoid cells. The otorrhea usually follows some of the exanthematous diseases.

Nose: "Ineffectual attempts to sneeze, with crawling and tickling in the nostrils; sneezing; dry coryza; bleeding several times daily, preceded and accompanied by pallor of the face."

For *epistaxis* in persons who have been overtaxed or have had prolonged debilitating diseases; especially in elderly people. Also for *nose bleed due* to *varicose veins* of the nose (Ammonium, Bovis.).

Mouth: "Teeth bleed when cleaned (Mercurius, Muriatic ac., Staphisagria); pure blood flows into the mouth after sucking the teeth; gums retracted (Silica and Mercurius); tongue coated white; also covered with dry, dark coating in typhoid fever, yellow and fissured in cholera."

Stomach: "*Aversion* to meat, especially *fat* meat (Pulsatilla); aversion to milk which makes him flatulent; *eructations* after eating or drinking agg. P.M.; violent; empty almost constant eructations; nausea in morning without vomiting; *contractions at night* extending into chest with distention of abdomen; pain in pit with sensitiveness to touch; the simplest food distresses; acidity when lying on the back and when walking."

That *Carbo veg. is homeopathic to flatulent dyspepsia* is proven by the fact that beneficial results are claimed for it whether used crude in large tablets or in the 30th. We use is, however, for the following symptoms: *stomach* swollen. *distended* like a drum; profuse, violent, sour *eructations; distress* which comes from 30 to 60 minutes after eating; complete *inertia* of the stomach so that the simplest food lies in stomach till it ferments; foul breath; a brown, slimy, putrid diarrhea; pulse small and weak; frequency of dyspnea; coldness of the extremities, sometimes of the whole body.

Stools: "Diarrhea, partly mucous; bloody."

The *stools of Carbo veg.* as described by the above symptoms usually *accompany low types of fevers*. They have a *putrid odor*, are often involuntary (Hyoscyamus), are brown or dark yellow, *often slimy*. There is coldness of the extremities, of the tongue and breath, especially if there are cholera symptoms. The *pulse* is *weak*, the *air hunger marked* and there is a tendency to complete collapse.

Female Generative Organs: "Aphthæ of pudenda; red sore places looking like ulcers; milky, *excoriating*, copious, thin, *leucorrhea*."

In addition to the above leucorrheal condition, the *mucous membrane of the vagina is studded with varicose veins*, oozing blood, which is offensive (Ammonium). The varicose condition and the leucorrhea are agg. just before the menses, which are early, profuse, thick, dark and offensive (Belladonna).

Respiratory Organs: "Roughness of the larynx with deep, rough voice which failed if he exerted it but without pain in the throat (Phosphorus); rawness and soreness in the evening from frequent clearing of throat; pain in region of the thyroid cartilage as if ulcerated; hoarseness so that speaking aloud was difficult; dryness in trachea not amel. by hawking: cough from itching in larynx with tenacious salty expectoration of pieces of green mucus."

For *chronic laryngeal catarrh* of old people, with rawness and soreness in larynx: also *chronic bronchitis* of old people, with *burning* in the chest and *strangulation on coughing*, amel. by heat. The *cough* is *spasmodic* as well as suffocative.

It has helped me in a few desperate cases of *pneumonia*, last stage, with *marked dyspnea, cold breath*, general coldness, weak pulse and a tendency to collapse. Finally for *pulmonary hemorrhage* with the burning pains in lungs, coldness of the skin and desire to be fanned.

Heart: " *Weakness of the chest* on waking; burning in chest as from glowing coals; pulse weak; palpitation."

Useful for the ***break in compensation*** and ***fatty degeneration*** when you have the dyspnea, the desire to be fanned, the cold sweat and coldness in general.

Skin.

"Fine itching on the hands; boils and ulcers surrounded by pimples; *offensive pus* from *ulcers* which are very ***sensitive*** (Asafœtida)."

When I began the study of medicine, pulverized charcoal and Stramonium leaves were the two ingredients for poultices for indolent ulcers with offensive discharges. I occasionally use them now, with Carbo veg. 30th internally.

Blood.

It is one of our tried remedies for certain types of low fevers and sepsis, *e. g., yellow, typhoid* fevers and ***puerperal sepsis.*** In all we have the ***putrid discharges,*** the ***coldness,*** the ***prostration.*** Let me give you a case as an illustration; was called with an old school physician to see Mrs. H., aged 24, who had been delivered of a child five days previous. There had been a good deal of hemorrhage due to retained placenta. On the third day a chill, followed by the usual septic temperature. I found the face pale, pinched and cold; the ***stomach*** and ***abdomen greatly distended;*** the pulse rapid, weak and intermittent; stools involuntary and very offensive; lochia scanty but foul; varicose veins of right leg; urine very scanty, and the nurse fanning the patient though the windows of the room were all open.

I suggested Carbo veg. The Dr. said, "Good, have you any with you?" When I took out my vial of the 30th, he exclaimed, "*Hell! white charcoal.*" She was given a gr. of powder every hour for 12 doses and then began to improve.

She is alive after 25 years and has in her possession a most beautiful obituary written because her old school Dr. went from her to her aunt's home just after the first powder was given and reported that the patient would be dead in less than an hour. I am thankful that this remedy is seldom indicated for outside of the dyspepsia all conditions for which it is indicated are desperate ones. I never use any but the 30th except the crude for poultices.

BERBERIS VULGARIS.

Make-up: *Rheumatic* and lithic diatheses.

Loc.: Urinary and digestive tracts; liver.

Sen.: Shooting; sticking; colicky; spasmodic; sharp.

Mod.: Agg. from motion; *jarring;* rising from sitting position.

Leaders: Pains following the ureter and the reddish, sandy or mucous sediment in urine.

Urinary Organs.

"*Drawing in bladder,* extending into female *urethra,* often arising in the lumbar region and extending along the *ureter;* burning pains *in bladder* whether empty or full; sensation as if some urine remained after urinating; smarting, *stitching, burning* in the *urethra; urine blood red* or pale yellow, soon becomes *turbid* and deposits a thick *mucous* and bright red, mealy *sediment;* clay-like white or whitish-gray sediment."

Berberis is one of the quartet of great remedies for patients who suffer from what is known as the "*lithic diathesis.*" The above is a complete picture of renal calculi and their effect upon the mucosa of the urinary tract. When using Berberis the patient should cut out hard waters, using if possible only distilled. Coffee and condiments of all kinds should be used sparingly.

Digestive Tract.

Stomach: "Appetite variable; *eructations* without bad taste or *smell;* aching, *burning,* shooting, sticking pains in region of stomach; bilious risings."

Liver: "*Stitches in* region of *gall-bladder* worse from pressure; in left hepatic region near border of false ribs extending into region of stomach."

Rectum: "Urging to stool; long continued sensation after stool, as if one had just been to stool or had just recovered from pain in the anus."

Anus and Stool: "*Burning pain as if parts around* it were sore (Silica, Sulph.); crawling, burning and itching in and about it; tearing extending around anus; stool clay colored; diarrheic."

With the above symptoms you have the sallow complexion (Iodium, Sepia) and the tenderness of the liver extending out over the abdomen and around the back.

Sexual Organs: "Soft, pulpy swelling of the spermatic cord. lower part, when walking, with, at times, drawing, burning, smarting or tearing pains sometimes extending into the testicles when sitting and into epididymis (Gelsemium, Clematis). drawing pain extending into testicle (Pulsatilla) or abdomen: *burning pain* in *vagina* (Kreosote), especially anteriorly, even extending to labia; menses scanty with pain preceding the flow which is scanty and irregular."

Back and Extremities: For *neuralgia* of spermatic *cords* and *testicles* (Clematis, Actea and Pulsatilla). For dysmenorrhea with *pain radiating* down the thighs and *every other direction. Vaginismus* associated *with* leucorrhea and the *bladder symptoms.*

"Stitching, tearing, crushed, bruised pains in loins with stiffness (Rhus), making it difficult to rise from seat, at times numbness."

One of our *leading remedies* for *lumbago,* with some or all of the urinary symptoms.

COLOCYNTHIS.

Make-up: Neurotic, bilious, easily offended.

Loc.: Nerves; mucous membranes; sexual organs.

Mod.: *Amel.* rest, *by pressure,* by *warmth,* by bending forward.

Agg. by motion, eating and drinking, evening and night.

Sen.: *Cutting; griping; pinching;* twisting; *squeezed;* sticking; shooting; colic.

Nerves.

Abdomen: "Distention and pain; *pinching,* as if the bowels were pressed inward. *Amel.* by *pressure* and *bending* forward, with cutting extending towards pubic region so severe that facial muscles were distorted and eyes drawn together; pain as if *squeezed* between stones; *paroxysmal pains* obliging him to bend forward, amel. by soft *stool; cutting* pains after eating, with tenesmus; griping pain agg. after eating fruit, with cutting pains and chill; pain about the navel, amel. by frequent discharge of flatus; twitching, sticking pains extending from the umbilicus to loins and spine; acute pain agg. by walking; sensitivenees; sense of inflation after dinner with compression in throat and nausea."

Head: "*Tearing, digging* through brain, agg. by moving eyelids; *vertigo* which occasions falling on turning the head quickly; sudden sticking pains in forehead; boring, burning pains in right side; boring, sticking in right temple; confusion with pressing, burning pain in left orbit; temple, nose and teeth amel. by heat."

Eyes: "*Cutting* pains in eyeballs agg. by stooping; *twitching pains* in eyelids."

Face: "Tearing in cheeks; constriction in left molar bone extending into the left eye; sticking pain in upper jaw."

Urinary Organs: "Frequent urging to urinate, with scanty emission, alternating with copious, clear, water; sudden sticking pains in the bladder, along the urethra and ureters."

Extremities: "Cramp in middle of left thigh; *sticking; drawing; cutting;* pains from hip to knee amel. by sitting, lying on left side, and warmth; agg. by cold and by walking."

Colocynth is one of the best remedies for all forms of *algias* and for neuritis in a few locations. It has palliated the pains of *glaucoma* and *iritis.* Warmth and pressure relieve nearly all neuralgic pains. A light touch will agg. an algia, while hard pressure will amel. Many of the neuralgic pains are relieved by rest, but the pains compel the *patients* to *twist, turn,* and *wiggle.*

Membranes.

Intestines: "Fluid stools *agg. by eating* and *drinking;* fluid stools with discharge of flatus, with colic; stools which are thin, frothy, saffron-yellow, musty, offensive; bloody stool with nausea but cannot vomit; bloody stools with tenesmus."

Colocynth produces irritation, inflammation and functional changes of the membrane of the alimentary canal. It cures a *diarrhea caused* from *anger,* from *eating fruit;* from drinking *ice water* or *lemonade,* especially when the body is overheated. It is the great remedy for the result of a 4th of July picnic. It is also useful for *dysentery* from the same causes when you have the colic, pains and modalities of the drug, followed by bloody mucous stools always agg. by eating and drinking.

Sexual Organs.

Cramp-like pains in left ovary and uterus, pains as if the parts were *squeezed* in a vise; paroxysms of acute pain in abdomen, pelvis, sacrum and hips; amel. by *flexing thighs* on pelvis; lochia suppressed; menses suppressed with cramping pains, amel by bending double."

Colocynth has cured ovaralgia and ovaritis. The *ovaralgia* is *agg.* by *slight* pressure but *amel.* by *hard pressure.* The ovaritis is generally due to cystic tumor. The 3rd if continued will in many cases absorb the systs, or if some of the cystic tumors are removed it will prevent their return or the development of others. Colocynth is the best known antidote to lead poisoning. When called to a case of painter's colic give five drops of the 3rd in four ounces of as hot water as the patient can drink. Repeat in fifteen minutes. This will obviate the use of opium in three out of four cases. Between the attacks give five drops of the 30th before each meal and at bedtime.

EUPATORIUM PERFOLIATUM.

Make-up: Of *bilious temperament* and irritable stomach.
Loc.: *Bones;* liver; *muscles,* blood.
Sen.: *Broken;* bruised; *sore;* aching.
Mod.: *Agg. FROM MOTION: AT* 9 A.M.; cold air.
Amel. *vomiting* of *bile.*

Bones.

"*Soreness* in bones; *aching* of bones, with soreness of the flesh; bruised feeling in every bone preventing lying in bed and causing despair, moaning and crying out."

These "*bone pains*" are the *characteristics of* this ancient domestic *remedy* and are found in intermittent, relapsing and bilious fevers; dengue; also rheumatic and syphilitic pains.

Liver.

"*Soreness in* region of *liver* on moving or *coughing;* abdomen full and distended; *vomiting* of *bile,* with trembling and great *nausea* causing great prostration; *dark brown,* scanty *urine* depositing a whitish clay-like deposit; yellow jaundiced skin."

For symptoms like the above no remedy will bring more rapid and permanent results than Eupatorium perf. from 3x to 30x.

Muscles.

Chest: "Pain, soreness and heaviness behind sternum and in cardiac region worse from least motion."

Neck and Back: "*Beating* pain *in nape* and *occiput*, better after rising; aching in arms and forearms as if beaten; painful soreness of wrists as if broken or dislocated; soreness of lower limbs, with aching; calves of legs feel as if beaten."

Blood.

Intermittent Fever: "Chill in morning, 9 A.M., thirst and uneasiness precedes chill; chill severe with thirst for cold water; chill with nausea and vomiting after drinking; *nausea* and *vomiting* of bile just *as* the *chill goes off* and the heat begins; pungent heat; little sweat."

The *time* of day and the *vomiting* of *bile* are the *characteristics* of this condition of the drug. All the bone and muscle pains mentioned elsewhere are present with the intermittent fever. Rarely there may be profuse sweating.

Influenza: "*Eyeballs sore;* nose dry; thirst great; violent coryza; cough with soreness and heat in bronchi."

In this condition the cough is usually worse lying on back, better lying on face. The coughing hurts the head and chest (Bryonia). The general aching and bone pains are also present in the influenza of Eupatorium perf. I have found the 3x most useful.

SYPHILINUM.

Make-up: Dirty; disgusting to themselves; suppurative (Hepar).

Loc.: M.M.; glands; nerves; bones.

Sen.: All.

Mod.: Agg. night, sundown and sunrise; extreme cold or heat; damp weather.

Amel. change of position, *i. e.*, slow motion.

Leaders: All symptoms agg. at night; ulceration of M.M.;

skin and bones presenting a grayish base and having an offensive discharge; abscesses or boils coming in succession; copper-colored spots on the skin.

Mucous Membranes.

Eyes: "Profuse lachrymation; eyeballs covered with fungus-like growth (Thuja), with pain intense at night; marked redness and pain; both eyes glued together in morning."

For *chronic recurrent phlyctenular inflammation* of the *cornea* with marked photophobia; for *pustular conjunctivitis* of delicate, scrofulous children; for *scrophulous eruption of canthi.*

Ear: "Calcareous deposit on tympanum; otorrhea with acrid, watery or purulent discharge, rarely deafness."

Nose: "Nose stopped up and burning; fluent coryza; offensive, thick, yellow-green nasal discharge; scabs form in both nostrils during sleep; sore itching and scabbing over of nostrils."

For *chronic catarrhal rhinitis* of children of syphilitic parents; for ozena. *Burning, itching* and the *formation* of *scabs are* the three *leading symptoms* of the group (Kali bich., Mercurius, Hydrastis).

Mouth: "The tongue thickly coated, dirty; edges indented or serrated by teeth; tongue coated dirty white; ulcerations with very painful, smarting, burning as if on fire, on tongue, in mouth, nose and throat; profuse saliva."

For *herpetic eruption* of *mouth, tonsils;* and *stomatitis.*

It has helped *chronic hypertrophy* of the *tonsils* of persons with syphilitic history.

Stomach: "Heart-burn with pain and rawness from stomach to throat pit; vomiting of food, or dark grumous matter; painful spots over stomach region."

Useful for *ulceration* of the *stomach,* generally of herpetic origin, occasionally of syphilitic.

Abdomen, Anus and Stools: "Pain or distress deep in

abdomen as if in omentum; *fissures* at the *anus* also ulcers of the anus and rectum. Stools dark, bilious and offensive."

Several cases are on record in which *Syphilinum* high has cured the above group found in syphilitic patients.

Female Genital Organs: "Profuse, thick, yellow, offensive *leucorrhea,* with constant pain across the back; uterus and surrounding parts soft and flabby."

It has cured a few cases of *leucorrhea* with the above symptoms when the *backache agg. at night* was the *ranking symptom.* It helped clear up several cases of leuçorrhea in baby girls who were born in a maternity home. In some cases the mothers had syphilis, in others it was not proven that they had. With most of these there were the dark offensive stools. The 200th was used for these cases.

Nerves.

Eyes: "Neuralgia every night, gradually increasing from 8 P.M. till 3 A.M., continuing the same for two hours and gradually decreasing until it ceased at 10 A.M.; eye very red and closes because of pain; a horizontal bar across the pupil hindering the sight."

For *strabismus* and *iritis* also for *neuralgia* and *neuritis.* A few cases of *ptosis paralytica* have been cured by it when in addition there was drawing of the face, jerking of the lid and eye.

Face: "Face drawn to one side, with difficult speech and mastication."

Syphilinum has helped clear up *cerebral hemorrhage* with hemicrania, great mental depression, spasmodic twitching of muscles and *profuse saliva* which is very *offensive.*

Extremities: "Rheumatic pain and lameness of shoulder and arm, agg. by raising the arm laterally; excruciating pain in lower extremities banishing sleep, agg. by hot applications, amel. by pouring cold water on them; cannot sit in a low chair or squat down, owing to loss of control over knee and hip joints; tearing pain in knee and thighs agg. at night."

Skin.

"Pustular eruption on different parts of the body, with a *biting sensation* as if from bugs.

For *copper-colored maculæ* looking like smallpox; *pemphigus* with same smallpox appearance often confluent and persistently reappearing; use the 30th and 200th.

TUBERCULINUM.

Tuberculinum is the nosode which I have used most frequently of the 33 genuine nosodes which H. C. Allen includes in his Materia Medica of the Nosodes. H. C. Allen devotes 30 pages to the symptoms of Tuberculinum. In not more than one per cent. of the cases in which I have used it have I given Tuberculinum as the indicated remedy, with the expectation of curing with it alone. I give it as an intercurrent remedy when I feel sure that I have prescribed the indicated remedy but without results. I use it in many cases where I formerly used Sulphur. I must say, however, that in many cases where I gave it simply as an intercurrent, the patients began to improve and continued till normal. What are the indications for its use? I cannot give them with the accuracy that I can for Variolinum or Syphilinum, but the following will help you. I find that it is more often called for after the failure of such remedies as Phosphorus, Ferrum phos., Stannum, Iodium, Kali carb., Calcarea carb., Pulsatilla, Hepar, Hydrastis and Kreosote; remedies which have an elective affinity for the tissues which are most frequently attacked by the t. b. c. and scrofulous diathesis; remedies which act rapidly, deeply; remedies capable of producing not only functional but structural changes, such as enlarged glands, ulcers, phthisis, not only general loss of weight but waste of some special organ like the lungs.

Secondly you will find the *ranking symptoms of Tuberculinum* to be the *unexpected, uncommon symptoms of the t. b. c. group* of the above named remedies, *e. g.*, all the symptoms of the t. b. c. group found under Stannum are present except that the patient is very cheerful and hopeful; or all the symptoms of the throat are those of Phosphorus except that the hoarseness is amel. by talking and singing. I have neither the mind nor the time to group or grade the many symptoms which you may read in the 30 pages of H. C. Allen's Materia Medica or the nine and a half pages which Clark devotes to it in his Dictionary. In these volumes and in our Journals, desperate cases of almost every disease are reported cured by it. I do know that it helped me in many cases differing widely in their etiology, diagnosis and prognosis.

VARIOLINUM.

Make-up: Nothing definite.

Loc.: Skin; nerves.

Sen.: Aching; lancinating; throbbing.

Mod.: Agg. motion.

Leaders: *Backache* and other *pathognomonic symptoms of smallpox* are the *characteristics* of Variolinum. In addition to the backache, severe chill and coldness and chilliness as if cold water were trickling down the back; high temperature with extremely hot skin; nausea; violent headache; pains in bones of the limbs.

There is no doubt in my mind about the power of Variolinum to prevent and abort smallpox. That was proven on the best of authority in innumerable cases. But failure has also been attributed to its use in as many cases. The causes of failure are two, 1st the preparation, 2nd the patient. The preparation should be fresh, the potency not too high—6th or 12th. The dose, three to five grains, repeated three times daily for three or four days. The patient should report every day for examination, and the symptoms carefully recorded. The reason Variolinum has been discredited is because many people who do not wish to be vaccinated by the old method get Variolinum from some physician and never take it. They report symptoms which never existed and by so doing get a certificate from the careless or crafty physician.

Skin.

"Small, sharp, pointed *pimples,* suppurating, dry, resting on small read areolæ, frequently interspersed with spots of red color; severe itching; petechial eruption."

The skin condition for which Variolinum has proven most useful in my hands is that of *herpes zoster.* The eruption is like that stated above, is usually found on the trunk of the body. The nervous symptoms are marked and the pain and temperature prominent symptoms of the group. There are neuralgic pains following the eruptions (Mezerium).

I have also found it helpful for *scarlet fever* with an irregular eruption, a hot, dry skin and high temperature. One case was of t. b. c. diathesis and had suffered from eczema during dentition. She was seven years old. The outset was severe, first a *chill;* the *temperature 104* within 36 hours; severe *back* and headache; *eruption slow* in developing; severe sore throat and scanty urine. Variolinum 6th brought out the eruption; brought down the temperature and improved the patient within 36 hours.

Brain and Nerves.

Mind: "Delirium with high temperature."

Head: "Severe, lancinating, throbbing pains through head agg. with every pulsation; intolerable pain in the occiput; crazy feeling through the brain, hard to describe."

Back: "Intolerable aching in the lumbar and sacral region; pain in muscles of the back like rheumatism, agg. on motion."

Most of the above symptoms accompany or follow the skin conditions, especially herpes. Use from 6th to 30th.

VERATRUM VIRIDE.

Make-up: Plethoric, full-blooded.

Loc.: Vaso-motor centers; medulla; chest; kidneys.

Mod.: Agg. Rising up, lying on back.
Amel. Rubbing.

Sen.: Griping; throbbing, cramping.

Leaders: *Bloated, livid* face; *congestion; faintness, dry, red streak* along *center* of *tongue.*

Brain and Nerves.

Mind: "*Delirious;* quarrelsome, striking and kicking with hands and feet (Hyoscyamus)."

The *delirium* of Veratrum vir. is a most furious one and is *found in* many of the conditions cured by the drug. You will find it in bronchitis, pneumonia, nephritis and metritis, calling for Veratrum vir.

Head: "*Fullness and heaviness* (Gelsemium) in the morning, vertigo in morning on rising, amel. closing the eyes and resting the head, with photophobia; vertigo on rising from bed with nausea and vomiting (Cocculus)."

Veratrum vir. is frequently useful for *congestive headaches* rarely in neuralgia. With the *fullness* and *weariness* you have the *flushed face* which is nearly always bloated; diplopia; *vertigo;* nausea; vomiting. When, as is frequently the case, the headache is due to, or associated with, lung or kidney troubles you have the additional symptoms of those groups plus a "*dry, red streak through the center of the tongue.*"

Cerebral hyperemia and *apoplexy* occasionally call for Veratrum vir., also *cerebro-spinal meningitis.*

Kidneys.

Although we have very little from the provers for this locality, I feel that a thorough proving would put it in the class with Arsenicum and Apis for *acute nephritis* following the exanthemata when convulsion was the ranking symptom.

Years ago Dr. C. W. Eaton called me to see a boy of 8 years who was suffering from nephritis following scarlet fever. The boy had a *flushed face* and was *drowsy* (Apis); was very restless (Arsenicum); urine scanty, only a few drops at a time and loaded with albumin; temperature 104; pulse full; some edema of the feet (Arsenicum); very thirsty but vomited as soon as he drank (Arsenicum); convulsions with much regularity every two hours. Dr. Eaton had given Arsenicum 6th and 30th. I could see no other remedy, so advised Arsenicum 3rd. As we were leaving the house the father of the child arrived with an eclectic physician and discharged Dr. Eaton. The eclectic physician had an office next mine so the next day I went in to inquire after the boy. The Dr. replied, "Oh, better! he will be all right in a few days." I asked for the remedy, the dose and frequency of repetition of same. The doctor said, "I put one drop of Norwood's tincture of Veratrum vir. into two-thirds of a glass of water and ordered a teaspoonful every half hour for six hours. After that at longer intervals."

I have used it several times since in the same way for the same symptoms which as you see from the above were a mixture of Arsenicum, Apis and Belladonna.

Sexual Organs: Here again we have very little from the provers. However, Clark in his Dictionary gives us a long list of clinical symptoms and groups them under the headings of "*rigid os; pelvic congestions; puerperal fever* and *convulsions; suppressed menses and dysmenorrhea.*" I have verified only one of these conditions, viz., puerperal convulsions.

Over 30 years ago I offered to act as physician for a maternity home. It was a charity institution for which physicians donated their services. There had been three cases of deaths from "child bed fever" in two days. I delivered my first case about 8 P.M. Forty-eight hours afterwards I was called and found the woman with a flushed, hot face, staring eyes, anxious look and both hands in constant motion while she was screaming, "I've got the fever, I've got the fever." The pulse was rapid but there was but little temperature, no tenderness of the abdomen and the lochia was normal. I concluded the case was one of fear and gave Ignatia. During the next 12 hours all the above symptoms grew worse and the temperature went up to 100.5. The stools had become thin and offensive, one was involuntary; no sleep. I changed from Ignatia to Hyoscyamus. Twelve hours later the temperature was 104.8; puse 140, full and soft; face almost purple; pupils dilated and she had had two severe convulsions. The urine was very scanty. I made up my mind the patient would die. However, the post-scarlatinal convulsion case came to mind, and I gave Veratrum vir. as was given in that case. There was one more convulsion, after the third dose, after which all the symptoms gradually subsided and a complete recovery followed.

Respiratory Organs.

"Breathing heavy, difficult, slow, short, convulsive, almost to suffocation; constriction of chest."

Not many symptoms and general rather than specific are given by the provers, but Veratrum vir. has prevented and *cured* many *cases* of *penumonia, bronchitis* and *pulmonary congestion* (Aconite, Ferrum phos. and Belladonna). *Congestion* not only of the *lungs* but *also* of the *brain* is the *ranking* symptom of all three groups. The *full pulse,* marked *dyspnea,* hot head, *cold* extremities, *dry tongue* and *high temperature* are other prominent symptoms.

APIS.

Make-up: Dropsical; edematous.

Loc.: Mucous and serous membranes; brain; skin; kidneys.

Sen.: *Stinging;* burning; aching; piercing; weakness; full or swollen; sore; *stiff,* etc.

Mod.: Agg.: 5 P.M.; heat of bed; warmth.

Amel: Cold water; sitting.

Mucous and Serous Membranes.

Brain and Cord: The action upon the membranes of these two organs ends in *edema*. We have "stupor; short cries (cephalic); *screaming; hot head;* boring of head into pillow." With the above you also find "*strabismus;* scanty urine; and watery, painless stool."

Eye: "Lids *swollen, red, edematous; stinging; itching;* smarting; aching; and agglutination. Amel. from cold water."

Nose: "Sneezing; watery discharge worse in the evening."

Throat: "*Swelling; redness;* dryness with heat; constriction; white spots (edematous) on glottis; hoarseness; difficult swallowing and breathing; *diphtheritic exudate; stinging pains; mottled eruption* (scarlatina)."

With both scarlatina and diphtheria you have the mental conditions: "drowsy, stupid" and frequently the delirium.

Stomach and Intestines: "No thirst; nausea and vomiting; pain; soreness; and *sensitiveness* worse in the morning, when sneezing, on pressure or when lying in the horizontal position."

Rectum, Anus and Stools: With the above we have "*diarrhea* with a *raw* sensation in the *anus;* brown, *yellow,* bloody, *painless* stools."

In *cholera infantum* the stools are *profuse, watery* and accompanied by vomiting. The exception to the above is that with hydrocephalus you may have constipation.

Bladder: "Inflamed; *irritable; frequent,* sometimes involuntary *micturition; stinging pains;* strangury."

Respiratory Organs: "*Sensation as if he could not breath; suffocation,* as if he could not bear anything about the throat; hoarseness; breathing hurried and difficult; severe cough worse from lying and sleeping."

This cough is unusually short, dry, spasmodic, suffocative. The irritation is in the supra-sternal fossa. The attack may be started by pressing the larynx. Apis will cure edema of the larynx, also hydrothorax whether originating from the kidneys or pleura.

Heart: "Stinging pain in region of the heart."

Apis will help you in pericarditis when in addition to the above symptom you have great soreness over region of the heart, scanty urine, marked dyspnea, blue lips, stiffness of the abdominal muscles (Ab. walls feel like a board) and swollen legs.

Joints: "Edematous swelling."

The synovitis which Apis will help is usually accompanied by dropsy of the extremities due to kidney lesions or to some rheumatic condition.

Skin.

"*Stinging; swelling;* pricking; itching; burning; red and white blotches; cellular inflammation ending in suppuration; nettle rash over whole body stinging and pricking; large furuncles with stinging, burning pain."

With all *skin* affections of Apis whether *urticaria* or *erysipelas, swelling, edema, stinging and stiffness* are very prominent. These E. swellings you will find most marked about the face and genitals.

Kidneys.

Although we have but few symptoms from the provers and they call attention only to the *function* of the kidneys, we find from clinical experience that Apis does cause *irritation, inflammation* and *structural changes* as well as functional. For *acute nephritis* following any of the exanthemata, Apis shares the honors with Arsenicum for being the most frequently indicated remedy. The symptoms are as follows: "urine *scanty, high colored,* rarely bloody, *and loaded with casts;* the patient is drowsy, the "*stupor*" and "*dropsy*" come early, the latter seen in the puffed face. The patient has no thirst, is usually *quiet,* very rarely restless. Coma threatens. In the *chronic nephritis* the edemas mentioned under membranes frequently occur and may be relieved, rarely cured by Apis. There is one peculiar action of Apis on the function of the kidneys, viz., that there *is* frequently *with diphtheria, scarlet fever, erysipelas, NO INFLAMMATION,* but a *profuse, pale urine.*"

Female Generative Organs: "Bearing down, with sensation as before menses; metrorrhagia with heaviness of the abdomen; faintness and yawning."

It has cured *pelvic cellulitis* (Terebinthina); *ovarian cysts, metritis,* with enlarged uterus, following pregnancy. It has *checked threatened abortion;* also used successfully for *dysmenorrhea* when the organs are swollen and tender and there is a puffed, waxy appearance of the face.

TEREBINTHINA.

Make-up: *Dark;* fleshy.

Loc.: M.M.; kidneys; lungs, cellular tissue.

Sen.: *Stinging;* bruised; *sore; burning.*

Mod.: Agg.: Dampness; touch; pressure.
Amel. passing flatus; motion.

Leaders: *Distention of abdomen; smoky urine;* passive hemorrhages.

Mucous Membranes.

Stomach: "Eructation, rancid, *flatulent,* acrid; nausea; vomiting of mucus, food and blood; *excessive sensitiveness* in the region of the stomach to touch, *amel.* by *belching* or *passing flatus;* burning sensation in the stomach."

Abdomen: "Distention of ab. (Carbo veg.): obliging him to rest, *meteorism;* griping colic; cutting, sticking, tearing pain all through the abdomen."

I have used Terebinthina for *pelvic peritonitis* in a great many cases from various causes, *e. g.,* typhoid fever; extending from a *metritis, resulting* from *retained secundines* or *gonorrhea.* I cited several cases in the Medical Century, Vol. 1, Page 70, giving groups under these conditions. Since then

I *have had* many similar cases and *two* in which the *cause* was *extension* from *specific pelvic cellulitis.* The *ranking symptom* in all cases has been: *enormously distended* ab. which was very *sensitive to pressure, e. g.*, extending the legs was unbearable; also the retraction of the upper lip over the teeth; cold sweat of the extremities; *rapid, feeble pulse; thin, offensive stools;* thin, *offensive* acrid *lochia* (after miscarriage or childbirth) and *anxiety.*

Let me detail my last case. A graduate of this college asked me to go to a certain hospital in D. M. to see his sister who was in charge of an old school physician, a woman. I found the patient, an unmarried woman, light, fleshy, a seamstress by trade, already prepared for the operating room. In reply to my "What for?" the Dr. replied: "For ruptured appendix." Examination revealed all the symptoms mentioned above except the offensive discharges, in place of which there was constipation and in addition the cellular tissue of the entire pelvis was hot, much swollen and extremely sensitive. Heat, pain and fullness in the vagina and pelvis had preceded the abdominal symptoms. There had been no shock. I disagreed in the diagnosis and objected to the operation. The patient was turned over to me and treated as follows: Five drops of Terebinthina 6th every two hours. Turpentine stupes a little hotter than the temperature of body applied to the abdomen; ten drops of spirits of Terebinthina in a pint of hot water for enemas and vaginal douches. The douches to be given in large amount and retained as long as possible. The douches were given every three hours at first but at longer intervals later. The woman made a slow but complete recovery.

Urinary Organs.

"*Strangury*, bloody urine, then soreness of baldder (Cantharis); strangury and total suppression of urine (Stramonium); *incontinence of urine; dysuria;* urine bloody (Cantharis, Phosphorus, Erigeron) and scanty; smelling of violets."

Very helpful for *acute nephritis due* to exposure to *cold rains,* with the *severe burning, drawing in* the *kidney region* going down the ureters to the bladder; the *constant desire to urinate;* chilliness (Capsicum); the smoky or bloody urine and high temperature are the symptoms of this group. Also for *acute cystitis* when you have the strangury instead of the pain in back and down ureters.

Lungs.

"*Expectoration streaked with blood;* breathing difficult and lungs seem distended; breathing short, hurried, anxious."

Occasionally useful for *capillary bronchitis* when you have scanty, bloody urine in addition to the above.

Although I have used it in a few cases of typhoid I doubt if Terebinthina can cause changes in the blood simulating the changes resulting from typhoid. *Ulceration* and perhaps *perforations* with *peritonitis* are the only symptoms of typhoid I ever used it for.

CANTHARIS.

Make-up: Passionate; excitable.

Loc.: Genito-urinary organs; mucous membranes; skin.

Mod.: Agg. *urinating, drinking;* from bright objects and sight and sound of water.

Leaders: Acute, rapid and destructive inflammation, fearful tenesmus, much exudate.

Genito-Urinary Organs.

Urinary Organs: "Pain in bladder with *frequent urging and intolerable tenesmus;* burning, cutting pain in neck of bladder extending to navicular fossa; tenesmus and urging after discharge of urine; burning in the urethra better lying quietly on the back, worse standing and walking; constant urging, micturition painful and in drops; cutting before, during and after micturition; urine scalding and is passed in drops; *bloody urine.*"

Cantharis produces and cures most violent *cystitis* with marked inflammation, chills, urging to urinate, *intense tenesmus, urine bloody* and scanty. Useful for *irritation* of renal calculi.

Sexual Organs: "*Priapism;* drawing pains in the spermatic cord while urinating; desire disturbing sleep; *painful erections* most severe at night with contraction and pain in whole of the urethra; also strong, *persistent painless erection* without voluptuous sensation; swelling of vulva with irritation."

Will cure *urethritis specific* and non-specific, when the urethritis is due to the irritation of renal calculi. Male children constantly pull at the penis. For *ovaritis with* burning pains, especially during the menses when the ovaries are extremely sensitive to touch. For *puerperal metritis* with constant discharge from the uterus, the bladder pains and the peculiar sexual mania of the drug.

Mucous Membranes.

In addition to the condition described under genito-urinary organs we also have the following:

Throat: "*Burning* soreness with *inflammation* of *pharynx;* constriction at back part with pain, inflammation and covering with plastic lymph; aphthous ulcers covered with whitish crusts; swallowing difficult."

For *simple inflammation* of the throat which is bright red and feels like fire. For *aphthous ulcerations* with the soreness and spasmodic contraction causing deglutition. Also for *diphtheria* when there is much inflammation and thick, light-colored membrane. With the diphtheria you usually have *nephritis with albuminuria.* The inflammation, constriction and profuse exudate often threaten suffocation.

Respiratory Organs: "*Burning* pain in *larynx;* voice low, with sensation of weakness of the vocal cords; expectoration bloody, frothy."

The most frequent use I have made of the above symptoms has been for *edema* of the remi-glottis. The only remedy which has served me as well for edema of the glottis is Apis. The marked irritability and burning of Cantharis is easily differentiated from the apathy and stinging of Apis. Many of our authors say "It is useful for croup in children" but by no stretch of the imagination can I see any resemblance between the picture of Cantharis and that of exudative laryngitis (genuine membranous croup) while the constriction at back of throat is the only symptom which can be mistaken for spasmodic laryngitis (false croup).

The 3rd and 6th have served me the best for this condition. Give every half hour. Edema of the glottis is a difficult, dangerous condition to handle successfully.

Intestines: "Abdomen distended and tympanitic; *burning*, crawling *in rectum;* tenesmus; burning in rectum after diarrhea; stools consisting of blood and mucus, of white, tough *mucus, like* the *scrapings of the intestines* with streaks of blood."

Useful for both *diarrhea* and *dysentery* with the above symptoms. With the dysentery you usually find the burning pain of the drug in the perineum, throat and mouth. The mouth is sometimes dry and red, later may be edematous. There are a great many aphthous patches. In two cases of peritonitis following metritis with the badly distended abdomen and stools of Cantharis the remedy cured. In both cases Terebinthina had been tried and failed.

Skin.

"Itching *vesicles with burning* pains on being touched."

By grouping the other symptoms around this one found under the heading "Skin," we have formed *pictures* which correspond to those of *eczema* and *erysipelas*. The latter of the vesicular type. The *eczema* on backs of feet and hands was better from cold and worse from warmth. For many years I used a dilution of Cantharis for burns, especially sunburns. Lately, however, I use *Picric acid* unless there is marked vesication.

HELLEBORUS NIGER.

Make-up: Want of reaction; semi-paralytic.

Loc.: Brain and nerves, motor and sensory; mucous and serous membranes.

Sen.: Blunted; sluggish.

Mod.: Agg.: Cold air; suppressed eruptions; evening.
Amel.: Attracting their attention.

Leaders: Constant motion of one hand or foot or both; blunted sensibilities so that they can neither see, hear, or feel.

Brain and Nerves.

Mind: "Reflective; taciturn; do not wish to speak or to be spoken to; stupefaction, with slow answers (Phosphoric ac.)."

The *mental symptoms are* the *ranking ones in every group of the drug,* viz., stupor so marked that it is difficult for the patient to be aroused and when aroused still more difficult for the mind to control the body. The cause of the condition is *serous effusion* which is also a prominent symptom of most groups (Apis). We have *melancholia* with fear of death, and a low, stupid, muttering delirium (Baptisia).

Head: "Confusion; heaviness; congestion of the brain; vertigo; paroxysmal pains in occiput agg. motion, amel. pressure; nausea and vertigo agg. stooping, amel. on becoming erect."

Helleborus is our leading remedy for *hydrocephalus* and its sequellæ. The patient is *stupid; unconscious;* the eyes are fixed but cannot see; there is a constant *chewing motion, also automatic motion of* one *hand* or *foot;* sudden screams and *boring* of the *head* in *pillow;* usually suppression of urine. The above condition is usually preceded or accompanied by *convulsions.* The causes are concussion of the brain and repressed eruptions, especially of the exanthemata. Rarely the cause of the convulsions is meningitis. Helleborus saved a child for me who had 236 convulsions in 36 hours, the cause being tubercular meningitis.

With the sequellæ, the child is often idiotic, has no desires or aversions and frequently suffers from strabismus.

Serous and Mucous Membranes.

Mouth: "Dryness of palate with cutting scraping in it on moving the mouth to swallow."

Occasionally for aphthæ of the mouth.

Stools: "Stools only clear, tenacious, colorless mucus (Colchicum); white, gelatinous-like.

For *diarrhea* with the above symptoms frequently with tenesmus (Colchicum) rarely alternating with constipation. You will find these symptoms the ranking ones in the hydrocephalic group.

Urinary Organs: "*Frequent urging with scanty discharge;* urine in drops, no desire, no stream."

For sub-acute nephritis with suppression of the urine (Stramonium) and the dropsical symptoms (Apis). This kidney condition is accompanied by *inflammation* of the *mucosa* of the *bladder.*

Heart and Respiratory Organs: "Pulse rapid; or *slow;* 30 to 50, small and tremulous; sudden constant hacking cough; difficult breathing; constriction so that he gasps for breath but cannot breathe; feeling as if the chest could not expand."

Abdomen: "*Distention;* rumbling in; *colic* with pallor, sunken features and staggering walk; lips blue and covered with clammy sweat."

The weak heart action, in fact all the symptoms of the three sections are the result of dropsical effusions of the various organs of this locality. In this group is often found the only marked skin symptom of the drug, viz., "*Sudden dropsical swelling.*"

Blood and Thermic Center.

"*Coldness,* internal, between 5 and 6 P.M. Agg. lying down with shivering over body agg. shaking in the morning with goose flesh; heat in head; with usual warmth of body."

Occosionally useful for a low form of *typhoid* with the muttering delirium, the foul breath, great apathy (Opium); feeble pulse; general coldness and cold sweat. Use 30th rarely 6th.

VERATRUM ALBUM.

Make-up: Neurotic.

Loc.: Brain and nerves; intestinal canal; heart.

Sen.: Vomiting, *cramping,* trembling, thirst, *coldness,* weakness and *fainting.*

Mod.: Amel.: Heat; *hot water;* stimulants.

Leaders: The *vomiting and purging at the same time,* fainting after profuse, *watery stools and vomiting;* marked coldness.

Brain and Nerves.

General: "Trembling; spasms; weakness on going to stool. *with sinking down;* weakness paralytic, rapid; faintness."

One of our best remedies for *cholera Asiatic* or ***infantum,*** rarely cholera morbus, with the violent vomiting and purging, and the *intense coldness.* We also have some *cramping* and *pain* in the intestines, especially in the *cholera infantum* and *morbus, convulsions* with *violent* tonic spasms when the hands and feet draw inward. With the cholera you also have rigidity of the muscles of the face and cramps in the calves of the legs. The amount of water discharged through mouth and anus is enormous. For this reason you should use plenty of liquid as enemas. Take equal parts of milk and water of the temperature which you find in the rectum and inject in large quantities and often.

Mind: "Inconsolable over fancied misfortune, howls and screams; wails and weeps; sits brooding in corner; *anxious;* despondent." For *delirium* in cholera; *melancholia,* usually after great disappointment or religious excitement.

Head: "Vertigo; *pressing* on vertex in morning after waking which becomes *throbbing* on motion; crawling and bristling sensation as if a bunch of hair were electrified."

For *persistent vertigo* with *cold sweat* on forehead and *great weakness,* often *fainting* (Nux, Cocculus). For two forms of *neuralgic headache.* First, with feeling as if ice were on the vertex; second, *convulsive shocks* as soon as the patient raises the head, accompanied by vomiting, amel. by pressure on vertex.

Stomach: I am going to put the stomach symptoms under the location of brain and nerves because the choleras for which Veratrum alb. is useful are largely of nervous origin. The verified symptoms are: "*Violent hunger* and thirst, thirst for cold drinks; nausea and vomiting (Aconite, Capsicum); with the vomiting, pale sunken face covered with cold sweat, also purging, violent at first, slimy liquid with some food, later watery."

For cholera when you have the above symptoms plus the *coldness,* the *faintness,* the blue pinched face, the intense thirst.

Heart: "*Palpitation,* with anxiety and rapid, audible respiration (Aconite); pulse rapid, slow, irregular, at times intermittent."

Veratrum alb. is occasionally used in *cardiac* debility with the above symptoms. The *face* is usually *flushed* when lying down but becomes pale and covered with cold sweat from the least exertion. The pulse varies as the patient is quiet or in motion.

Mucous Membrane.

Although our text-books give us many symptoms and conditions under stomach, intestines and the respiratory organs I have never verified any except those which belong to the nervous cholera group or whooping cough.

Do not forget to use enemas of milk and hot water in all cases of purging.

Use the 6th and 30th, very rarely the 3rd, as it is a rank poison.

EUPHRASIA.

Make-up: *Tearful* though *not sad.*

Loc.: M.M. of *eyes* and nose.

Sen.: Smarting; burning; itching.

Mod.: Agg.: Sunlight, warm wind or in warm room.
Amel.: In open air; wiping eyes.

Leaders: For *watery eyes* (Cepa, Thuja). Abundant, acrid, hot, smarting tears with bland coryza. (Cepa the reverse.)

Mucous Membranes.

Eye: "*Cornea feels as if covered with mucus,* which obscures the vision and causes him to press the lids together; *biting; water runs from* the *eyes;* frequent biting and burning obliging winking; *burning* and *swelling* of the *lids* (Apis, Sulphur); frequent inclination to blink; sensitiveness to light especially candle light."

The virtues of Euphrasia (Eye bright) for eye troubles, especially blurred vision, were sung by Milton.

Before and since Milton's time Euphrasia has been successfully used for *CONJUNCTIVITIS, blepharitis, inflammation of the cornea* and even *iritis.* All the above conditions were chronic, subacute in character. The discharges were *PROFUSE, thick* at times, *watery* at others, *ACRID causing soreness* and sometimes *ulceration.* One of the ranking symptoms of the drug is the *tendency to accumulation* of *sticky mucus* over the *cornea* which obscures the vision, thereby causing frequent wiping, either with the lids or handkerchief. *Acrid tears* is another ranking symptom.

Most of the eye symptoms are accompanied by a "Profuse, fluent coryza, especially in the morning; also by profuse expectoration of mucus which comes up easily by a little hacking cough." Use the 3rd internally and a solution of 1 part tincture of Euphrasia to 9 parts of saturated Boric acid, freely applied to the eyes.

ALLIUM CEPA.

Make-up: Catarrhal; take cold easily.

Loc.: M.M. of eyes, *nose*, larynx; nerves.

Sen.: Sharp; burning; smarting; rawness.

Mod.: Agg. *in warm room;* getting wet feet.
Amel. in open, clear air.

Leaders: Frequent, violent sneezing with profuse acrid discharge; feeling as if the mucous membrane of the throat and lungs would split or were being pulled out when coughing.

Mucous Membranes.

Eyes: "Lachrymation with redness of the ball; L. with coryza agg. in evening and warm room."

For a *conjunctivitis* with *smarting, burning* profuse but bloody discharge, accompanying nose and throat trouble. This condition is usually acute and is very common. You probably have all heard of, if not used, onion syrup.

Nose: "Frequent sneezing on entering a warm room; catarrh with headache evenings, agg. in a close room; C. with lachrymation, also with a *copious acrid watery* discharge, amel. in open air."

Throat: "Constrictive pain in region of os hyoides extending downwards."

For *rhinitis* and *laryngitis* the result of taking cold from exposure to raw cold weather. The discharge is copious, *acrid,* with much sneezing, usually accompanied by the *conjunctivitis* which has the same profuse but *bloody discharge.*

Respiratory Organs: "Hoarseness (Phosphorus, Kali

bich.); hacking cough on inspiring cold air (Bromium); constant inclination to hack to relieve the tickling in larynx; stitching, tearing pains in the chest on inspiration."

The cough of Cepa is accompanied by severe pain. One patient expressed it as follows: "It seems as if there were a score of fish hooks in my lungs all on one line, and every time I cough or take a deep breath some one jerked the line." With the catarrhal condition of nose, etc., we have a frontal (sinus) headache with the dull, full pain extending into temples and eyes, with the modalities of Cepa (Kali bich., Pulsatilla, Hydrastis).

Nerves.

Cepa has often been *used* for *neuralgia* of the stump after an amputation or for *injuries* to the *nerves* (Arsenicum, Hypericum). The pains are fine shooting but not burning like Arsenicum. Use the 6th to 30th.

HYDRASTIS.

Make-up: *CATARRHAL;* dyspeptic; debilitated.
Loc.: *Mucous membrane* and glands; liver; skin.
Sen.: Sharp; sticking; burning.
Mod.: Agg.: Warmth; inhaling cold air; touch.
Amel.: Rest; pressure.

Mucous Membranes.

Eyes: "Smarting and burning of the eyes and lids; lids agglutinated in the morning; thick mucous discharge; dark, greenish-yellow conjunctiva."

Useful for *acute catarrhal ophthalmia* when the *lids* are *swollen* and the discharges profuse, with *smarting* and *burning*. Also for *chronic* ophthalmia of scrofulous patients when in addition to the symptoms found under the acute you have *opacity,* rarely *ulceration* of the *cornea.*

Ears: "Eustachian tubes stopped, partly or wholly; roaring, whirring and ringing."

Hydrastis has cured many cases of *otorrhea* following scarlet fever. There is usually impairment of hearing, the drum perforated and the discharge thick mucus (Kali bich.). The throat symptoms usually accompany this group.

Nose: "Sneezing from tickling in nostrils, then excoriating watery discharge from the nose, later the discharge becoming thick yellow."

For *catarrh* with the discharge as stated above. With most cases the catarrhal condition extends up into the sinuses and causes a severe frontal headache.

Note the modality of this condition. As the patient goes out into the cold air the M.M. becomes irritated, the discharge becomes much freer and the headache amel. by relieving the pressure in the sinuses (Pulsatilla, Kali bich.). The nasal catarrh is always posterior and the secretions fall into the throat.

For *hypertrophic* catarrh with the thick, yellow-green discharge which is often offensive. You find the same modalities as in the acute form. Then there is *ulceration* with the *bloody* discharges added to the above, and sharp, sticking pains.

Mouth: "Tongle large and marked by teeth (Mercurius); aphthæ; yellow coating."

Hydrastis is one of the four leading remedies for aphthous stomatitis (Borax, Muriatic ac., Mercurius) of women and children. It is one of the antidotes for the abuse of Chlorate of Potash when the latter has been taken for sore throat.

Give the third internally and the tincture, one part to nine of water, for a gargle or wash. Follow the directions given under Kali chlor.

Throat: "Hawking from increased mucus (Stannum, Iodium); sticky mucus about fauces which cannot be swallowed (Pulsatilla); rough, sore feeling in the morning on waking, agg. by swallowing."

There is no doubt about Hydrastis being used when not indicated. Many use Hydrastis as they do every "cure all" which comes along. For this reason it may not cure in all cases, but Hydrastis is indicated for *catarrhal sore* throat with a *free mucous discharge* with *burning* and *rawness.* The condition extends up into the nose and down into the chest. The entire mucous *membrane* is *covered* with *protruding points.* There are also some *ulcers.* The membrane is very *red* and irritable, agg. from least exposure to cold (Kali carb.).

Stomach and Abdomen: "Nausea; acute pain; sticking in the epigastrium; intermittent, acute pains in region of the liver extending to the scapula."

Clinical experience has shown that Hydrastis is far more useful in this section than these few symptoms would indicate.

Gastritis with frequent vomiting, loss of appetite, distress after eating and marked soreness has often been cured by the remedy. The vomited matter was mucus and blood in addition to the food. Many such cases have been called cancer but I have never considered the condition other than ulceration.

For *gastro-duodenal catarrh* Hydrastis shares the honors with Kali bich. You have constipation, sinking in the stomach region, palpitation of the heart, *vomiting,* often of *blood,* general weakness and frontal headache.

Often for the so-called torpid liver (Chelidonium, Podophyllum) with tenderness in region of liver, light-colored stool, yellow skin and sclera, and itching.

Chronic enteritis with feces covered by mucus.

For *ulceration* of the rectum, *fissures* of the anus and for *prolapsus* of the *rectum,* especially for children. It is second only to Podophyllum for the prolapsus.

Hydrastis is one of our most frequently called for remedies for *constipation.* It cured constipation of pregnancy when hemorrhoids complicated the condition; constipation of children when there was a general catarrhal condition of the M.M. but especially snuffles (Nux, Alumina), obstinate constipation with the dull frontal headache due to catarrh of the sinuses, with a weak, all-gone feeling of the stomach. Finally for constipation of the patients who have taken Sal hepat. and all sorts of nostrums but who are worse instead of better.

Dr. Pettitt of Waterloo had a pill called Pettitt's pill which won such a reputation for curing constipation that most of our pharmacies are now using it, adding or subtracting some of the Hydrastis Dr. Pettitt used, and adding Podophyllum or Strychnia, but are still selling it under the head of Pettitt's Pills. The indication for it is a large, dry stool *with no desire for an evacuation.*

Urinary and Sexual Organs: Clinically we find it useful for *chronic catarrh* of the *bladder* with *thick, ropy mucus in* the *urine* (Kali bich.). The most frequent use I have made of it is *inflammation* and *ulceration* of the cervix. You have itching and burning in the vagina, sometimes a fungoid growth (Thuja) and a profuse irritating discharge from the parts.

For this condition I use it in the form of *pulverized* root, four parts, Sanguinaria one part. After thoroughly cleansing the parts, dust them over with this compound and order a douche of hot, normal salt solution after 24 hours. This should be repeated at intervals of three or four days.

For *chronic gonorrhea* with a muco-purulent discharge with pain in certain points indicating chronic ulceration.

The *claims* made for its having cured *cancerous* ulceration *are not proven.* However, that many cases of *hard, nodular tumors* of the breasts have been cured by Hydrastis I do know. They were found in connection with the ulceration of the cervix. Finally for vaginal leucorrhea.

Respiratory Organs: "Hoarseness; desire to cough increased to nausea; cough with sweetish mucous expectoration."

We have already given the symptoms for its use in *laryngeal* and *bronchial* catarrh, *i. e.*, the pallor of the mucous membrane which is studded with red, ulcerating points about the remiglottis and the yellow tenacious mucus coughed up after some effort.

Skin.

We have not much from the provers under this section, but clinically Hydrastis has shown that it will cure *eczema, lupus, ulcers* and *epithelioma.*

CLEMATIS ERECTA.

Make-up: Rheumatic; herpetic.

Loc.: M.M., especially of eyes and urethra; glands; testicles; ovaries; mammæ; skin of scalp.

Sen.: Burning; itching; stinging; crawling.

Mod.: Agg. night; heat of bed; suppressed gonorrhea; washing in cold water.

Amel. sweating.

Leaders: Very hard, painful, swollen glands, the result of venereal infection.

Mucous Membranes.

Eyes: "Red; glittering; dry; burning as if fire streamed out of them (Aconite, Rhododendron); dryness and heat compelling him to close the lids (Aconite); sensation as of a veil before them."

For *pustular conjunctivitis* with great sensitiveness to cold air. This condition often accompanies simple or syphilitic iritis when you have the pressing pains, marked photophobia and profuse lachrymation. Agg. at night is also marked (Mercurius).

Glands and Glandular Organs.

Sexual Organs: "Testicles swollen (Pulsatilla, Rhododendron), sensitive, enlarged and dragging on the cord; bruised pain on slightest touch (Spongia, Rhododendron), with drawing and tension in the inguinal region."

One of our three most frequently called for remedies for *orchitis* due to suppressed gonorrhea, with pain greatly agg. at night, a feeling as if the urethra were contracted, so that he has to strain to pass a few drops and dribbling after micturition.

For *indurations* and *tumors* of the breasts which are very painful to touch, in a woman who had an eruption which came on just before the menses and disappeared about a week after. The woman menstruated regularly every 28 days just before the full of the moon. I also had another woman, a cousin of the one mentioned above, who came to me for relief from an acrid leucorrhea which came just before the menses. The menses were regular every 28 days. The leucorrhea was very annoying, agg. after urinating. About every fourth menstrual period instead of the leucorrhea there appeared an eruption at the base of the brain. There was a great deal of moisture, much itching and crawling, greatly aggravated at night when warm in bed. When the eruption was present there was no leucorrhea and vice versa. However, there was the severe shooting pain in the breast with both conditions. Use 3rd and 6th.

CANNABIS INDICA.

Make-up: Extremely sensitive; emotional.

Loc.: Mind, nerves, genito-urinary organs.

Sen.: Spasmodic, syncope.

Mod.: Agg.: Urinating; darkness; *noises,* talking; exertion.

Leaders: *Excessive exaltation followed by equally marked depression;* great mental excitement and the agg. by noise.

Brain and Nerves.

Mind: "*Imagines that he hears music, shuts his eyes and is lost in delicious thought; exaltation of spirits; anguish* with oppression *amel.* in open air; loquacity, with incoherent talk; *uncontrollable laughter* until the face is purple and the back aches; fear that he should become insane (Actea); *fixed ideas;* absentminded; unconscious every few minutes."

The drug has been used as a remedy in various forms of

delirium, especially delirium tremens with the above conditions.

Head: "Frequent involuntary shaking, *heaviness* with *unconsciousness* and falling; *shocks through brain on regaining consciousness, vertigo* on rising with stunning pain in occiput."

For two conditions, *migraine* with the *sensation* as if the head were *opening* and *shutting; uremic* headache with the same sensation.

Ears: "*Throbbing* and *fullness; buzzing* and *ringing;* noise like boiling water, music is very agreeable (Tarantula)."

Extremities: "Weakness of, amounting to paralysis; *pain across* the *shoulder and spine,* forcing him to stoop; *agreeable thrill* in arm, hand, and from knee down, with a *sensation as if a bird's claw were clasping the knee.*"

It has helped *threatening paralysis.*

Mucous Membranes.

Urinary Organs: "Urging after micturition, with much straining; *dribbling* after stream ceases; must wait a long time before urine flows; *stitching* and *burning* in the urethra before, during and after urinating copious colorless urine. Oozing of white, glossy mucus on squeezing the gland."

Sexual Organs: I have used it for gleet but prefer the Cannabis sativa for symptoms like the above. Use 30th.

MEZEREUM.

Make-up: Dirty, unhealthy skin; low vitality.

Loc.: *Skin;* M.M.; brain and nerves; bones.

Sen.: Itching; burning; smarting; chilliness.

Mod.: Agg. *night; warmth of bed;* suppressions; cold air; touch; mercury.

Amel.: Radiated heat.

Leaders: Pus forming into scabs; *neuralgia following* herpes.

Brain and Nerves.

Mind: "Everything seems dead, nothing makes a vivid impression on the mind; sad weeping mood (Pulsatilla, Ignatia, Mercurius). Anger with desire to say vexatious things (Anacardium); stupid; forgetful."

The most frequent use I have made of the mental symptoms of Merzereum is to counteract the effects of mercury and syphilis, on the mind. There is that same disgust for self and everything that Mercurius produces.

Head: "*Aching, with pain on slightest touch, after vexation* (Chamomilla), after moving about and talking, much agg. in open air, warm room, more in temples and sides of vertex; dizzy as if intoxicated, as if he had been up all night (Nux, Cocculus); stupefying pain through right side of brain to forehead."

For *neuralgic headaches* caused by syphilis or the abuse of mercury or both. The pains are boring, burning, extending from occiput over the whole brain, also downward to shoulders, leaving the parts very sensitive to touch (China).

Eyes: "Pressing and tearing pains in and about the eyes; jerking of muscles of the upper lids (Agaricus); inclination to blink."

It has helped many cases of *ciliary neuralgia* after operations (Cepa), when the pains shoot downwards accompanied by coldness and followed by soreness in bone.

The most frequent use I have made of Mezereum is for *supra-orbital* neuralgia following *herpes*. The herpes has caused falling out of all the eyebrows, sometimes the eyelashes. The part looks red and shiny and feels hot. The pains are sharp, come in paroxysms, agg. night and by heat.

Ears: "Tearing, boring, burning pain in and about the ears; sensation as if wind were blowing in ear; roaring."

Violent otalgia, involving the teeth and face, with constant *chilliness* (Cepa), generally *after* the *abuse* of *mercury*. For deafness after the *suppression* of an *eruption*.

Face: "Jerking in zygomatic muscles, *tearing below the eye* into the left side and teeth waking her from sleep; boring with burning in left cheek; tearing, drawing in the lower jaw."

For *facial neuralgia* arising from the teeth, especially in the infra-orbital region, so much agg. by washing the face that it brought tears, also agg. at night and by heat. Violent neuralgia of face and head with the same symptoms stated under eye. Numbness frequently follows these attacks of neuralgia.

Chest: "Sharp, constricting pains transversely across the abdomen, especially about the heart."

Here again for *intercostal neuralgia* following herpes zoster when the constriction is agg. night and by heat.

Skin.

"Usual liver spots on chest and arms become very dark, with desquamation; *ulcers on bony protuberances, covered with thick, whitish-yellow scabs under which thick yellow pus collects;* itching and burning *vesicles* around the ulcers which dry into scabs which are painful to remove; ichor, from scratched face, excoriates the other parts; honey-like scabs around the mouth, white, elevated over whole body; the child scratches its face continually; it becomes covered with blood and scabs which on being torn off leave a raw surface on which large pustules form."

Mezereum cures both *herpetic* and *eczematous* eruptions. The ranking symptoms are: *ulceration* and *formation* of *scabs over* thick *pus,* especially is this true *on* the *head; itching* which is greatly *agg.* by *scratching; agg.* at night and by heat. For *eczema impetiginoides* of the *whole face* covered with *THICK scabs,* with the same modalities as above stated.

For syphilitic colored spots on thighs and body. Varicose ulcers of the leg surrounded by a bluish-red discoloration extremely sensitive to touch, the slight touch causing bleeding (Asafœtida).

Finally for *pruritus* of old people with *terrible itching* of the *parts most shriveled, e. g.,* neck, etc., *with* intense formication.

Mucous Membranes.

Ear: "*Sensation* as if air were distending external meatus with a stopped up sensation in ears."

Chronic otitis with this feeling as if the ears were stopped up, usually with eczema behind the ear (Graphites) and pains shooting down into the face and teeth (Verbascum).

Nose: "Sneezing with fluent coryza; discharge of yellow, at times bloody, water which causes soreness and burning pain; discharge of thin mucus sometimes streaked with blood, which makes the nostrils sore."

There are two conditions for which it has been used with success: *chronic ozena, syphilitic* or from the abuse of Mercury with loss of smell and burning pain in the bones of the face and nose; for *ulcerations* of the septum with the same symptoms plus the blood-streaked mucous discharge.

Throat: "Feeling as if full of mucus, not amel. by expectoration; scraping, rawness and burning in pharynx, fauces and esophagus; dryness in fauces and irritation, causing dry, fatiguing cough."

For an *ulcerative, syphilitic sore throat* with the above symptoms, the burning relieved by cold air but the air caused aching of the gums.

Stomach: "Pain in epigastric region in the evening and at night, agg. pressure; vomiting of green, bitter mucus, sometimes streaked with blood."

Mezereum has cured gastric *ulcers* with the *marked burning* and uneasiness in stomach temporarily amel. by eating, which fact causes the patient to eat to excess (Iodium). A few cases of *supposed malignant ulceration* of the stomach have been relieved and some cured in which we had burning, drawing and distress of the entire stomach with vomiting of blood and also large quantity of blood from the bowels.

Stools: "Diarrhea constant with pain in the abdomen; brown feces containing white, shiny grains (Iodium, Phosphorus)."

The stools of the Mezereum patient vary with the different conditions, *e. g., sour, undigested, liquid stools* with much *colic* followed by *chilliness,* showing *functional changes* of the *stomach;* mucous stools streaked with blood and accompanied by tenesmus showing *ulceration* of *rectum,* or dysentery. Very rarely we may find a very hard, dry stool with prolapsus ani (Hepar).

Sexual Organs: "Mucous discharge from vagina; leucorrhea like white of an egg (Alumina); menses too frequent and lasting too long."

We find that in *ulceration* of the vagina with the above discharge there is often a *sensation* of *dryness,* which is marked, and some burning.

Bones.

As you have noticed in several of the above groups there is much inflammation and ulceration of the bones of the face especially the jaws and the long bones, just the ones most frequently affected by syphilis. There is *intense periostitis,* with extreme soreness and marked swelling also burning and agg. at night, which causes loss of sleep and its long train of symptoms. As in Mercurius the muscles and skin above the ulcerated bones also suppurate and leave chronic ulcers which bleed easily (Nitric ac., Mercurius). Mezerium is one of the best antidotes for the skin and bone effects of mercury, and it shares with Mercurius the honors for curing the same conditions the result of syphilis.

THUJA.

Make-up: Sycotic; hydrogenoid.

Loc.: M.M.; kidneys; *genito-urinary organs; skin;* glands.

Sen.: Sharp as from a nail; stitching; tensive.

Mod.: Agg.: *cold, damp;* tea; warm bed; gonorrhea; night.
Amel.: Moist heat; sneezing.

Leaders: A dirty, brown spotted or hairy skin; exuberant, warty or fungoid tissues; sleepless.

Mucous Membranes.

Ear: "Buzzing, roaring; creaking like the turning of a wooden screw, when swallowing saliva."

The most frequent use of Thuja is for *otorrhea* with a *discharge* which *smells* like *putrid meat.* There is an unhealthy polypoid tissue about the opening in the drum which bleeds very easily.

Nose: "Ulceration half an inch within the nostrils where there are scabs (Aurum, Nitric ac., Mercurius), swelling with induration and tensive pain; feeling of soreness in nostril agg. by pressure on alæ; sensation of dry catarrh and stoppage in the upper part agg. evening; dryness better in open air."

For *nasal catarrh,* when the discharge is large in amount, is thick, green or yellowish green and may be mucus, pus, or blood or all three of them. The discharges seem to come from the frontal sinuses (Mercurius, Pulsatilla, Kali bich.). There are also painful scabs in the nostrils, *scabs* and *warts* on the *margin* of the mucous membrane and skin.

Mouth: "White blisters on side of tongue close to the root; burning, agg. warm food; *tip painful to touch;* mouth filled with blisters as if burned."

For *aphthous sore* mouth. Also for retraction of the gums from the teeth, leaving a red, spongy *growth about* the *roots* of the teeth.

I had such a case in a young woman of 20 with dark, muddy skin, which would never heal if injured. She had a tooth extracted because it was decayed and ached. The pain was greatly agg. by cold drinks. Soon after the extraction there appeared in the site of the extracted tooth a red vascular substance which bled on the least provocation. The dentist called in a physician and the growth was curetted and cauterized. It returned in that locality and around the root of the adjoining tooth. That tooth was extracted but the growth continued to spread. Being told that all her teeth must be extracted and the jaw curetted, she came to me for help. The dentist told her the growth was cancerous in nature. Because of the appearance of the growth and skin the patient was put upon the 30th of the drug, five drops four times daily. The growth was bathed three times daily with a 1 to 2000th of the tincture of Thuja. Improvement began after ten days and continued till the growth was all gone, the skin greatly improved and the patient in better health than ever. Lest you be misled by the statement of the dentist, I will say that our pathologist found no evidence of cancer, and when I told him it was *scorbutic*, he simply said, "I don't know what scorbutic is."

Respiratory Organs: "A hacking, dry, short, interrupted cough; *convulsive* cough agg. at night."

I never knew the real significance of these symptoms till a patient was brought to me with a cough which fitted the description completely. She was dark, aged 23, had had muscular rheumatism, had a yellowish-green acrid leucorrhea, also nasal polypi and ulceration of the nostrils. Notwithstanding all the symptoms of the mucous membrane the cough was so harrassing and not only "*convulsive*" but *explosive, shattering,* that I put her upon Drosera and promised results. The next day she reported worse and on questioning stated that the cause of the cough was irritation about the vocal cords. I took her to our throat specialist, who found the cords and remi-glottis studded with little vascular growths. I turned the case over to the specialist but the next day she came to the office, saying the specialist burnt her mouth and throat so she would not see him again. I gave placebo for 48 hours to await the result of the 23 per cent. solution of Argentium nit. which the specialist had used. The cough had not improved; I then put her upon Thuja 1000 B. and T.'s preparation, five drops night and morning. I also had her use as a gargle the 1 to 2000th solution of the tincture. The restlessness and sleeplessness began to improve at once. The cough did not subside for a week and did not cease till after six weeks when the growths had been absorbed. The patient had no more rheumatism and the catarrhal symptoms greatly improved, although the leucorrhea continued in a mild form after each menstrual period.

Although I have tried Thuja many times and with the same preparations that were used in the two cases cited above, I never saw any benefit from it in a purely catarrhal cough.

Sexual Organs: "Glans secreted thin mucus, causing moisture; itching and intermittent burning between glands and prepuce; *red growth like condylomata on inner surface of prepuce;* sweat on scrotum, perineum and thighs; *itching* and *biting* of *labia* during and after micturition; burning and biting in vagina when walking and sitting; yellow-green leucorrhea."

Thuja has the credit of curing *secondary syphilis; chancroidal ulcer* of genitals; *epithelioma* of *vagina* and cancer of *uterus.* Also *uterine polypi, chronic gonorrheal ovaritis, leucorrhea* which *made* the *vagina* very *sensitive* (Kreosote, Sulphur). I have verified the efficacy of Thuja for all of the above conditions, but the one for which I have most frequently used it is for "cock's comb excrescences." In over *90 per cent.* of the cases they *are found* in the *scar tissue* of *lacerations* of the *os.* They are *redundant, red, vascular,* bleed at least touch and discharge a green or yellow excoriating substance. For these cases use the remedy internally in any potency, and also locally. I give the patient a copious douche of the 1 to 2000 solution of the tincture and after the douche apply soft sponges saturated in the same to the os about the excrescences. The treatment should be continued for some time after the growths have disappeared.

Anus and Stools: "Swelling of hemorrhoidal veins; moisture; discharge of bloody slime day and night, sticking; burning when sitting or when touched; soreness after the slimy discharge as if the skin were cracked; constriction of anus with almost every stool; diarrhea watery, painless (China)."

For *warts, fistulas* and *hemorrhoids.* The only use I have made of the remedy in this section has been for the growths and diarrhea. One case of each as an illustration. A business man about 50, dark and sluggish, came to me with the statement, "Can you permanently get rid of my rat tail?" and proceeded to undress to show me what he meant. About the anus was a row of bleeding hemorrhoids and in addition a combination polypus and wart which hung down about two inches. The base was about half an inch up the rectum. I replied that I could cut it off. This he refused to have me do because an orificialist had operated on his brother and destroyed the sphincter ani. So I put him on Thuja 30th internally and gave him a solution 1 part tincture to 3 parts water to apply locally. The "rat tail" and hemorrhoids all disappeared in six weeks and never returned.

The only form of *diarrhea* I ever use it for is one following *improper vaccination.* The stools are *watery,* greasy, *copious,* often green, *expelled with* much *flatus, agg.* after *eating* especially after breakfast. Use the 30th.

Skin.

"*Wart-like excrescences* on any part of the body, red itching spots as from flea bites, agg. evening; ***candylomota*** at juncture of skin and mucous membrane *which bleed easily.*"

Aside from the warts and excrescences already mentioned it has been used successfully for *lupus, varicose ulcers* and pemphigus *eczema.* Following Boenninghausen's suggestion, I have used it many times for *smallpox* if the patient was of the Thuja make-up. Give it as soon as the vesicles begin to fill.

Brain and Nerves.

Mind: "*Loathing of life* (Arsenicum, Mercurius), ***ill humor; sadness*** (Pulsatilla, Sulphur), with disposition to weep; could scarcely collect his senses for half an hour after waking."

Like all drugs useful for venereal diseases Thuja produces an unhappy condition. You will find the mental symptoms of high rank in every group. We sometimes find great emotional sensitiveness; weeping when listening to music (Ignatia), etc. Thuja has two fixed ideas with its *melancholia,* 1st, That they are made of glass which will break easily; 2d, That they have something alive in the abdomen, *i. e.,* some animal or that they are pregnant.

Head: "Sticking pains; transitory sensation as if a nail were driven into the skull, agg. touch."

This symptom has been verified many times in the *neuralgic* headache which has been caused by drinking tea to excess (Coffea). The pains extend from vertex over the whole head, agg. at night.

Eyes: "Feeling in lids as if swollen; and as if a foreign body were in the eye; burning in the edges, with stinging; agg. evening; vision dim in the open air with confusion of head; pressure in eyes as if they were too large and would be pressed out; luminous disc like a firefly before the eyes."

For *syphilitic iritis* with gummata on the iris when the pains are very severe, agg. night. For *ciliary neuralgia* when the pains extend all over the head and face causing great soreness, agg. by chewing or lying on face. Also for *kerato-iritis* with excessive *photophobia* and some *opacity,* agg. night.

Extremities: "Drawing pains in back and legs; drawing pains in sacrum, coccyx, and thighs which after his sitting long prevented his standing erect; trembling of hand and foot; crawling in tips of fingers; weakness in legs when sitting, changing to cutting in muscles of calf when walking."

The only use I have ever made of it was for *gonorrheal rheumatism* for which I consider Thuja the most frequently indicated remedy. Use all potencies.

ANACARDIUM.

Loc.: Brain and nerves; skin.

Sen.: As of a plug; pressure.

Mod.: Agg.: Mental exertion; *emotions, especially anger.*
Amel.: While eating.

Leaders: Failing memory; dull pressure; irresistible desire to swear.

Brain and Nerves.

Mind: "Memory weak in morning, especially as regards single names; loss of comprehension with confusion and empty feeling in head; he is separated from the whole world and despairs of doing what is required of him; apprehensive; anxiety with suspicion of everything about him; excessive anger at slight offense, breaking out in personal violence."

Extremely valuable for *brain fag* and *melancholia* with fixed ideas of demons; at times inclination to swear. He fears he is being pursued; is suspicious, which leads him to attempt to escape (Belladonna) or refuse to eat for fear of being poisoned (Hyoscyamus).

Head: "*Pressure on vertex as from a plug;* vertigo as if turning in a circle, agg. stooping."

The *headaches* are *deepseated, digging, throbbing,* amel. eating but very much agg. by mental exertion.

Stomach: We have but one symptom but that of high rank, viz., *vomiting of ingesta during pregnancy,* amel. by eating but which leaves the sensation of a lump (plug) in stomach.

Abdomen: Enteralgia with feeling around the umbilicus as if a blunt plug were squeezed into the intestines.

Rectum and Anus: "*Tenesmus* but he cannot expel anything and the *rectum seems plugged* up; urging to stool after eating, more in the upper part of the intestines."

The *characteristic symptom* of the drug, viz., sensation of a *plug* is often found in these sections.

Skin: "Dry feeling in hands and fingers; burning and stinging; blisters and pustules."

Anacardium is an extremely valuable remedy for *eczema* with the *above symptoms plus an irritable mind.* The *itching* and *burning* are marked (Rhus). Use 3rd and 6th.

AGARICUS.

Make-up: *Nervous;* anemic; *frostbitten.*

Loc.: *Nerves* (spinal axis); heart and *skin.*

Sen.: *Twitching;* jerking; trembling; *burning;* itching; drawing; cutting; griping; *cramping.*

Nerves.

Head: "Tearing; *twitching;* shooting; *piercing;* aching."

Agaricus cures two varieties of headaches, one a dull, the result of prolonged office work, the other the *result* of *anemia* of the spine. The 3x of Agaricin given three times daily cured a most violent case of *Tic Douloroux* of the left side of face after Arsenicum, Magnesia phos. and Belladonna had failed. A *slight touch* would *cause* the paroxysms to recur.

Eye: "*Twitching* of balls; spasmodic pains in lids while reading; contraction of lids; trembling; burning in left canthus; agglutination of canthi; motion of type with flickering when reading."

Very frequently cured *asthenopia* caused by prolonged strain; also for *spasm* of accommodation with twitching of both eyeballs and lids. The muscles are *weak* as well as *irritable.*

Face: "Pale with *bluish appearance* about the eyes, nose and mouth; itching and burning as after freezing; upper lips chapped with burning and smarting; dryness of lips; burning pimples with yellow serum; stitching as if splinters were forced between skin and flesh."

For *neuralgia* of the face with the above symptoms. For *chorea* of the face of *children.* It is with the latter that the *eruptions* about the mouth occur.

Mouth: "Tearing; gnawing; pulsating; stitching; burning pains in tongue; soreness of tongue; sensation of *dryness yet profuse saliva* with constant spitting."

Has cured *neuralgia* of the teeth when worse in open air; also neuralgia of the tongue of choreic children when there was profuse vitiated saliva causing soreness of the lips.

Abdomen: "Emission of much inodorous flatus; distention; trembling; cutting; griping; stitching; drawing."

The gastric *enteralgias* of Agaricus are usually catarrhal in origin and the patient passes a great deal of odorless flatus. The stools are usually watery accompanied by "violent pinching pain."

Bladder: "Frequent *urging* to urinate; burning; stitching."

The nervous Agaricus patients pass but *little urine* which is of a clear, lemon color.

Sexual Organs: "Profuse, early menses with violent tearing, pressive pains in back and abdomen with *itching* of external *genitals*."

Respiratory Organs: "Constriction of larynx; *convulsive* cough; *paroxysmal* cough; constant irritation to cough, sudden, violent attacks of *cough;* respiration difficult, deep, sighing, noisy at night."

The Agaricus patient suffers from a spasmodic, convulsive, nervous cough. The cough is usually dry but exceptionally there may be loose mucus. The cough has been so severe as to cause hemorrhages.

Chest: "*Stitching;* tearing; pinching; sprained; bruised; aching; drawing; burning; shuddering; *anxiety;* constriction; tension; oppression; heaviness; rawness."

All these sensations are due to two conditions, *i. e., uncomplicated neuralgias* due to abnormal circulation of the blood caused by *spasmodic contraction* of the *blood vessels*, poor oxygenization of the blood. Exercise aggravates and eating aggravates. I have found Agaricus helpful for patients whom Stannum iod. was benefiting, when there was a sudden aggravation of the Stannum symptoms (viz., weakness of the chest, expectoration of small hard lumps of mucus and the night sweats).

Back: "*Bruised* feeling in *muscles; aching* along *spine* and limbs; stitching; deep-seated burning; aching along spinal cord when stooping; *soreness* to touch; drawing; boring; tension; weakness."

All of the above symptoms have been repeatedly verified in patients suffering from *spinal anemia,* lumbago or the "lightning like pains" of *locomotor ataxia.* All of these pains are worse walking in the open air, especially in cold weather.

Extremities: "*Trembling; twitching;* splinter-like; burnt; tearing."

The peculiarity of these pains is that they seem to be just beneath the skin, shift from place to place and are worse from motion.

Skin.

Ears: "*Redness;* burning and itching as if they had been *frozen.*"

Face: "Blueness of the tip of nose; redness of face with itching and *burning* as after *freezing.*"

Extremities: "Feet feel frost bitten; *redness* of the fingers with *burning, itching,* as if *frozen.*" Apply a dilution of the tincture and give the 3x internally for frost bite.

Heart.

"*Palpitation;* aching; oppression; *anxiety.*"

For irritable heart caused by excesses in venery, use of tea, coffee or tobacco.

Use in from tincture to 1m, most often 30th.

FERRUM PHOSPHORICUM.

Make-up: *Anemic;* fair; florid; emotional.

Loc.: Circulation; blood; heart; lungs; brain and nerves; mucous membranes; bones; thermic centers.

Sen.: Dull; heavy; sharp; shooting; pinching; tearing; drawing; stitching; sore.

Mod.: Agg.: Motion; at night; eating.

Amel.: cold; rest; lying down.

As we began with a remedy which was useful at the beginning of inflammatory conditions (Aconite), so we will close with another remedy, which if given at the outset of diseases which are inflammatory in character, especially of the circulatory pulmonary organs, will abort the conditions. Unlike Aconite, however, Ferrum phos. is useful in many conditions for the last as well as the first stage. It is one of Schuessler's twelve tissue remedies and you have a more exhaustive study of it in Boericke & Dewey's study of those tissue remedies.

Respiratory organs: "Acute, short, spasmodic cough, which is very painful; cough agg. in open air, touching larynx, at night; sharp stitching pains in chest on deep inspiration." We get prompt results with it in several conditions of the lungs: 1st, *congestion with* a peculiar *swishing sound* like the waves against the side of a boat in quiet water; a very *rapid pulse; flushed face;* scanty blood-streaked expectoration; *high temperature* and marked restlessness. 2nd, *pneumonia* with the same symptoms as for congestion, plus heaviness of the *chest* and dullness over certain areas, also a dry, hacking cough. Ferrum phos. was one of the most frequently indicated remedies for *Flu-pneumonia.* 3rd, *Pleurisy* with the sharp stitching pain with every breath; *high temperature,* dry *cough and rapid pulse.* I have found it especially useful for bronchitis of young children and old people with the above symptoms. Not only will you find it helpful in acute but in *chronic bronchitis* when a fresh exposure causes the above symptoms. 4th, *Whooping cough with hoarseness or complete loss of voice;* vomiting; epistaxis and a rapid pulse. The *rapid pulse* and *bloody sputum* are the *ranking symptoms* of *all conditions* of this locality.

Heart and circulatory organs: "Full, bounding pulse; dull, aching pain about the heart and extending to back and spine; palpitation of heart." In the first stage of *carditis, endocarditis, peri-carditis* and *cardiac arteritis,* I have verified all these conditions. In all I have found a rapid pulse with tension between Aconite and Gelsemium.

There is one other condition in which the rapid pulse has been the ranking symptom, and that is exophthalmus. The symptoms of this condition rank in the following order if Ferrum phos. is indicated: *rapid pulse, protrusion of eyes, tremor with the enlarged thyroid,* last but often not present. In several such cases all the symptoms except the protrusion of the eyes have disappeared from the use of the 30th, a dose twice daily.

Blood: Decrease in number of blood cells, tendency to hemorrhage; marked weakness; yellow, watery stools; poor appetite; frequent vomiting and irritability of the heart, constitute a group of symptoms which we call *pernicious anemia* which *have been helped by Ferrum phos.* By helped, I mean life prolonged and the patient made more comfortable. For this condition I use the 3x.

Head: "Violent throbbing pain in head amel. by nosebleed; violent headache during the menses; head and scalp extremely sensitive to touch." For *congestive headaches* which come just *before* the *menses* (Actea), also at the *climacteric,* amel. when the flow is established (Lachesis) and by epitaxis.

Stomach: "Vomiting, at irregular times, of green vomita, sometimes of blood; poor appetite; weight and fullness in stomach; pain in stomach after eating and from pressure."

Dyspepsia in anemic patient.

Eyes: "Eyes red; burning; suffused; pain in eye ball agg. by motion." For *neuralgia* of eye balls (Agaricus) and *conjunctivitis.*

Ears: "Ringing and buzzing; hardness of hearing; redness and soreness over mastoid."

The remedy has been useful for *otitis* and ***mastoiditis.***

Male Sexual Organs: "Dull aching in the testicles; frequent desire to urinate with pain in urethra." It has been curative in the first stage of orchitis and urethritis.

Female Sexual Organs: "Bearing-down in uterus with pain in ovaries; dryness of the vagina; dysmenia with flushed face and rapid pulse; menses too frequent and too profuse."

One of our best remedies for congestive dysmenorrhea. Also useful for vaginismus when the parts are dry and hot. It has also cured the cough of pregnancy when the cough was accompanied by spurting of urine.

Thermic centers: We find inflammatory conditions and a high temperature with all pulmonary diseases.

INDEX OF REMEDIES.

GENERAL INDEX AND REPERTORY.

BONES AND BLOOD.

Bones.

Blood.

Secondary Anemia: Arsenicum, 202; Arsenicum iod., 202; Ferrum phos., 25; Phosphoric ac., 260; China, 211; Nux vom., 115.

Hemorrhages from anus: Mercurius, 128; Arsenicum alb., 199; Capsicum, 13; Ipecac, 253; Lachesis, 195; Hamamelis; Aloe, 239.

Hemorrhage from kidneys: Hamamelis; Cantharis, 322; Terebinthina, 321; Arsenicum alb., 200; Mercurius cor., 128; Phosphorus, 255.

Hemorrhage from lungs: Phosphorus, 257; Ferrum phos., 25; Ferrum, 144; Aconite, 1; Sanguinaria, 263; Tuberculin, 311; Ipecac, 251.

Hemorrhage from nose: Bryonia, 108; Arnica, 99; Hamamelis; Phosphorus, 255; Mercurius, 124.

Hemorrhage from stomach: Phosphorus, 256; Ipecac, 253; Arsenicum alb., 200; Argentum nit., 131; Hydrastis, 332; Kali bich., 37; China, 214.

Hemorrhage from uterus: China, 215; Phosphorus, 255; Sanguinaria, 262; Ergot; Secale, 193; Trillium, 197; Nitric ac.; Calcarea carb., 63; Belladonna, 20; Chamomilla, 191; Platinum, 148; Sabina, 196.

Blood and Infectious Diseases.

Sepsis: Arsenicum, 202; Rhus tox., 103; Arnica, 100; Echinacea, 217; China, 211; Chininum ars., 205; Arsenicum iod., 205; Lachesis, 218; Baptisia, 206; Mercurius, 121; Hepar, 110; Terebinthina, 319; Carbo veg., 302.

Erysipelas: Rhus tox., 102; Belladonna, 21; Arsenicum, 200; Graphites, 94; Apis mel., 323; Hepar sulph., 114; Kali iod., 52; Cantharis, 323; Lachesis, 219.

Diphtheria: Lachesis, 221; Lycopodium, 93; Arsenicum, 202; Mercurius, 125; Phytolacca, 294; Baptisia, 206; Nitric ac.; Muriatic ac., 289; Gelsemium, 208; Capsicum, 14; Apis, 317; Mercurius cor., 128; Mercurius cyn., 129; Cantharis, 322; Bromium, 168; Echinacea, 217; Ignatia, 272.

Measles: Pulsatilla, 182; Bryonia, 110; Gelsemium, 207; Kali bich., 39; Arsenicum, 200.

Pertussis: Ipecac, 251; Drosera, 99; Kali bich., 39; Sambucus; Moschus, 280; Mephitis; Sanguinaria, 263; Hepar, 110; Rumex, 264; Spongia, 175; Belladonna, 21; Hyoscyamus, 24; Graphites, 99; Arnica, 100; Cuprum, 138; Zinc m., 164; Cina, 247.

Scarlet fever: Belladonna, 21; Arsenicum alb., 202; Ammonium carb., 269; Lachesis, 219; Apis, 317; Mercurius, 117; Lycopodium, 93; Rhus, 102; Bryonia, 109; Chininum ars., 206; Tuberculinum, 313; Echinacea, 217; Muriatic ac., 290.

Rheumatic fever: Colchicum, 281; Bryonia, 109; Rhus tox., 103; Actea rac., 175; Arnica, 100; Sulphur, 4; Caulophyllum; Pulsatilla, 179; Natrum sulf., 78; Phytolacca, 295; Rhododendron, 296; Syphilinum, 310; Variolinum, 313; Mercurius sol., 121; Thuja, 343; Iodium, 173.

Influenza: Gelsemium, 209; Ferrum phos., 35; Arsenicum alb. and iod., 202; Baptisia, 206; Rhus tox., 102; Bryonia, 106; Eupatorium perf., 308; China, 211; Tartar emet., 266; Chininum, 205; Strychnia phos.; Antimonium ars.; Ipecac, 254; Pulsatilla, 179.

Small-pox: Arsenicum, 200; Tartar emet., 267; Belladonna, 21; Thuja, 343; Variolinum, 312; Crotalus; Phosphorus, 260; Lachesis, 218; Rhus, 102; Syphilinum, 311.

Typhoid: Bryonia, 109; Baptisia, 206; Rhus tox., 102; Gelsemium, 209; Muriatic ac., 290; Arsenicum, 202; Phosphoric ac.; China, 211; Carbo veg., 302; Nux vom., 120; Nitric ac., 290; Lycopodium, 93; Terebinthina, 319; Helleborus, 326; Lachesis, 218.

Dysentery: Mercurius cor., 128; Arsenicum, 199; Capsicum, 13; Colocynth, 306; Ipecac, 253; Nux vom., 117; Hyoscyamus, 24; Mercurius sol., 125; Argentum nit., 132; Cantharis, 323; Secale, 195.

Chicken-pox: Rhus tox., 102; Tartar emet., 269; Antimonium crud,; Apis, 318.

Mumps: Aconite, 1; Mercurius, 127; Belladonna, 19; Phytolacca, 294; Hepar, 110.

Yellow fever: Gelsemium, 209; Aconite, 1; Crotalus; Arsenicum, 202; Veraturm alb., 326; Carbo veg., 302.

Malaria: China, 215; Quinine, 216; Natrum mur., 73; Gelsemium, 209; Eupatorium, 308; Arsenicum, 202; Nux vom., 115; Bryonia, 109; Capsicum, 14; Arnica, 100; Rhus, 103; Arsenicum iod., 296; Gelsemium, 209; Chininum sulph., 216; Cactus, 230; Ipecac, 254.

Cholera: Camphor; Cuprum, 139; Veratrum alb., 326; Arsenicum, 202; Carbo veg., 302; Cuprum ars., 141; Crotalus; Naja.

Cerebro-spinal fever: Actea, 17; Cicuta, 225; Belladonna, 15; Zinc. phos., 164; Opium; Veratrum vir., 314.

Infantile Spinal Paralysis: Gelsemium, 207; Belladonna, 15; Aconite, 1; Calcarea carb., 60; Secale, 193; Phosphorus, 250; Plumbum, 152.

Pulmonary Tuberculosis: Tuberculin, 311; Arsenicum iod.; Kali carb., 45; Iodium, 172; Silica, 157; Ferrum phos., 35; Stannum, 158; Stannum iod., 160; Sanguinaria; Kali iod., 50; Spongia, 175; Ars. iod., 204.

Syphilis: Syphilinum, 308; Kali iod., 48; Phytolacca, 295; Mercurius, 122; Mezereum, 338; Nitric ac., 341; Alumina, 235.

BRAIN AND NERVES.

Irritation.

General Neuralgia: Arsenicum, 198; Belladonna, 15; Colocynth, 305; Plumbum, 149; Zinc., 161; Verbascum; Capsicum, 12; Pulsatilla, 179; Magnesia phos., 84; Ranunculus bulb., 298; Spigelia, 227; Aconite, 1; Mezereum, 336; Arnica, 101; Rhus tox., 105; Allium cepa, 330.

Neuralgia of eye: Arsenicum alb., 195; Cedron; Spigelia, 22; Belladonna, 19; China, 212; Ignatia, 269; Rhus, 105; Actea, 177; Agaricus, 347;

Ranunculus bulb., 298; Natrum mur., 72; Magnesia mur., 85; Mezereum, 337.

Neuralgia of ear: Verbascum; Capsicum, 12; Belladonna, 18; Chamomilla, 190; Pulsatilla, 179; Kali phos., 55; Mezereum, 337.

Neuralgia of teeth: Chamomilla, 190; Belladonna, 17; Phosphorus, 259; Causticum, 57; Mercurius, 122; Coffea, 297; Nux vom., 118; Arsenicum, 198; Rhododendron, 297; Colocynth, 305; Pulsatilla, 180; Magnesia phos., 86.

Neuralgia of glottis: Belladonna, 19; Hyoscyamus, 23; Moschus, 280; Acetic ac.; Bromium, 16.

Neuralgia of face: Arsenicum, 198; Kali phos., 57; Natrum phos., 74; Phosphorus, 258; Magnesia carb., 80; Colocynth, 305; Syphilinum, 310; Hepar, 118; Mezereum, 338; Cham., 190; Spigelia, 228; Phos., 259; Magnesia phos., 85.

Neuralgia of stomach: Arsenicum alb.; Argentum nit., 132; Hydrastis, 332; Ipecac, 258; Colocynth, 305; Phosphorus, 256; Iris, 249; Podophyllum, 241; Nux vom., 119; Magnesia phos., 86.

Neuralgia of intestines: Colocynth, 305; Plumbum, 150; Dioscorea; Arsenicum, 199; Magnesia phos., 87; Magnesia mur., 81; Cina, 246; Nux vom., 118; Magnesia carb., 80; Chamomilla, 190.

Neuralgia of ovaries: Zincum, 163; Colocynth, 309; Actea, 178; Aconite, 3; Platinum, 148; Staphisagria, 291; Conium, 224; Belladonna, 20; Plumbum, 151; Crotalus; China, 215; Apis, 317; Magnesia phos., 88.

Neuralgia of heart: Spigelia, 228; Cactus, 229; Nux vom., 12; Actea rac., 177; Kalmia; Magnesia phos., 83; Lachesis, 220; Gelsemium, 207.

Neuralgia of testicles: Zincum, 163; Berberis, 303; Pulsatilla, 183.

Neuralgia of uterus: Actea, 177; Colocynth, 309; Cocculus, 277; Viburnum; Plumbum, 151; Belladonna, 20; Magnesia phos., 83; Conium, 224; Platinum, 148; Ignatia, 271; Nux vom., 119; Sepia, 186; Sabina, 196.

Neuralgia of intercostal nerves: Ranunculus bulb., 298; Actea, 177; Rhododendron, 296; Nux vom., 115; Mezereum, 338; Rumex, 265; Arnica, 101; Gaultheria; Kali carb., 42; Spigelia, 228; Paris quad.

Neuralgia of lumbar plexus: Bryonia, 110; Rhus, 103; Actea, 177; Rhododendron, 296; Arnica, 101; Belladonna, 17.

Neuralgia of coccyx: Belladonna, 17.

INFLAMMATION.

General remedies for Neuritis: Aconite, 4; Belladonna, 17; Arsenicum, 197; Phosphorus, 258; Rhus tox., 105; Chamomilla, 190; Causticum, 12; Syphilinum, 310.

Neuritis of teeth: Chamomilla, 190; Belladonna, 18; Coffea, 276; Pulsatilla, 179; Staphisagria; Magnesia carb., 80; Magnesia phos., 86.

Neuritis of glottis: Belladonna, 19; Hyoscyamus, 23; Moschus, 280; Acetic ac., 16.

Neuritis of ear: Verbascum; Capsicum, 12; Belladonna, 18; Chamomilla, 190; Pulsatilla, 179; Kali phos., 55; Mezereum, 337.

Neuritis of eye: Arsenicum alb., 198; Cedron; Spigelia, 22; Belladonna, 19; China, 212; Rhus, 105; Ignatia, 269; Ranunculus bulb., 298; Actea, 177; Agaricus, 347; Natrum mur., 72; Magnesia mur., 85; Mezereum, 337.

Neuritis of face: Arsenicum, 198; Kali phos., 57; Natrum phos., 74; Phosphorus, 259; Magnesia carb., 80; Colocynth, 305; Syphilinum, 310; Hepar, 118; Mezereum, 338; Spigelia, 228; Phosphorus, 259; Chamomilla, 190.

Neuritis of heart: Spigelia, 208; Cactus, 229; Nux vom., 120; Actea rac., 177; Kalmia; Magnesia phos., 93; Lachesis, 220; Gelsemium, 207.

Neuritis of intestines: Colocynth, 305; Plumbum, 150; Dioscorea; 'Arsenicum, 199; Magnesia phos., 87; Magnesia mur.; Cina, 246; Nux vom., 118; Magnesia carb., 80; Chamomilla, 190.

Neuritis of testicles: Zincum, 163; Berberis, 303; Pulsatilla, 183.

Neuritis of ovaries: Colocynth, 306; Actea, 178; Belladonna, 20; Lachesis, 220; Platinum, 148; Apis, 317; Chamomilla, 191; Cocculus, 277; Zinc. val.; Kali phos., 56.

Neuritis of uterus: Actea, 177; Colocynth, 309; Cocculus, 277; Viburnum; Plumbum, 151; Belladonna, 20; Magnesia phos., 83; Conium; Platinum, 148; Ignatia; Nux vom., 119; Sepia, 186; Sabina, 196.

Neuritis of stomach: Nux vom., 116; Chamomilla, 190; Ignatia, 270; Iris, 249; Sanguinaria, 262; Lycopodium, 90; Belladonna, 19; Magnesia phos., 87; Plumbum, 150; Arsenicum, 199; Colocynth, 305; Magnesia phos., 87.

FUNCTIONAL.

Mind.

Active: Coffea, 276; Opium; Scutellaria; Belladonna, 15; Hyoscyamus, 23; Kali phos., 54.

Amative or amorous: Hyoscyamus, 23; Cantharis, 321; Veratrum alb., 327; Platinum, 146; Lachesis, 220; Phosphorus, 255 and 258.

Cross, Angry: Chamomilla, 189; Antimonium crud.; Nux vom., 116; Bryonia; Colocynth, 306; Cina, 245; Sulphur, 4; Lycopodium, 89; Calcarea carb., 62; Nitric ac.; Anacardium, 345; Zinc. met., 160; phos., 258; Petrol., 293.

Anxious: Arsenicum, 198; Aconite, 1; Ignatia, 269; Calcarea carb., 62; Moschus, 280.

Capricious, Changing: Pulsatilla, 179; Chamomilla, 189; Platinum, 146; Lachesis, 220; Ignatia, 269; Alumina; Ferrum met.; Zincum, 160.

Confusion: Hyoscyamus, 22; Phosphorus, 258; Phosphoric ac.; Gelsemium; Rhus tox., 105; Calcarea carb.

Delirium: Belladonna, 15; Hyoscyamus, 22; Stramonium, 25; Lachesis, 220; Bryonia; Veratrum v., 314; Baptisia, 206; Petroleum, 293;

Graphites; Arsenicum, 198; Cannabis ind., 335; Muriatic ac.; Veratrum alb., 327; Gelsemium; China, 212; Mercurius col., 122; Zinc. m., 169; Secale, 193; Coffea, 276; Kali brom., 40.

Dull, Stupid: Baryta carb.; Calcarea carb., 62; Natrum carb., 69; Phosphoric ac.; Picric ac.; Baptisia, 206; Gelsemium, 207; Lycopodium; Rhus tox., 105; Sepia; Opium; Kali brom., 40; Tobacco, 27; Kali phos., 54; Natrum mur., 71; Apis, 317; Nux vom., 116; Anacardium, 346; Zincum phos., 164; Phosphorus, 258.

Excited: Hyoscyamus, 22; Tarantula; Nux vom., 116; Stramonium, 25; Cannabis ind., 335; Lachesis, 220; Coffea, 276; Aconite, 3; Chamomilla, 190; Cantharis; Platinum, 146; Ferrum phos.

Fear of Death or some Misfortune: Arsenicum, 198; Aconite, 2; Nux vom., 115; Mercurius, 122; Calcarea carb., 62; Pulsatilla, 183.

Fear of Falling: Borax; Gelsemium, 208.

Fear of ghosts: Pulsatilla; Stramonium, 25; Carbo veg.; Phosphorus, 258.

Fear he will not succeed: Argentum nit., 133; Gelsemium; Arnica; Phosphorus, 258; Natrum mur., 70; Sulphur.

Fear, effects of: Glonoine, 235; Gelsemium; Opium; Silica, 153.

Fear of becoming insane: Actea rac., 176; Calcarea carb., 62; Cannabis ind., 335; Veratrum vir., 314.

Foolish, Silly: Hyoscyamus, 22; Argentum nit., 133; Baryta carb.; Belladonna, 15; Natrum carb., 69; Anacardium, 346; Phosphoric ac.

Grief, effects of: Ignatia, 270; Pulsatilla, 183; Staphisagria; Causticum, 57; Phosphoric ac.; Lachesis, 220; Chamomilla, 189.

Homesickness: Capsicum; Ignatia, 270; Bryonia, 106; Hyoscyamus, 22.

Imagination too vivid: Platinum, 146; Coffea, 276; Belladonna, 15; Hyoscyamus, 22; Cocculus, 277; Sabina.

Impatient: Tarantula; Belladonna, 15; Nux vom., 115; Ignatia, 269; Arsenicum.

Irritable: Nux vom., 144; Silica, 153.

Impulsive: Platinum, 144; Pulsatilla; Coffea, 276; Ignatia, 269; Chamomilla, 189.

Intoxicated, as if: Gelsemium, 208; Opium; Nux vom., 116; Capsicum; Conium, 221; Cocculus, 277.

Jealous: Hyoscyamus, 22; Lachesis, 220.

Loquacious: Hyoscyamus, 22; Actea rac., 175; Stramonium, 25.

Moral Perversion: Hyoscyamus, 22; Stramonium, 25; Veratrum alb., 326; Platinum, 146; Belladonna, 15; Anacardium, 346.

Proud, arrogant: Platinum, 146; Ignatia, 269; Veratrum alb., 326; Sulphur; Lycopodium, 89.

Restless: Aconite, 1; Arsenicum, 198; Chamomilla, 189; Belladonna, 15; Rhus, 105; Nux vom., 116.

Sad: Natrum mur., 70; Sepia; Actea rac., 175; Ignatia, 269; Aurum, 135; Argentum nit., 133; Stannum, 159; Calcarea carb.; Lilium tig.; Mercurius sol., 122; Pulsatilla, 183; Sulphur; Kali phos., 54; Nux vom.,

116; Anacardium, 346; Ferrum, 142; Zinc. m., 160; Conium, 222; Moschus, 280.

Sensitive: Coffea, 276; Chamomilla, 190; Ignatia, 269; Nux vom., 115; Arsenicum, 198; Belladonna, 15; Hepar sulph., 111; Magnesia phos., 84.

Sighing: Ignatia, 269; Stramonium, 25; Stannum, 169.

Suicidal tendency: Arsenicum, 198; Mercurius, 122; Thuja, 344; Aurum, 135.

Suspicious: Hyoscyamus, 22; Ignatia, 269; Pulsatilla; Causticum, 57; Actea rac., 176.

Unconscious: Nux, 274; Belladonna, 15; Phosphoric ac.; Cocculus, 277; Gelsemium, 208; also see Epilepsy; Gels., 237.

Weak memory: Zincum m., 160; Conium, 22.

Convulsions, general: Belladonna, 14; Aconite, 1; Stramonium, 25; Hyoscyamus, 22; Actea rac., 176; Apis, 317; Zinc., 160; Zinc. phos., 16; Cuprum, 13; Cuprum ars., 141; Helleborus, 325; Veratrum vir., 315; Gelsemium, 207; Passiflora; Arsenicum alb., 198; Opium; Cicuta, 225; Nux vom., 116; Cina, 245; Veratrum alb., 226; Glon., 236.

Convulsions, Apoplectic: Belladonna, 15; Arnica, 100; Glonoine, 235; Baryta carb.; Opium; Nux vom., 116.

Convulsions, Choreic: Actea, 176; Cuprum, 140; Hyoscyamus, 24; Calcarea carb., 60; Kali ars.; Tarantula; Zinc., 164; Zinc. val., 164; Belladonna, 16; Gelsemium, 207; Arsenicum, 198; Nux vom., 116; Ignatia, 273; Argentum nit., 134; Cuprum ars., 141.

Convulsions, Epileptic: Amyl nit.; Zinc. phos., 164; Argentum nit., 133; Calcarea carb.; Lachesis, 220; Silica, 153; Hyoscyamus, 22; Cicuta, 225; Cocculus, 277; Nux m., 276; Cuprum, 140; Kali brom., 40; Causticum, 57; Plumbum, 149; Tarantula; Lilium tig.; Sulphur; Kali phos., 52.

Convulsions, Hydrocephalic: Apis, 317; Calcarea phos., 66; Zinc., 162; Helleborus, 325.

Convulsions, Hysterical: Ignatia, 270; Chamomilla, 189; Nux vom., 116; Nux m., 276; Cuprum, 140; Kali brom., 40; Causticum, 57; Plumbum, 149; Tarantula; Lilium tig.; Sulphur; Kali phos., 52.

Convulsions, Meningeal: Helleborus, 325; Tuberculinum, 312; Iodium, 169; Iodoform; Apis, 317; Actea rac., 176.

Convulsions, Puerperal: Veratrum vir., 315; Mercurius cor., 128; Gelsemium, 210; Belladonna, 15; Arsenicum, 198; Chamomilla, 191; Hyoscyamus, 22; Stramonium, 25; Opium; Glonoine, 235.

Convulsions, Uremic: Veratrum vir., 314; Arsenicum alb., 198; Cuprum ars., 141; Mercurius cor., 128; Plumbum, 149; Ammonium carb.; Cuprum met., 140; Phytolacca, 293.

Convulsions from Cholera Morbus: Belladonna, 15; Cuprum ars., 141; Veratrum alb., 326; Cuprum, 139; Veratrum vir., 314.

Convulsions from Fright: Stramonium, 25; Opium; Hyoscyamus, 22; Zinc., 160; Ignatia, 269; Gelsemium, 208.

Convulsions from Suppressed Eruptions: Sulphur; Zinc., 160; Cuprum, 138; Veratrum vir., 314; Apis, 317; Bryonia; Helleborus, 425; Gelsemium; Stramonium, 25.

Convulsions from Teething: Chamomilla, 189; Belladonna, 16; Scutellaria; Passiflora.

Convulsions from Tetany: Stramonium, 25; Rhus tox., 105; Hypericum; Belladonna, 15; Cicuta, 225; Hyoscyamus, 22.

Convulsions from Worms: Cina, 245; Cicuta, 225; Cuprum, 138; Ignatia, 269; Sabadilla.

Convulsions from Whooping Cough: Cuprum, 139; Zinc. phos.; Zinc., 164; Arnica; Belladonna, 21.

Convulsions from Tic: Agaricin, 349; Belladonna, 15; Strychnia phos., 258.

Convulsions of the Diaphragm (Hiccough): Belladonna, 15; Cicuta, 226; Ignatia, 270; Veratrum alb., 326; Nux vom., 115; Tabacum, 27; Colchicum, 281; Magnesia phos., 84; Kali brom., 40; Secale cor., 193; Pulsatilla, 181.

Trembling: Cocculus, 279; Gelsemium, 207; Actea rac., 177; Mercurius, 122; Lycopus; Conium, 221; Natrum mur., 70; Nitric ac.; Opium; Zincum, 160; Stramonium, 25; Sulphuric ac.; Belladonna.

Paralysis: Gelsemium, 207; Lachesis, 220; Causticum, 57; Plumbum, 149; Strychnia phos.; Rhus, 103; Belladonna, 20; Kalmia; Zinc. phos.; Conium, 221; Phosphorus, 260; Cuprum ars., 141; Secale, 193.

Paralysis Agitans: Mercurius, 122; Hyoscyamus, 22; Gelsemium, 207; Plumbum, 149; Nux vom., 115; Zincum brom.

Structural Changes.

Ataxia Paraplegia: Cuprum ars.; Zinc. val.; Ustilago.

Locomotor Ataxia: Cuprum iod.; Alumina, 235; Argentum nit., 144; Nux vom., 120; Causticum, 57; Plumbum, 152; Zinc., 161; Agaricus, 347; Berberis; China, 212; Plumbum iod., 149; Oxalic ac.; Thallium.

Headaches.

Anemic: China, 212; Calcarea carb., 63; Calcarea phos., 66; Ferrum, 144; Ferrum phos., 351; Natrum mur., 72; Cyclamen; Mercurius, 121; Sanguinaria, 261; Kali brom., 40; Anacardium, 346; Agaricus, 347.

Congestive: Bryonia, 106; Cactus, 230; Ignatia, 270; Glonoine, 235; Amyl nit.; Gelsemium, 207; Belladonna, 15; Stramonium, 26; Magnesia mur., 84; Veratrum vir., 314; Nux vom., 117; Ferrum phos., 351.

Rheumatic: Rhus tox., 105; Phytolacca, 293; Thuja, 345; Actea, 176; Sarsaparilla; Bryonia.

Syphilitic: Kali iod., 49; Mercurius iod.; Nitric ac.; Hepar; Phytolacca, 293; Asafœtida; Aurum, 136.

Frontal: Nux vom., 117; Natrum mur., 73; Bryonia, 106; Arsenicum, 197; Belladonna, 15; Ignatia, 270; Mezereum, 337; Phosphorus, 258; Hyoscyamus, 22.

Occipital: Picric ac.; Bryonia, 106; Gelsemium, 208; Actea rac., 176; Cocculus, 278; Agaricus, 347; Silica, 154; Zinc. phos., 164; Lachesis, 220;

Temporal: Belladonna, 15; China, 212; Pulsatilla; Argentum nit., 164; Lycopodium; Nux vom., 117.

Platinum, 147; Phosphorus, 258; Lachesis, 220; Cactus, 230; Helonias; Ipecac.

Vertex: Calcarea phos., 66; Ranunculus bulb., 298; Zinc. phos., 164; Platinum, 147; Phosphorus, 258; Lachesis, 218; Cactus, 230; Helonias; Ipecac, 250.

Menstrual: Actea, 176; Cocculus, 279; Belladonna, 20; Nux, 275; Calcarea phos., 66; Ferrum phos., 350; Pulsatilla, 179; Glonoine, 235; Veratrum vir., 314; Sanguinaria, 261; Sepia, 186; Lachesis, 218; Amyl nit.; Crocus; Gelsemium, 207; Graphites, 93; Natrum mur., 73.

Habitual: Actea, 176; Bryonia, 106; Gelsemium, 207; Sanguinaria, 261; Ferrum phos., 251; Magnesia phos., 84; Nux vom., 116; Glonoine, 235; Pulsatilla, 179; Chamomilla, 187.

Headache, reflex from:

Eyes: Gelsemium, 207; Lachesis, 217; Hepar, 110; Paris quad.; Croton tig.; Spigelia, 227; Rhododendron, 297.

Stomach: Nux vom., 116; Pulsatilla, 207; Nux m., 275; Bryonia, 107; Iris, 248; Cocculus, 279; Ipecac, 250; Sanguinaria, 261; Cyclamen; Argentum nit., 134; Antimonium crud.; Lycopodium, 90.

Liver: Iris, 248; Bryonia, 106; Chelidonium, 244; Nux vom., 120; Podophyllum; Sepia, 186; Magnesia mur., 82; Carduus; Sulphur, 5.

Kidneys: Cannabis ind., 336; Arsenicum, 201; Baptisia, 206; Phosphorus, 258; Mercurius cor., 128; Plumbum, 151.

Nasal catarrh: Pulsatilla, 207; Kali bich., 36; Hydrastis, 331; Kali iod., 48; Magnesia mur., 82; Alumina, 234; Mercurius prot., 130.

MUCOUS MEMBRANE.

General Remedies: Hydrastis, 330; Kali bich., 35; Pulsatilla, 179; Mercurius sol., 123; Gelsemium, 208; Arsenicum alb., 198; Arsenicum iod., 202; Euphrasia, 328; Allium cepa., 329; Zinc. sulph., 166; Sanguinaria, 262; Lachesis, 218; Lycopodium, 89; Ipecac, 250; Capsicum, 12; Bryonia, 106; Calcarea carb., 63; Cantharis, 322; Phosphorus, 255; Mercurius, 123; Arsenicum, 198; Argentum nit., 131; Hydrastis, 330; Kali bich., 35; Muriatic ac., 288; Kali chlor., 46; Nitric ac.; Hepar.

INFLAMMATION.

Conjunctivitis: Euphrasia, 328; Gelsemium, 208; Sepia, 187; Pulsatilla, 179; Allium cepa, 329; Arsenicum iod., 203.

Otitis: Belladonna, 18; Chamomilla, 190; Verbascum.

Rhinitis: Allium cepa, 329; Gelsemium, 208; Belladonna, 18; Mercurius sol., 124; Kali carb., 43; Alumina, 234; Causticum, 59; Bryonia, 108; Chamomilla, 191; Sulphur, 7.

Stomatitis: Belladonna, 18; Argentum nit., 131; Lycopodium, 92; Pulsatilla, 180.

Glossitis: Belladonna, 18; Acon., 1; Lachesis; Apis; Cantharis.

Pharyngitis: Belladonna, 19; Cantharis; Phytolacca, 294; Ferrum phos., 350; Alumina, 234; Apis, 317.

Laryngitis: Belladonna, 21; Sanguinaria, 263; Phosphorus, 255; Rumex, 264; Causticum, 59.

Gastritis: Nux vom., 116; Arsenicum alb., 199; Chamomilla; Sanguinaria, 262; Lycopodium, 90; Sepia, 188; Ipecac, 253; Carbo veg., 300; Pulsatilla, 181.

Enteritis: Colocynthis, 306; Arsenicum alb., 199; Bryonia, 107; Nux vom., 118; Cuprum ars., 140; Cantharis, 323; Terebinthina, 319; Calcarea carb., 64.

Proctitis: Mercurius sol.

Urethritis: Cantharis, 321; Mercurius cor., 128; Apis, 317; Arsenicum alb., 199; Capsicum, 14; Cannabis sat., 336; Chimaphila; Thuja, 343; Cannabis ind., 336; Mercurius cor., 128; Mercurius sol., 126; Argentum nit., 132; Pulsatilla, 183; Sulphur, 9.

Vaginitis: Pulsatilla, 182; Thuja, 343; Kreosotum, 286; Sepia, 185; Calcarea carb., 63; Iodium, 171; Mercurius, 126; Sanguinaria nit., 262; Phosphorus, 255; Alumina, 234; Syphilinum, 310; Magnesia mur., 82; Graphites, 97; Carbo veg., 301; Hydrastis, 333; Clematis, 335; Ferrum, 144; Sabina; Conium, 224.

Appendicitis: Belladonna, 19; Bryonia, 108; Mercurius sol., 125; Echinacea, 218; Hepar, 110.

Functional Changes.

Altered Excretions and Secretions:

Of Eyes: Euphrasia, 328; Arsenicum alb., 198; Mercurius cor., 128; Mercurius nit., 130; Sulphur, 6; Pulsatilla, 179; Hydrastis, 330; Graphites, 98; Kali bich., 35; Mercurius sol., 123; Hydrastis, 330; Clematis, 334; Gelsemium, 208.

Of Ears: Pulsatilla, 179; Mercurius sol., 124; Calcarea carb., 63; Tellurium, 55; Kali bich., 37; Phosphorus, 259; Silica, 155; Hepar, 112; Capsicum, 12; Kali carb., 45; Kali phos., 56; Carbo veg., 300; Syphilinum, 309; Mezereum, 339; Thuja, 341.

Of Nose: Allium cepa, 329; Gelsemium, 208; Arsenicum alb., 198; Mercurius sol., 124; Hydrastis, 331; Sanguinaria, 262; Causticum, 59; Phosphorus, 255; Alumina, 234; Arsenicum iod., 202; Kali carb., 43; Sulphur, 7; Natrum carb., 69; Graphites, 98; Bryonia, 108; Chamomilla, 191; Syphilinum, 262; Causticum, 59; Phosphorus 255; Alumina, 234; Arsenicum iod., 202; Kali carb., 43; Sulphur, 7; Natrum carb., 69; Graphites, 98; Bryonia, 108; Chamomilla, 191; Syphilinum, 309; Hepar, 112.

Stools, Watery: Aloe, 239; Veratrum alb., 321; Podophyllum, 240; Ferrum, 143; Natrum sulph., 76; Ipecac, 253; Antimonium tart., 267; Magnesia carb., 79.

Stools, Green: Ipecac, 253; Mercurius dulc., 129; Pulsatilla, 181; Magnesia carb., 79.

Stools, Frothy: Elaterium; Magnesia carb., 79; Rheum; Kali bich, 37.

Stools, Alternating Constipation and Diarrhea: Chelidonium, 248; Podophyllum, 240; Aloe, 239; Nux vom., 116; Sulphur, 8.

Stools of Cadaverous Odor: Sulphur, 8; Carbo veg., 301; Arnica, 100; Lachesis; Bromium; Staphisagria.

Stolls agg. drinking: Croton tig.; Veratrum alb., 326; Argentum nit., 132; Arsenicum.

Stools agg. eating: China, 215; Aloe, 239; Croton tig.; Natrum sulph., 76; Ferrum, 143; Thuja, 344.

Stools agg. excitement (emotional): Gelsemium, 209; Ignatia, 270; Argentum nit., 132; Coffea; Pulsatilla, 181.

Stools with tenesmus: Mercurius cor., 128; Colchicum, 282; Capsicum, 13; Rhus tox., 105; Alumina, 234.

Structural Changes.

Ulceration—Growths of:

Eye: Arsenicum alb., 198; Nitric ac.; Hydrastis, 330; Kali iod., 48; Silica, 155; Kali bich., 38; Mercurius, 123; Zinc. sulph., 166; Ars. iod., 202.

Ear: Capsicum, 12; Silica, 155; Hepar, 112; Mercurius, 124; Calcarea phos., 66; Tellurium; Kali bich., 35.

Nose: Kali bich., 36; Mercurius, 124; Phosphorus, 255; Sanguinaria, 262; Bovista; Hydrastis, 331; Zinc. phos., 165; Calcarea carb., 63; Carbo veg., 30; Mezereum, 339; Sepia, 187; Arsenicum iod., 202; Petrol., 292.

Mouth: Kali chlor., 47; Mercurius, 124; Arsenicum, 198; Hydrastis, 331; Muriatic ac., 288; Phosphorus, 256; Borax, 284; Kali bich., 36; Carbo veg., 300.

Throat: Kali bich., 37; Mercurius sol., 125; Hydrastis, 329; Petrol., 292.

Lungs: Phosphorus, 257; Silica, 57; Stannum iod., 158; Kreosote, 288; Hepar, 113; Carbo veg., 301; Arsenicum iod., 202; Antimonium ars.; Tuberculinum, 311.

Stomach: Arsenicum, 19; Kali bich., 37; Hydrastis, 332; Argentum nit., 131; Ipecac, 253; Kreosote, 287; Phosphorus, 256; Calcarea carb., 64; Syphilinum, 309; Mezereum, 339.

Intestines: Arsenicum, 199; Kali bich., 37; Nitric ac.; Muriatic ac., 28; Rhus, 105; Baptisia, 206; Calcarea iod., 68; Bryonia, 108; Calcarea carb., 64; Pulsatilla, 181.

Rectum and Anus: Silica, 156; Sulphur, 8; Hepar, 113; Mercurius, 125; Arsenicum alb., 199; Aloe, 239; Podophyllum, 240; Muriatic ac., 290; Mercurius cor., 128.

Bladder: Argentum nit., 132; Mercurius, 126; Cannabis sat., 335; Chimaphila; Hydrastis, 333; Kali bich., 38; Thuja, 345; Sepia; Sulphur, 9; Syphilinum, 310; Mercurius cor., 128.

Urethra: Argentum nit., 132; Mercurius, 126; Cannabis sat., 335; Chimaphila; Hydrastis, 333; Kali bich., 38; Thuja, 345; Sepia; Sulphur, 9; Syphilinum, 310; Mercurius cor., 128.

Vagina: Thuja, 343; Kreosote, 286; Sanguinaria, 262; Alumina, 234; Hydrastis, 333; Phosphorus, 255; Kali bich., 38; Argentum nit., 132; Borax, 286; Arsenicum alb., 199; Cantharis, 322; Iodium, 171; Natrum mur., 74; Hepar, 110; Mercurius sol., 126; Arsenicum iod., 203.

SKIN.

Leading Remedies: Arsenicum alb., 200; Sulphur, 5; Graphites, 96; Rhus tox., 102; Apis, 218; Thuja, 344; Kali brom., 42; Cantharis, 323; Arsenicum iod., 204; Croton tig.; Kali ars., 34; Mezereum, 338; Petroleum; Tartar emet., 267; Clematis, 335; Pulsatilla; Ranunculus bulb., 298; Zinc. sulph., 166; Urtica u.; Natrum mur., 74; Picric ac.; Belladonna, 21; Hepar, 114; Mercurius sol., 127.

Irritation.

Dermatalgia-Hyperesthesia: Belladonna, 21; Secale, 193; Sulphur, 5; Kalmia; Arnica, 101; Zinc. sulph., 166.

Itching: Sulphur, 5; Urtica u.; Aresnicum alb., 200; Staphisagria; Lycopodium, 92; Agaricus, 349; Causticum, 59; Silica, 153; Alumina, 233; Pulsatilla; Rumex, 265; Arsenicum iod., 204; Clematis, 335; Cantharis, 323; Ledum.

Inflammation.

Dermatitis: Picric ac.; Cantharis, 323; Arsenicum, 200; Belladonna, 21; Carbolic ac.; Kali mur., 52; Rhus, 102; also see remedies under Eczema.

Functional Changes.

Dry: Lycopodium, 92; Sulphur, 5; Alumina, 233; Nux m., 273; Sepia, 189.

Moist: Graphites, 96; Arsenicum alb., 200; Rhus tox., 102; Arsenicum iod., 204; Sulphur, 5; Tartar emet., 267; Mzereum, 338; Cantharis, 323; Calcarea carb., 60; Psorinum; Staphisagria, 290.

Acne: Kali brom., 42; Caulophyllum; Sulphur, 5.

Erythema: Belladonna, 21; Rhus, 102; Arsenicum, 200; Phytolacca, 295.

Urticaria: Arsenicum alb., 200; Apis, 318; Rhus, 102; Urtica; Kreosote, 287; Natrum mur., 74; Cocculus; Rumex, 265.

Structural Changes (including cracks and growths).

Boils and Carbuncles: Anthrac.; Arsenicum, 200; Lachesis, 219; Rhus tox., 102; Silica, 157; Apis, 218; Carbo veg., 302; Tarantula; Kreosotum, 285; Muriatic ac., 290; Phytolacca, 295; Sulphur, 5; Belladonna, 21; Hepar, 114.

Eczema: Graphites, 96; Arsenicum alb., 200; Rhus tox., 102; Arsenicum iod., 204; Sulphur, 5; Tartar emet., 267; Mezereum, 338; Cantharis, 323; Calcarea carb., 60; Psorinum; Staphisagria; Croton tig.; Kali ars., 34; Kali iod., 52; Natrum mur., 74; Hepar, 114; Mercurius sol., 127; Sepia, 189; Cicuta, 227; Petrol., 291.

Epithelioma: Arsenicum alb., 200; Arsenicum iod., 204; Hydrocotyle; Kreosote, 287; Hydrastis, 334; Kali mur., 52; Kali chlor.; Carbolic ac.; Sepia, 189; Muriatic ac., 290.

Gangrene: Lachesis, 219; Secale, 193; Arsenicum alb., 200; Carbo veg.; Kreosote, 287; Capsicum, 14.

Herpes, Circinatus and Zoster: Ranunculus bulb., 298; Rhus tox., 102; Arsenicum alb., 200; Graphites, 96; Cantharis, 323; Mezereum, 338; Hepar, 114; Thuja, 344; Sulphur, 5; Kali ars., 34; Kali iod., 52; Tuberculinum, 313; Petrol., 291; Tellurium; Barium; Clematis, 335; Graphites, 96; Calcarea carb., 60.

Impetigo: Arsenicum, 200; Sulphur, 5; Rhus tox., 102; Clematis, 335; Graphites, 96; Calcarea carb., 60.

Keloids: Calcarea fluor., 68; Fluoric ac.; Nitric ac.; Graphites, 96.

Leucoderma: Aresnicum, 200; Sulphur, 5; Zincum, 163; Nitric ac.

Lichen: Natrum mur., 74; Arsenicum alb., 200; Arsenicum iod., 202; Mercurius, 127; Berberis, 304; Calcarea carb., 60; Kali carb., 42; Mezereum, 338; Staphisagria; Hydrastis, 334.

Lupus: Natrum mur., 74; Graphites, 94; Rhus tox., 102; Sepia, 189; Apis, 318; Hydrocotyl; Hydrastis, 334; Petroleum; Fluoric ac.; Kali bich., 39.

Prurigo: Zinc., 166; Calcarea phos.; Ledum; Rumex, 265; Arsenicum iod., 204; Alumina, 233; Zinc. phos., 166.

Psoriasis: Kali ars., 34; Ars. iod., 204; Petrol., 291.

Ulcers: Mercurius sol., 127; Asafœtida; Nitric ac.; Arnica, 101; Arsenicum alb., 200; Echinacea; Hamamelis; Phytolacca.

Warts: Thuja, 344; Staphisagria; Causticum, 59; Mercurius sol., 127.

Cracks and Fissures: Petroleum, 291; Graphites, 96; Alumina, 233; Sulphur, 5; Silica, 157; Hepar, 114; Sepia, 189; Æsculus.

Ecchymoses and Petechiæ: Arnica, 101; Lachesis, 2199; Crotalus; Baptisia, 207; Rhus tox., 102; Arsenicum, 200; Echinacea.

Eruptions.

Psoriasis: Arsenicum iod., 204; Kali ars., 36; Petroleum, 291.

Scabs and Crusts: Mezereum, 338; Calcarea carb., 60; Sulphur, 15; Conium; Arsenicum, 200; Cicuta, 227.

Unhealthy (heals slowly): Hepar, 114; Sulphur, 5; Silica, 157; Petroleum.
Excrescences and Growths: Thuja; Staphisagria; Mercurius sol., 123; Arsenicum iod., 204; Nitric ac.; Silica, 157; Lachesis, 217; Zinc. sulph., 166.
Ulceration: Kali bich., 39; Arsenicum, 200; Asafœtida; Kali iod., 204.

GLANDS AND GLANDULAR ORGANS.

Glands.

Induration of: Iodium, 169; Baryta carb.; Calcarea carb., 60; Phytolacca, 294; Conium, 224; Calcarea iod., 68; Arsenicum iod.; Baryta iod.; Calcarea fluor., 68; Mercurius iod.; Kali mur., 52; Hepar, 111; Lapis alb.
Inflammation of: Aconite, 2; Belladonna, 19; Hepar, 30th; Mercurius sol., 124; Apis, 317; Lachesis; Phytolacca, 294; Lycopodium, 91; Thyroidin; Kali bich., 38; Calcarea iod., 68; Calcarea phos.; Baryta iod.; Iodium, 169; Tuberculinum, 311; Graphites, 94; Spongia, 174; Bromium, 167; Lycopus; Ferrum phos.; Echinacea, 217.
Suppuration of: Hepar, 3rd, 110; Mercurius sol., 121; Silica, 156; Sulphur; Kali iod., 48; Phytolacca, 294; Lachesis, 218; Tuberculinum, 311.

Glandular Organs.

Hepatalgia: See section under Nerves.
Nephralgia: See under Nerves.
Ovaralgia: See section under Nerves.
Splenalgia: Bryonia, 107; Ceanothus; Arnica, 101; Anacardium; Sulphur, 5.

INFLAMMATION.

Hepatitis: Bryonia, 107; Belladonna, 19; Hepar, 111; Silica, 153; Mercurius, 127; Kali iod., 40; Arsenicum iod., 202; Chionanthus, 238; Kali carb., 44; Calcarea carb., 61; Natrum sulph., 76; Lycopodium, 90; Eupatorium perf., 307; Nux vom., 120; Sepia, 188; Aloe, 239; Podophyllum, 240; Iris, 249.
Lienitis: Ceanothus; China, 214; Quinine, 216; Lachesis, 218; Bryonia, 107; Carbo veg.; Arsenicum, 197; Natrum mur., 70; Silica, 156; Iodium, 170.
Mastitis: Bryonia, 109; Phytolacca, 294; Belladonna, 19.
Nephritis: Aconite, 2; Belladonna, 20; Cantharis, 321; Colchicum, 282; Plumbum, 153; Arsenicum, 201; Bryonia, 110; Terebinthina, 321; Phytolacca, 294; Apis, 318; Veratrum alb.; Calcarea ars., 67.
Orchitis: See male generative organs.
Lymphangitis: Mercurius, 127; Belladonna, 19; Apis, 317; Arsenicum iod.; Hepar, 111; Calcarea carb., 61; Graphites, 94; Aurum, 135; Calcarea ars., 67; Natrum mur., 70.

Ovaritis: See female generative organs.

Parotitis: Mercurius, 124; Belladonna, 19; Pulsatilla, 183; Clematis; Hepar, 110; Arsenicum alb., 201; Sulphur, 5; Calcarea iod., 68; Conium, 221; Silica, 156; Rhus, 105; Bromium, 168.

Pancreatitis: Belladonna, 19; Arsenicum, 201; Phosphorus, 256; Mercurius iod.; Iris, 248.

Tonsillitis: Belladonna, 19; Mercurius sol., 127; Mercurius iod.; Phytolacca, 294; Hepar, 112; Lachesis; Baryta carb.; Calcarea iod., 68; also see Diphtheria.

Functional Changes.

Liver.

Icterus, catarrhal and neonatorum: Podophyllum, 240; Mercurius sol., 127; Arsenicum alb., 201; China, 214; Nux vom., 120; Chelidonium, 243; Lachesis, 218; Crotalus; Chionanthus, 238; Carduus.

Biliary Calculi: Chelidonium, 246; Belladonna, 19; Berberis, 304; Myrica, 232; China, 214; Carduus m.; Chionanthus, 237; Podophyllum, 240; Calcarea ren.

Kidneys, Urine decreased: Apis, 318; Cantharis, 321; Arum tri.; Helleborus, 325; Nitric ac.; Nux vom., 119; Opium; Sepia; Kali brom., 40; Stramonium, 26; Aconite, 3; Lachesis; Arsenicum alb., 201; Digitalis, 232; Veratrum vir., 314.

Kidneys, Urine increased: Ignatia, 271; Phosphoric ac.; Equisetum; Gelsemium, 207; Lactic ac.; Syzygium; Kali acet., 33; Chionanthus, 238.

Kidneys, brick dust sediment: Lycopodium, 91; Berberis, 303; Natrum sulph., 77; Arsenicum, 197; Mercurius cor., 128; Veratrum vir., 314; Sepia; Senecio; Borax, 284.

Kidneys, blood in: Arnica, 99; Mercurius cor., 128; Terebinthina, 321; Hamamelis; Arsenicum, 201; Ipecac, 250; Platina; Cantharis, 322; Kali chlor., 33; Nitric ac.; Calcarea ars., 67.

Kidneys, pus in: Arnica, 100; Arsenicum, 201; Mercurius cor., 128; Phosphorus; Cantharis, 322; Berberis, 303.

Kidneys, casts in: Cantharis, 322; Mercurius cor., 128; Apis, 318; Arsenicum alb., 201; Phosphorus; Argentum nit., 133; Plumbum, 151; Natrum ars.

Testicles, Emission of Semen: See under Male Generative Organs.

Prostate: Chimaphilla; Natrum sulph., 77; Zinc. pic., 166.

Structural Changes.

Liver, Hyperemia of: Bryonia, 107; Chionanthus, 238; Mercurius, 127; Myrica, 232; Digitalis, 231; Apis, 317; Carduus.

Liver, Cirrhosis of: Arsenicum alb., 199; Phosphorus, 257; Apocynum; Apis; Mercurius, 127; Hydrastis, 332; Podophyllum, 240; China, 214; Chelidonium, 243.

Liver, abscess of: See Glands, Suppuration of.

Spleen: Ceanothus; China, 214; Quinine; Lachesis, 218; Bryonia, 107; Carbo veg.; Arsenicum, 199; Natrum mur., 70; Silica, 156; Iodium, 170.

Kidneys: Mercurius cor., 128; Arsenicum, 201; Phosphorus, 255; Plumbum, 153; Berberis, 303; Cantharis, 321.

Testicles, Atrophy of: See same under Male Sexual Organs.

Testicles, Indurated: See Male Sexual Organs.

Goiter: Calcarea carb., 60; Spongia, 174; Iodium, 169; Calcarea iod., 68.

Mammary: Bryonia, 109; Hepar, 111; Phytolacca, 295; Mercurius, 127; Phosphorus, 256; Silica, 156; Conium, 224; Graphites, 96; Iodium, 171; Clematis, 335; Sepia, 187.

Mesenteric: Calcarea iod., 68; Phytolacca, 294; Syphilinum, 309.

MUSCLES.

Irritation.

Chorea: See section under Nerves.

Cramps: Cuprum, 138; Cuprum ars., 141; Camphor; Veratrum alb., 326; Causticum, 56; Viburnum; Actea rac., 175; Secale, 192.

Inflammation.

General Myalgia: Bryonia, 106; Actea, 175; Colchicum, 281; Aconite, 1; Gelsemium, 210; Rhus, 103; Rhododendron, 296; Ruta; Arsenicum iod., 202; Eupatorium perf., 308; Phytolacca, 295; Ferrum phos., 252; Zincum; Sanguinaria; Prunus spin.

Functional Changes.

Any of the remedies which produce irritation, inflammation or the structural changes may be useful in functional changes.

Structural Changes.

Atrophies: Plumbum, 151; Kali iod., 48; Aurum iod., 135; Strychnia phos.; Phosphorus; Arsenicum iod., 202.

The Dystrophies: Plumbum, 151; Cuprum, 138; Cuprum ars., 141; Zinc., 16; Arsenicum alb., 197.

JOINTS.

Irritation.

Neuralgia: Ferrum, 143; Ferrum phos., 352; Bryonia, 106; Prunus spin.

Inflammation.

Serous Membrane: Bryonia, 106; Iodium, 173; Apis, 318; Calcarea fluor., 68; Sticta; Causticum, 58; Ledum; Rhus, 104; Sanguinaria, 261.

Functional Change.

Weakness: Gelsemium, 207; Argentum nit.; Kali carb., 45.

Structural Changes.

Bryonia, 106; Silica, 153; Rhus tox., 104; Hepar sulph., 120; **Mercurius**, 123; Lithium carb.; Calcarea carb., 62; Ledum.

ARTERIES.

Arterio-Sclerosis and Aneurysm: Kali iod., 48; Baryta carb.; **Plumbum** iod., 149; Glonoine, 235; Lycopodium, 89; **Aurum** mur., 135; **Secale**, 192; Zinc. phos., 164; Digitalis, 230; Bryonia, 108; **Arsenicum** alb., 197.

VEINS.

Congestion of: Gelsemium, 207; Arnica, 100; Carbo veg., 299; **Digitalis**, 23; Baptisia, 230; Ammonium carb., 267; Crotalus; **Phytolacca**, 293; Secale, 192.

Hemorrhoids: Thuja, 344; Aloe, 239; Podophyllum, 240; Sulphur, 8; Æsculus; Hamamelis; Sepia, 18; Muriatic ac., 290; Natrum mur.; Nux vom., 115; Silica, 156; Petroleum, 293; Collinsonia.

Phlebitis: Pulsatilla, 184; Hamamelis; Arnica, 100; Ledum; **Lachesis**, 219; Millefolium; Calendula; Carduus; Ferrum phos., 352; Fluoric ac.; Carbo veg., 301; Bovista.

Varicose Veins and Ulcers: Pulsatilla, 184; Hamamelis; Carbo veg., 301; Lachesis, 219; Ferrum phos., 252; Calcarea fluor., 68; Zinc. sulph., 166; **Mezereum**, 338; Ledum; Nitric ac.; Bovista; Carduus.

THERMIC CENTERS.

Chilly and Cold: Heloderma; Camphor; Veratrum alb., 326; Silica, 153; Natrum mur., 73; Moschus, 279; Nux vom., 116; Rhus tox., 101; Eupatorium, 308; Antimonium tart., 266; China, 213; Causticum, 56; Arsenicum, 201; Agaricus, 349; Calcarea carb., 67; Capsicum, 14; Cactus, 230; Cina, 247; Carbo veg., 299; Helleborus, 326; Pulsatilla, 184; Sepia, 188; Secale, 192; Gelsemium, 209.

Fever, heat: Aconite, 1; Secale, 192; Belladonna, 14; Arsenicum, 201; Phosphorus, 255; Lachesis, 218; Bryonia, 109; Sulphur, 11; Chamomilla, 192; Rhus, 101; Sepia, 188; Gelsemium, 209; China, 215.

Sweat: Chininum ars., 205; Veratrum alb., 326; Carbo veg., 299; Chamomilla, 191; Opium; Mercurius, 121; China, 213; Calcarea carb., 67; Sepia, 188; Silica, 153; Antimonium tart., 266; Hepar, 115; Cuprum ars., 141.

Mixed chill, fever: Arsenicum, 201; Ipecac, 354; Ignatia, 273; Nux vom., 115; **Pulsatilla**, 179.

Sweat in Sepsis: Chininum ars., 205; China, 213; Mercurius, 121; Silica, 153; Hepar, 115; Carbo veg., 299.

Sweat in Tuberculosis: Chininum ars., 205; Stannum; Silica, 153; China, 213; Calcarea carb., 67; Kali carb., 42; Tuberculinum, 311.

Sweat, excessive local: Bryonia, 109; Belladonna, 14; Calcarea carb., 67; Chamomilla, 191; Mercurius, 121; Silica, 153.

Sweat in Malaria: China, 213; Rhus, 101; Chininum ars., 205; Arsenicum alb., 201; Kali carb., 42; Gelsemium, 209; Bryonia; Natrum mur., 73.

Sweat, cold: Veratrum alb., 327; Carbo veg., 299; Tartar emet., 266; Calcarea carb, 67; Mercurius, 121; Secale, 192.

Sweat, hot: Chamomilla, 191; Belladonna, 14; Opium; Ignatia; Hepar, 115; Iodium, 172; China, 213.

Climacteric, hot flushes: Actea; Sanguinaria, 261; Sepia, 185; Lachesis, 221.

EYE.

Neuralgia: See section under Nerve.

Inflammation.

Conjunctivitis: Euphrasia, 328; Arsenicum, 198; Apis, 317; Rhus, 105; Mercurius cor., 128; Pulsatilla, 179; Aconite, 2; Allium, 329; Argentum nit., 131; Belladonna, 16; Kali bich., 35; Clematis, 334; Graphites, 98; Hepar, 111; Sulphur, 6; Kali iod., 52; Petrol., 292; Natrum sulph., 77; Syphilinum, 309; Mercurius nit., 130; Zinc. sulph., 166; Alumina, 233.

Iritis: Colchicum, 281; Rhus tox., 105; Bryonia, 106; Clematis, 334; Kalmia; Spigelia, 228; Terebinthina, 319; Syphilinum, 310.

Blepharitis: Pulsatilla, 179; Sulphur, 6; Mercurius sol., 127; Staphisagria; Mezereum, 337; Causticum, 59; Graphites, 98; Apis, 317; Hepar, 111.

Retinitis Albuminurica: Mercurius cor., 128; Phosphorus, 259; Arsenicum alb., 198; Gelsemium, 208; Crotalus; Apis, 317.

Rhinitis Hemorrhagica: Phosphorus, 259; Crotalus; Lachesis, 218; Mercurius cor., 128; Apis, 317; Arnica, 99; Belladonna, 16; Gelsemium, 207.

Functional Changes.

Asthenopia: Ruta; Gelsemium, 208; Sulphur, 6; Agaricus, 347; Causticum, 57; Carbo veg., 300; Calcarea carb., 63; Cedron; Kali carb., 45; Lachesis, 218; Natrum mur., 72; Hepar, 117; Conium, 223.

Black spots before: Physostigma; Lycopodium, 92; Lachesis, 218; Carbo veg., 300; China, 212; Phosphorus, 259; Cyclamen, 334; Kali phos., 55.

Black, suddenly becoming: Stramonium, 25; Belladonna, 16; Phosphorus, 256; Natrum mur., 72; Pulsatilla, 179; Conium, 223; Mercurius, 123; Silica, 154; Hyoscyamus, 23; Glonoine, 236; Kali phos., 55.

Blindness: Hyoscyamus, 23; Stramonium, 25; Opium; Silica, 154; Pulsatilla, 179; China, 212; Lycopodium, 89; Phosphorus, 259.

Dim vision: Phosphorus, 259; Euphrasia, 328; Causticum, 57; Cannabis ind., 236; Conium, 223; Hepar, 111; Calcarea carb., 63.

Diplopia: Gelsemium, 208; Causticum, 57; Aurum; Hyoscyamus, 23; Nitric ac.; Stramonium, 25; Magnesia mur., 85; Zincum, 162.

Dryness: Lycopodium, 89; Sulphur, 6; Alumina; Graphites, 98; Belladonna, 16; Causticum, 59; Mezereum, 337.

Hemiopia: Lithium carb.; Aurum, 135; Lycopodium, 89.

Illusions of animals or bugs: Stramonium, 25; Hyoscyamus, 23; Actea, 177.

Illusions of black: Stramonium, 26; Phosphorus, 259.

Illusions of red: Belladonna, 16; Phosphorus, 259.

Illusions of yellow: Sepia, 187.

Light, flashes of: Belladonna, 16; Cyclamen, 334; Digitalis; Lachesis, 218; Physostigma; Phosphorus, 259; Silica, 154.

Objects, large: Argentum nit., 131; Nux m., 275; Hyoscyamus, 23; Photophobia; Conium, 223; Gelsemium, 208; Kali bich., 35; Lachesis, 218; Nux vom., 117; Hepar, 111; Rhus tox., 104; Ipecac, 252.

Pupils contracted: Opium; Calcarea carb., 63; Nux com., 117; Zinc., 162; Cocculus; Ignatia.

Pupils dilated: Belladonna; Gelsemium.

Structural Changes.

Atrophy of Nerve: Strychnia; Nux vom., 117.

Corneal ulceration: Mercurius cor., 128; Kali bich., 35; Argentum nit., 131; Hepar, 111; Sulphur, 6; Graphites, 98; Ipecac, 252; Natrum mur., 72; Rhus tox., 104; Silica, 154.

Crusts on lids: Petroleum; Sulphur, 6; Staphisagria; Graphites. 98.

Ptosis: Gelsemium, 208; Rhus tox., 104; Causticum, 57; Alumina; Sepia, 187; Kalmia.

Styes: Staphisagria; Pulsatilla, 179; Hepar, 111; Calcarea pix.

EAR.

Irritation.

Otalgia: See section under nerves.

Inflammation.

Otitis: Belladonna, 16; Capsicum, 12; Chamomilla; Pulsatilla, 179; Verbascum.

Functional Changes.

Hearing acute: Coffea, 276; Aconite, 2; Belladonna, 16; Chamomilla, 190; Spigelia, 227.

Deafness from catarrh: Kali mur., 51; Aresnicum alb.; Hydrastis, 330; Graphites, 93; Gelsemium, 207; Iodium, 167; Mercurius, 124; Pulsatilla, 179; Kali bich., 35; Petroleum, 292; Hepar, 118.

Hearing Dull: Pulsatilla, 179; China, 212; Chininum sulph.; Lycopodium,

89; Nitric ac.; Kali mur., 51; Calcarea carb., 63; Sulphur, 4; Silica, 155; Capsicum, 12; Kali bich., 35; Causticum; Phosphorus, 259.

Humming and Buzzing: China, 212; Pulsatilla, 179; Calcarea carb., 63; Causticum, 57.

Echoing: Causticum, 57; Phosphorus, 259.

Frost bitten: Agaricus, 349; Causticum, 57.

Deafness from catarrh: Kali mur., 51; Arsenicum alb.; Hydrastis, 330; Graphites, 94; Gelsemium; Iodium; Mercurius, 124; Pulsatilla, 179; Kali bich., 35; Petroleum, 292; Hepar, 118.

Structural Changes.

Furuncles: Calcarea phos.; Calcarea pix.; Hepar, 114; Mercurius sol., 124; Picric ac.

Mastoid: Capsicum, 12; Tellurium; Aurum, 136; Silica, 155; Hepar, 118; Mercurius sol., 124; Ferrum phos., 251.

Otorrhea: See section under mucous membrane.

Polypi: Thuja, 341; Sanguinaria, 261; Calcarea carb., 63; Lycopodium, 89; Phosphorus, 259.

Paralysis of Nerve: Chininum sulph., 216; China, 212; Silica, 155; Belladonna, 16; Hyoscyamus.

Atrophy of Nerve: China, 212; Chininum sulph., 216.

Menier's Disease: Kali phos., 57; Quinine; China, 212; Rhus; Natrum sali., 78.

RESPIRATORY ORGANS.

Irritation.

Spasm of Larynx: Hyoscyamus, 23; Spongia, 175; Bromium, 167; Stramonium, 25; Belladonna, 21; Cuprum, 139; Chlorine; Sambucus; Moschus, 280.

Inflammation.

Bronchitis: Aconite, 1; Bryonia, 107; Causticum, 59; Phosphorus, 257; Ferrum phos., 351; Mercurius sol., 126; Terebinthina, 321; Belladonna, 21; Ipecac, 251; Hepar sulph., 113 and 114; Pulsatilla, 182; Kali bich., 39; Arsenicum iod., 201; Iodium, 172; Sulphur, 11; Kali carb., 45; Calcarea carb., 64; Hydrastis, 333; Natrum sulph., 77; Magnesia carb., 80; Veratrum vir., 316; Cina, 247; Terebinthina, 321; Allium cep., 329.

Broncho-pneumonia: Aconite, 3; Ipecac, 251; Tartar emet., 266; Bryonia, 107; Tuberculinum; Arsenicum iod., 201; Kali bich., 39; Grindelia rob.; Ammonium carb., 268.

Laryngitis: Aconite, 1; Spongia, 175; Kali bich., 39; Belladonna, 21; Alumina, 234; Causticum, 59; Hepar sulph., 113; Phosphorus, 257; Sanguinaria, 262; Argentum nit., 132; Drosera; Apis, 120; Acetic ac.; Kali iod., 50; Black oxide of lime; Carbo veg., 301; Nux vom., 120;

Bromium, 167; Chamomilla, 191; Conium, 225; Alum, 234; Rumex, 264.

Pleuritis: Bryonia, 107; Aconite, 3; Kali carb., 45; Ranunculus bulb., 297.

Pneumonitis: Aconite, 1; Bryonia, 107; Ferrum phos., 350; Chelidonium, 244; Veratrum vir., 316; Phosphorus, 257; Sulphur, 10; Ammonium carb.; Tartar emet., 266; Grindelia rob.; Stannum iod., 158; Sulphur, 11; Kali iod., 50; Carbo veg., 301; Hepar, 114; Spongia, 175; Digitalis, 232; Sanguinaria, 263.

FUNCTIONAL CHANGES.

Aphonia: Gelsemium, 207; Hyoscyamus, 23; Belladonna, 21; Argentum nit., 134; Sanguinaria, 263; Spongia, 175; Acetic ac.

Asthma: Arsenicum, 199; Tartar emet., 266; Lobelia; Ipecac, 251; Moschus, 280; Grindelia rob.; Nux vom., 119.

STRUCTURAL CHANGES.

Laryngitis with Exudation: Kali bich., 38; Hepar, 112; Oxide of lime, 68.

Pulmonary Atelectasis: Strychnia phos.; Ammonium carb., 268; Tartar emet., 266.

Pulmonary Congestion: Aconite, 3; Ferrum phos., 350; Veratrum vir., 316; Gelsemium, 207; Belladonna, 21.

Pulmonary Edema: Apis, 317; Cantharis, 32; Antimonium ars.; Adrenalin; Kali iod., 50; Sanguinaria, 265; Digitalis, 232.

Pulmonary Emphysema: Strychnia phos.; Arsenicum alb., 199; Antimonium ars.

Pulmonary Gangrene, Pyemia: Capsicum, 14; Arsenicum iod., 202; Silica, 157; Hepar, 113; Kreosote, 288; Carbo veg., 301.

Pulmonary Tuberculosis: See section under Blood and Infectious Diseases.

Pleurisy with effusion: Arsenicum iod., 201; Cantharis, 323; Iodium, 172; Kali iod., 50; Sulphur, 11; Apis, 318; Ferrum phos., 352; Mercurius, 127; Silica, 157; Hepar, 113; Chininum ars., 205; Apocynum can.; Digitalis, 232.

HEART.

IRRITATIONS.

Cardalgia: See section under Nerves.

INFLAMMATION.

Peri-carditis: Bryonia, 107; Aconite, 1; Apis, 318; Colchicum, 281; Spigelia, 228; Arsenicum, 197; Arsenicum iod., 20; Iodium, 173.

Endo- and Myo-Carditis: Cactus, 229; Aconite, 1; Iodium, 173; Spigelia, 229; Aurum, 137; Bryonia, 107; Camphor; Arsenicum alb.; Arnica, 99; Apis, 318; Digitalis, 231; Strychnia phos., 173; Cratægus; Arsenicum iod.; Phytolacca, 295.

Functional Changes.

Angina Pectoris: Amyl nit.; Glonoine, 237; Spigelia, 228; Gelsemium, 207; Natrum nit.; Lithium carb.; Kali iod., 50; Cactus, 229; Naja; Nux vom., 120; Lachesis, 220.

Bradycardia: Kalmia; Gelsemium, 207; Digitalis, 231; Apocynum can.

Tachycardia: Ferrum phos., 352; Spigelia, 228; Coffea; Aconite; Ammonium val.; Nux vom., 120; China, 211; Moschus, 281.

Sensations of coldness about: Camphor; Natrum mur., 73; Petroleum; Kali bich., 35.

As if grasped or squeezed: Cactus, 229; Amyl nit.; Lilium tig.

As if stopped beating: Tabacum, 28; Aurum, 137; Digitalis, 231; Cicuta.

As if turned over: Lachesis, 220; Tabacum, 28; Crotalus; Calcarea carb.

Causing cold sweat: Tabacum, 28; Veratrum alb., 327; Cactus, 229; Digitalis, 231; Carbo veg., 302; Spigelia, 228.

Intermittent pulse: Digitalis, 231; Natrum ars.; Muriatic ac., 288; Lycopus; Secale, 192.

Pain from heart to arm: Spigelia, 228; Naja; Actea, 177; Kalmia; Lachesis, 220; Rhus tox., 104; Tabacum, 28; Magnolia.

Palpitation, general: Arsenicum; Lycopus; Coffea crud., 176; Strophanthus; Phosphorus, 258; China, 211; Platinum, 145; Natrum mur., 73; Lycopodium, 89; Cactus, 229; Nux vom., 120; Pulsatilla, 184; Rhus tox., 104; Phosphoric ac.; Spigelia, 227, 228; Agaricus, 347; Ferrum phos., 252; Lilium tig.; Actea, 177; Sepia, 185; Cactus, 229; Digitalis, 231; Naja; Gelsemium, 207; Glonoine, 237; Coca; Moschus, 280; Kalmia; Physostigma.

Palpitation, nervous: Gelsemium, 207; Argentum nit., 130; Arsenicum; Lycopus; Spigelia, 228; Phosphorus, 255; Lilium tig.; Cactus, 229; Rhus tox., 104; Nux vom., 273.

Heaviness about: Aurum, 137; Bryonia, 106; Amyl nit.; Digitalis, 231; Colchicum, 281; Lycopus; Moschus, 279; Spigelia, 228; Gelsemium, 207; Ferrum phos., 351.

Small and Wiry: Aconite, 1; Veratrum alb., 327; Muriatic ac., 288.

Weakness: Arsenicum alb., 197; Carbo veg., 302; Muriatic ac., 288; Tartar emet.; Rhus tox., 104; Ammonium carb., 267.

Structural Changes.

Aneurism: Baryta carb.; Veratrum vir., 313; Lycopodium, 89.

Dilatation: Digitalis, 231; Strophanthus; Adonis; Agaracine, 349; Nux vom., 120; Strychnia; Strychnia phos., 173; Convallaria; Argentum nit., 130; Tabacum, 28.

Fatty degeneration: Strychnia phos., 173; Arsenicum alb., 197; Arsenicum iod., 202; Phosphorus, 258; Carbo veg., 302; Iodium, 173.

Valcular lesions: Digitalis, 231; Strychnia phos., 173; Strychnia; Colchicum, 281; Lithium carb.; Caffeine; Cratægus; Strophantus; Glonoine, 237; Spartium; Convallaria.

Modalities of.

Agg., Pressure about: Lachesis, 220; Cactus, 229; Colchicum, 281; Pulsatilla, 184; Lycopodium, 89.

Agg., Use of Alcohol: Nux vom., 120; Argentum nit., 130; Strophanthus.

Amel., from sitting up: Cactus, 229; Spongia, 174; Grindelia; Arnica, 99; Natrum mur., 73.

Amel., Deep breathing: Digitalis, 231; Ignatia, 269; Moschus, 280; Cannabis ind., 335.

STOMACH.

Irritation.

Gastralgia: See section under Nerves.

Inflammation.

Gastritis: See section under Mucous Membrane.

Hemorrhages: See sections under Blood.

Functional Changes.

Acidity: Magnesia carb., 79; Robinia; Calcarea carb., 64; Lycopodium, 90; Nux vom., 118; Carbo veg., 300; Kali carb., 43; Iris, 249; Natrum carb., 70; Hepar, 113; Lithium carb.; Pulsatilla, 181; Sepia, 187; Natrum mur., 72; Sulphur, 7; Hydrastis, 332.

Appetite increased: Iodium, 169; China, 214; Cina, 245; Sulphur, 7; Lycopodium, 90; Graphites, 98; Sepia, 187; Calcarea carb., 64; Nux vom., 118; Stannum; Phosphorus, 256.

Appetite decreased: Colchicum, 282; Kali carb., 43; Arsenicum, 199; Lycopodium, 90; Pulsatilla, 181; Nux vom., 118; Chamomilla, 190; China, 214; Antimonium c.

Appetite variable: Cina, 245; Chamomilla, 190; Iodium, 172; Natrum carb., 70; Petroleum, 292; Lachesis, 218; Argentum nit., 131.

Aversion to food and drink: Arsenicum, 199; Antimonium crud.; Colchicum, 282; Kali carb., 43; Nux vom., 118; Pulsatilla, 181; Chamomilla, 190; Ipecac, 253; Sepia, 187; Natrum mur., 71; Lycopodium, 90; Graphites, 98; Cocculus, 278.

Aversion to meat: Pulsatilla, 181; Petroleum, 292; Sulphur, 7; Silica; Sepia, 187; Carbo veg., 300.

Aversion to milk: Sulphur, 7; Silica; Sepia, 187; Ignatia, 270; Carbo veg., 300.

Aversion to sweets: Causticum, 56; Sulphur, 7; Graphites, 98.

Aversion to tobacco: Ignatia, 270; Nux vom., 118; Calcarea carb., 64; Lycopodium, 90.

Craving for bitter: Natrum mur., 72; Digitalis; Graphites. 98.

Craving for coffee: Bryonia, 107; Nux vom., 118.

Craving for cold things: Arsenicum, 199; Bryonia, 107; Veratrum alb., 327; Phosphorus, 256; Rhus, 101; Bismuth; Graphites, 98.

Craving for fats: Calcarea phos., 65; Nux vom., 118; Nitric ac.

Craving for indigestible things: Calcarea carb., 64; Calcarea phos., 65; Natrum mur., 72; Nux vom., 118.

Craving for juicy things: Veratrum alb., 327; Phosphoric ac.; **Staphisagria**, 181; Graphites, 98.

Craving for salty: Natrum mur., 72; Causticum, 56; Veratrum alb.

Craving for sweets: Argentum nit., 131; Kali carb., 45; Lycopodium, 90; China, 214; Sulphur.

Flatulency: Carbo veg., 300; Asafœtida; Argentum nit., 131; Nux m., 273; Ignatia, 270; Nux vom., 118; China, 214; Pulsatilla, 181; Chamomilla, 190; Rumex, 265; Calcarea phos., 65; Calcarea carb., 64; Sulphur, 7.

Eructations: Carbo veg., 300; Argentum nit., 131; Lycopodium, 90; Nux vom., 118; Bryonia, 107; Berberis, 304; Pulsatilla, 181; Mercurius, 125; Natrum mur., 72; Arnica, 100; Cocculus, 278; China, 214; Sepia, 187; Ipecac, 253; Kali carb., 43; Natrum phos., 74; Graphites, 98; Terebinthina, 319; Chamomilla, 190; Chionanthus, 238.

Gastroptosis: Sepia, 187; Pulsatilla, 181; Hydrastis, 332.

Gastric headache: Nux vom., 117; Pulsatilla, 181; Iris, 248; Sanguinaria, 261; Ferrum phos., 351; Ipecac, 253; Cocculus, 278; Argentum nit., 131; Bryonia, 106; Chelidonium, 243; Cyclamen.

Nausea: Ipecac, 253; Arsenicum alb., 199; Æthusa; Antimonium tart., 267; Veratrum alb., 326; Sepia, 187; Iris, 250; Sanguinaria, 262.

Sensation, burning: Arsenicum, 199; Phosphorus, 256; Sulphur, 7; Iris, 249; Mercurius cor., 128; Lycopodium, 90; Sanguinaria, 262; Colchicum, 282; Hydrastis, 332; Mezereum, 339; Robinia; Secale, 194; Argentum nit., 131.

Sensation, heartburn: See Acidity.

Sensation, lump in: Pulsatilla, 181; Nux m.; Nux vom., 118; Bryonia, 107; Abies nigra; Argentum nit., 131; Bismuth; Gelsemium, 208; Kali carb., 43; Robinia.

Sensations, Paroxysmal: Colocynth, 305; Belladonna, 19; Kalmia; Dioscorea.

Sensations, Pulsating: Sepia, 187; Hydrastis, 332; Kali carb., 42; Spigelia; Asafœtida.

Sensation, shooting to arm: Dioscorea; Tabacum, 27.

Sensation, shooting to back: Belladonna, 19; Plumbum, 150; Robinia; Cuprum, 140; Chelidonium, 243; Rumex, 265; Phosphorus, 256; Platinum, 148; Carbo veg., 300; Calcarea phos., 66.

Sensation, shooting to chest: Argentum nit., 131; Nux vom., 118; Robinia; Rumex, 264; Colocynth, 305; Petroleum, 292.

Satiety, before eating: Lycopodium, 90; China, 214.

Satiety, while eating: Lycopodium, 90; Cyclamen; Ferrum, 143; Kali carb., 43; Nux v., 118.

Satiety, after eating: Lycopodium, 90; Argentum nit., 131; Graphites, 98;

China, 214; Cocculus, 278; Berberis, 304; Dioscorea; Calcarea phos., 65; Rumex, 264; Robinia.

Taste, bad: Pulsatilla, 180; Mercurius, 125; Nux vom., 118; Arnica, 100; Staphisagria; Carbo veg., 300; Colocynth, 305; Bryonia, 107.

Taste, bitter: Bryonia, 107; Nux vom., 118; Chamomilla, 190; China, 214; Iris, 250.

Taste, metallic: Mercurius, 125; Iris, 250; Cuprum, 139.

Taste, sour: Nux vom., 118; Lycopodium, 90; Calcarea carb., 64; Pulsatilla, 181.

Taste, sweet: Stannum, 159; Sabadilla; Phosphorus, 256.

Vomiting of bile: Podophyllum, 240; Sanguinaria, 261.

Vomiting, black: Arsenicum, 199; Nux vom., 118; Lachesis, 218; Phosphorus, 256; Argentum nit., 132.

Vomiting, blood: Hydrastis, 332; Ipecac, 253.

Vomiting, curds: Æthusa; Antimonium crud.; Ipecac, 253.

Vomiting, fecal: Nux vom., 118; Lycopodium, 90; Cocculus, 278; Opium; Veratrum alb., 327.

Vomiting mucous: Kali bich., 37; Ipecac, 253; Drosera; Hydrastis, 332; Podophyllum, 240.

Vomiting of pregnancy: Podophyllum, 242; Phosphorus, 256; Magnesia carb., 79; Kreosote, 287.

Vomiting and Purging: Veratrum alb., 327; Ipecac, 253.

Vomiting, violent: Veratrum alb., 327; Arsenicum, 199; Lobelia; Apomorphia; Antimonium tart., 267; Magnesia phos., 87; Colchicum, 282

Structural Changes.

Ulcerations: Argentum nit., 132; Phosphorus, 256; Sanguinaria, 262; Hydrastis, 332; Kali bich., 37; Mezereum, 339; Crotalus; Carbolic ac.; Sepia, 187.

Modalities.

Agg., Alcohol: Nux vom., 118; Phosphoric ac.; Lachesis, 218; Argentum nit., 131; Kali bich., 37; Ferrum phos., 251; Antimonium crud.

Agg., Anger: Chamomilla, 190; Nux vom., 118; Colocynth, 305; Staphisagria.

Agg., Coffee: Nux vom., 118; Sulphuric ac.; Fluoric ac.

Agg., Cold drink: Arsenicum, 199; Kali carb., 43; Staphisagria.

Agg., Warm drink: Bryonia, 107; Phosphorus, 256.

Agg., During menses: Pulsatilla, 181; Chamomilla, 190; Virburnum op.; Magnesia phos., 88; Cocculus, 278; Colocynth., 305; Kali carb., 43.

Agg., Eating: Carbo veg., 300; Lycopodium, 90; Kali carb., 44; Cocculus, 278; Nux vom., 118.

Agg., Eating fats: Pulsatilla, 181; Kali mur., 51; Natrum carb., 70; Cyclamen; Graphites, 98; Hepar, 113; Carbo veg., 300.

Agg., mixed rich foods: Nux vom., 118; Argentum nit., 131; Antimonium crud.; Ipecac, 253.

Agg., Pregnancy: Ammonium mur.; Cocculus, 279; Nux m., 273.

Agg., Suppressed menses: Ammonium mur.; Lycopodium, 92; Kali carb., 46; Cocculus, 279.

Amel., Bending double: Colocynthis, 305; Magnesia phos., 83; Natrum sulph., 76; Colchicum, 282; Rhus tox., 105; Petroleum, 292.

Amel., Cold drinks: Phosphorus, 256; Mercurius cor., 128; Bryonia, 107.

Amel., Eating: Anacardium; Sepia, 187; Calcarea phos., 66; Ignatia, 270; Iodium, 170; Graphites, 98; Chelidonium, 244; Sulphur, 7; Pulsatilla, 181; Mezereum, 339; Sabadilla.

Amel., Eructations: Argentum nit., 131; Lycopodium, 90; Calcarea phos., 65; Carbo veg., 300; Plumbum, 150.

Amel., Hard pressure: Colocynth., 305; Magnesia phos., 83; Cina, 244; Dioscorea; Nux vom., 118; Stannum, 159; Plumbum, 150.

MALE GENERATIVE ORGANS.

Irritation.

Neuralgia of testicles: See section under Nerves.

Inflammation.

Orchitis: Clematis, 334; Pulsatilla, 183; Mercurius sol., 126; Staphisagria; Rhododendron, 296; Spongia, 174; Jaborandi; Copaiva; Iodium, 170.

Epididymitis: Rhus, 101; Rhododendron, 296; Pulsatilla, 183; Gelsemium, 207.

Functional Changes.

Effects of enforced continence: Conium, 224; Phosphorus, 259; Agnus cast.; Graphites, 97.

Effects from sexual excesses: Kali brom., 41; Staphisagria; Picric ac.; Phosphorus, 259; Conium, 224; China, 216; Zincum phos., 165.

Erections while lying on back: Platinum, 224; Rhus, 101.

Seminal emissions too soon: Zinc., 163; Conium, 224; Graphites, 97; Phosphorus, 259.

Seminal emissions: Lycopodium, 91; Gelsemium, 207; Phosphoric ac.; Ferrum, 142; China, 211; Phosphorus, 259; Conium, 224; Sepia, 185; Kali phos., 56; Zinc. pic., 166.

Impotency: Causticum, 58; Lycopodium, 91; Sulphur, 6; Phosphorus, 259; Conium, 224; Agnus cast., 56; Caladium; Capsicum, 14; Kali brom., 41; Kali phos., 56; Iodium, 17.

Priapism: Cantharis, 322; Phosphorus, 259; Platina, 145; Carbo veg., 300; Silica, 192; Kali brom., 41; Nux vom., 119; Mercurius cor., 128; Thuja, 343; Argentum nit., 132; Iodium, 17.

Testicles, Atrophy: Aurum, 136; Staphisagria; Iodium, 170; Kali iod., 49; Capsicum, 14.

Testicles, Indurated: Conium, 224; Aurum, 136; Arnica, 101.

Testicles, swollen: Apis, 316; Cubeba; Arnica, 101; Rhododendron; Aurum, 136; Pulsatilla, 207; Conium, 224; Nitric ac.; Mercurius, 126; Hamamelis; Iodium, 17; Phosphoric ac.; Spongia.

Hydrocele: Aurum, 136; Iodium, 171; Pulsatilla; Clematis, 334; Hamamelis.

Penis, Ulcers and Excrescences: Thuja, 343; Hepar, 113; Mercurius, 126; Staphisagria; Argentum nit., 132; Mezereum, 336.

FEMALE GENERATIVE ORGANS.

Irritation.

Neuralgia of Ovaries: See section on Nerves.

Neuralgia of Uterus: See section on Nerves.

Inflammation.

Metritis, Simple: See section under Mucous Membrane.

Metritis, Puerperal: Arsenicum alb., 202; Lachesis, 218; Arsenicum iod., 205; Terebinthina, 319; Chininum ars., 205; Phosphorus, 260; Hepar, 110.

Ovaritis: Colocynth., 306; Plumbum, 151; Platinum, 148; Belladonna, 20; Conium, 224; Aconite, 3; Mercurius, 126; Hepar, 110; Hamamelis; Cantharis, 322; Bromium, 168; Iodium, 171.

Vaginitis: Plumbum, 151; Platinum, 148; Aurum, 137.

Functional Changes.

Amenorrhea: Pulsatilla, 183; Calcarea carb., 62; Sulphur, 9; Phosphorus, 260; Aconite, 1; Aurum, 137; Graphites, 97; Sepia, 186; Rhus tox.; Sanguinaria, 263; Nux m., 275; Ignatia, 272; Platinum, 148; Zinc., 163; Chamomilla, 191; Colocynth, 306; Ferrum, 144.

Dysmenorrhea, nervous: See section under Nerves.

Dysmenorrhea, membranous: Borax, 284; Sanguinaria, 262; Sulphur, 9; Natrum mur., 70; Graphites, 97; Calcarea carb., 63; Chamomilla, 190; Rhus tox.; Kali bich., 38; Lachesis, 218; Magnesia phos., 88; Nux vom., 119.

Menses, delayed: Pulsatilla, 183; Sepia, 185; Graphites, 97; Sulphur, 9; Sanguinaria, 262; Kali carb., 46; Magnesia carb.; Natrum mur., 70; Calcarea phos., 65; Viburnum op.

Menses, discharge black: Magnesia mur., 82; Cantharis, 322; Nux m., 275; Secale, 193.

Menses, discharge clotted: Belladonna, 20; China, 215; Actea rac., 178; Chamomilla, 191; Crocus; Cyclamen; Platinum, 148; Cocculus, 279.

Menses, too early: Belladonna, 20; Calcarea carb., 62; Chamomilla, 191; Nux vom., 119; Platinum, 148; Bromium, 168; Aloe, 239.

Menses, Epilepsy during: Lachesis, 218; Actea rac., 175; Plumbum; Causticum, 59; Argentum nit., 132.

Menses, Eruptions at time of: Sepia, 18; Graphites, 97; Manganum; Crotalus; Sulphur, 5; Caulophyllum.

Menses, Exhaustion from: China, 215; Picric ac.; Ferrum pic.; Phosphorus, 259; Alumina, 233; Arsenicum, 197; Helonias; Cocculus, 279; Calcarea carb., 62; Ipecac, 254; Ferrum, 144; Carbo veg., 301.

Menses, Fainting during: Cocculus, 279; Nux m., 275; Moschus, 280.

Menses, Flatulence during: Lycopodium, 92; Ammonium mur.; Cocculus, 279; Kali carb., 46.

Menses, Hysteria during: Actea rac., 178; Caulophyllum; Cocculus, 279; Magnesia mur., 82.

Menses, Profuse too: China, 215; Phosphorus, 260; Sabina, 196; Belladonna, 20; Calcarea carb., 62; Nux vom., 119; Ipecac, 254; Ferrum, 144; Ergot, 149; Platinum, 148; Kali carb., 46; Stannum, 159; Bromium, 168; Iodium, 171; Trillium, 197; Aloe, 239.

Menses, Suppressed: Sulphur, 9; Pulsatilla, 183; Lycopodium, 92; Phosphorus, 260; Silica, 157; Ignatia, 272; Glonoine, 236; Belladonna, 20; Veratrum vir., 315; Platinum, 146; Nux m., 275; Moschus, 280.

Menstruation, Delayed: Pulsatilla, 183; Sulphur, 9; Calcarea carb., 62; Phosphorus, 260.

Metrorrhagia: Trillium, 197; Hydrastis, 333; Nitric ac.; Phosphorus, 260; China, 215; Belladonna, 20; Iodium, 171; Ipecac, 254; Sanguinaria, 262.

Nymphomania: Hyoscyamus, 23; Platinum, 146; Cantharis, 322; Phosphorus, 260; Agnus c.

Threatened Abortion: Actea, 178; Kali carb., 46; Apis, 319; Plumbum, 152; Chamomilla, 190; Ipecac, 254; Ignatia, 272.

Vaginismus: Belladonna, 20; Colocynthis, 306; Plumbum, 152; Platinum, 148; Chamomilla, 191; Actea rac., 175; Zinc. phos., 164; Naja; Lillium tig.; Apis, 319; Bryonia, 109; Iodium, 170; Magnesia phos., 88; Ferrum phos., 35; Conium, 224; Aconite, 1; Hepar, 111; Hamamelis; Kali phos., 56.

STRUCTURAL CHANGES.

Uterus enlarged: Aloe, 239; Belladonna, 20; Sepia, 185; China, 215; Secale, 157; Arsenicum, 197; Veratrum alb., 326; Mercurius iod., 129; Mercurius rub., 129; Aurum mur., 137.

Uterus, Excrescences: Thuja, 343; Kreosote, 286; Graphites, 97; Hydrastis, 333.

Uterus, Fibroids: Trillium, 197; Calcarea iod., 68; Secale, 157; Kali iod., 49; Hydrastis, 333; Platinum, 148.

Uterus, Polypi: Phosphorus, 260; Sanguinaria, 262; Thuja, 343; Conium, 224; Hydrastis, 333; Pulsatilla, 183.

Uterus, Prolapsus: Sepia, 185; Belladonna, 20; Lilium tig.; Hydrastis, 333; Pulsatilla, 183; Trillium, 197; Helonias; Murex; Calcarea carb., 63; Calcarea iod., 68; Podophyllum, 242; Platinum, 148; Natrum mur.,

70; Thuja, 343; Arsenicum, 197; Nux vom., 119; Aloe, 238; Stannum, 159.

Uterus, Cancer: Arsenicum alb., 197; Conium, 224; Hydrastis, 333; Kreosote, 286; Secale, 157; Ergot.

BLADDER.

IRRITATION.

Cystoplegia: Belladonna, 19; Causticum, 58; Lachesis, 218; Gelsemium, 218; Opium; Rhus tox., 101; Zincum, 163; Tabacum, 27; Helonias.

Cysto-Spasms: Cocculus, 277; Cantharis, 322; Nux vom., 119; Capsicum, 14; Tarantula; Magnesia phos., 87.

INFLAMMATION.

Cystitis and Urethritis: Cantharis, 322; Aconite, 3; Terebinthina, 321; Capsicum, 14; Arnica, 99; Belladonna, 19; Cannabis sat., 336; Colchicum, 282; Erigeron; Causticum, 58; Chimaphila; Lithium carb.; Pulsatilla, 182; Hydrastis, 333; Kali bich., 38; Natrum sulph., 77; Lycopodium, 91; Berberis, 303; Apis, 34; Mercurius sol., 126; Mercurius cor., 128; Argentum nit., 132.

FUNCTIONAL.

Desire to urinate urgent: Cantharis, 322; Mercurius cor., 128; Nux vom., 119; Sulphur, 9; Staphisagria; Terebinthina, 321.

Micturition, difficult or ineffectual: Cannabis ind., 336; Cantharis, 322; Digitalis; Mercurius cor., 128; Magnesia mur., 82; Nux vom., 119.

Micturition, frequent: Mercurius, 125; Nux vom., 119; Lycopodium, 91; Causticum, 58: Argentum nit., 133.

Micturition interrupted: Clematis, 334; Conium, 221; Thuja, 343; Gelsemium, 207.

Micturition, involuntary: Causticum, 58; Cina; Belladonna, 19; Calcarea phos.; Phosphorus, 255; Pulsatilla, 181; Hyoscyamus, 23; Natrum sulph., 73; Magnesia phos., 87; Zinc. m., 163; Gelsemium, 207; Kreosote, 286.

Urine retained: Belladonna, 20; Aconite, 3; Opium; Cantharis, 322; Tarantula; Terebinthina, 321; Lycopodium, 91; Nux vom., 119; Zinc. m., 163; Ignatia, 271.

MODALITIES.

Because I find that the modalities play a very important part in determining the rank of the symptom or group of symptoms, I am giving a large space to this heading. I am, however, giving only those modalities which I have verified. In the arrangement, I have followed that found in Dr. C. M. Boger's Synoptic Key.

Time.

Periodicity: China, 211; Natrum mur., 70; Chininum sulph., 216; Cedron.

Aggravation, morning: Podophyllum, 240; Sulphur, 5; Lachesis, 218; the Kalis.

Forenoon: Natrum mur., 70; Eupatorium perf., 307; Sulphur, 5; Cedron.

Afternoon: Lycopodium, 89; Gelsemium, 207; Belladonna, 14; Pulsatilla, 179.

Night: Mercurius, 131; Arsenicum, 198; Kali carb., 42; Rhus, 101; Nux vom., 115; Sulphur, 5.

Aggravations.

Agg., from air, weather change and before storm: Rhus tox., 101; Rhododendron, 296; Arsenicum, 198; Silica, 153; Calcarea carb., 60; Ranunculus bulb., 297; Nux m., 273.

Cold: Hepar, 111; Aconite; Nux vom., 115; Kali carb., 42; Calcarea carb., 60; Moschus, 279; Rhus tox., 101; Hepar, 111; Causticum, 56; Capsicum, 12; Silica, 153.

Drafts of air: Hepar, 111; Silica, 153; Rhus tox., 101; Capsicum, 12; Calcarea carb.; Nux vom., 115; Belladonna.

Dry air: Hepar; Aconite; Causticum, 56; Nux vom.; Spongia, 174.

Uncovering and undressing: Secale, 192; Chamomilla, 189; Drosera; Mercurius; Ledum; Sabina, 196; Nux vom., 115; Silica, 153; Sulphur, 5.

Hot weather: Podophyllum, 240; Iris, 248; Pulsatilla, 179; Bryonia, 106; Æthusa.

Heat of bed and wraps: Mercurius, 121; Chamomilla, 189; Ledum; Secale; Sulphur, 5; Dioscorea; Muriatic ac.

Amelioration.

Air, open: Pulsatilla, 179; Kali bich.; Arsenicum; Sabina, 196; Magnesia carb., 78; Iodium, 169; Fluoric ac.; Carbo veg., 299; Aurum, 135; Arsenicum alb., 198; Kali iod., 48; Alumina, 233; Argentum nit., 131.

Bending: Colocynth, 305; Magnesia phos., 85.

Aggravation.

Breathing: Bryonia, 106; Aconite, 1; Rhus tox., 101; Colchicum, 280; Terebinthina; Spigelia, 227; Ferrum phos., 352.

Climacteric, at: Lachesis, 218; Sepia, 186; Actea, 176; Sanguinaria, 261.

Coughing by: Bryonia, 107; Drosera; Ipecac, 251; Belladonna, 23.

Debauch, agg. after: Nux vom., 116; Carbo veg., 299; Opium; Stramonium, 24.

Dentition, agg. during: Chamomilla, 191; Calcarea phos., 65; Calcarea carb., 60; Scutellaria; Kreosote, 286; Staphisagria.

Discharge, agg. by excessive: China, 211; Aconite; Calcarea carb., 62; Phosphorus, 255; Veratrum alb., 326.

Discharges, amel. by: Lachesis, 218; Nux vom., 115; Sulphur, 11; Kali bich., 35; Pulsatilla, 183; Bryonia, 106; Graphites, 97; Sepia, 186; Cuprum, 138.

Eating, agg. before, i.e., empty stomach: Sulphur, 7; Calcarea carb., 64; Fluoric ac.; Iodium, 169; Phosphorus, 255; Natrum carb., 70; Staphisagria.

Eating, agg. while: Carbo veg., 300; Conium, 221; Nitric ac.; **Mercurius**, 125.

Eating, agg. after: Lycopodium, 89; Calcarea carb., 64; Bryonia, 108; Causticum; Kali carb., 44; Natrum mur., 72; Sepia, 187; Silica; Sulphur, 11; Nux vom., 116.

Eating, amel. by fasting: Chamomilla, 189; Natrum mur., 72.

Eating, amel. while: Anacardium; Ignatia, 270; Lachesis, 218; Zinc.; Capsicum, 13.

Eating, amel. after: Natrum carb., 70; Phosphorus, 256; Plumbum, 150; Sepia, 187; Iodium, 169; Chelidonium; Silica, 154; Arsenicum alb., 198.

Excitement, agg. by: Chamomilla, 190; Colocynth., 306; Ignatia, 269; Pulsatilla, 179; Phosphoric ac.; Staphisagria; Nux vom., 115; **Lachesis**, 218; Gelsemium, 209; Argentum nit., 131; Opium; Stramonium, 24.

Exertion, mental agg. by: Picric ac.; Phosphorus, 258; Nux vom., 117; Rhus tox., 101; Calcarea carb., 60; Sulphur, 5; **Cocculus**, 277.

Exertion, physical, agg. by: Arnica, 100; Rhus tox., 101; Bryonia, 106.

Eructations, agg. by: Chamomilla, 190.

Eructations, amel. by: Argentum nit., 131; Lycopodium, 90; **Pulsatilla**, 181; Carbo veg., 300.

Food and Drinks.

Agg. by beer: Nux vom., 115; Kali bich.

Agg. by bread: Bryonia, 107; Pulsatilla, 181; Nux vom., 116; Sulphur.

Agg. by butter: Pulsatilla, 179; Carbo veg., 300.

Agg. by cabbage: Lycopodium, 86; Bryonia, 106; Petroselinum.

Agg. by coffee: Nux vom., 115; Chamomilla, 190; Ignatia, 269; Causticum; Cantharis.

Agg. by cold: Arsenicum, 197; Nux vom., 115; Rhus tox., 101; Lycopodium; Belladonna, 16; Sepia, 185; Chamomilla, 189.

Agg. by condiments: Nux vom., 116.

Agg. by farinaceous: Natrum sul., 74; Lycopodium, 91.

Agg. by fats: Pulsatilla, 179; Cyclamen; Ferrum, 143; Carbo veg., 310; Graphites, 98.

Agg. by fruits: Veratrum alb., 327; Arsenicum alb., 199; Pulsatilla, 181; Bryonia, 107; China, 214.

Agg. by any liquids: Arsenicum, 197; Phosphorus, 255; Veratrum alb., 327; Cocculus, 278; Rhus tox., 101.

Agg. by milk: Æthusa; Antimonium crud.; Calcarea carb., 64; Nitric ac., Pulsatilla, 181.

Agg. by alcoholics: Nux vom., 116; Zinc., 160; Sulphur, 7; Arsenicum alb., 199; Opium.

Agg. by strawberries: Sepia, 187.

Agg. by meats: Argentum nit., 131; Ignatia, 269.

Agg. by tobacco: Spongia; Ignatia, 269; Arsenicum alb., 199; Staphisagria.

Amel. by coffee: Chamomilla, 190.

Amel. by cold: Bryonia, 107; Belladonna, 15; Apis, 316; Causticum, 58.

Amel. by water: Phosphorus, 256; Sepia, 187; Causticum, 58.

Amel. by tobacco: Tarantula; Arnica.

Agg. by light: Belladonna, 14; Euphrasia; Calcarea carb., 60; Sepia, 187; Rhus tox., 105; Arsenicum alb., 198; Argentum nit., 131; Nux vom., 117; Phosphorus, 259; Mercurius cor., 128; Silica, 154; Glonoine, 236; Graphites, 98; Lycopodium, 89; Stramonium, 24.

Agg. looking at bright objects: Stramonium, 24; Belladonna, 14.

Agg. straining eyes: Ruta; Natrum mur., 72; Nux vom., 117; Calcarea carb., 60; Lycopodium; Argentum nit., 131; Rhododendron, 297; Silica, 154.

Menses, agg. before: Calcarea carb., 62; Pulsatilla, 183; Sulphur, 5; Veratrum alb.; Cuprum, 138; Kali carb., 46; Lycopodium, 92; Lachesis, 218; Natrum, 71; Actearac, 1.

Menses, agg. during: Natrum mur., 71; Ammonium carb., 267; Chamomilla, 190; Graphites, 97; Hyoscyamus, 22; Actea, 178; Nux m., 119.

Menses, agg. after: Borax; Graphites, 97; Kreosote, 286; Nux vom., 119.

Mercury, agg. by: Hepar, 110; Nitric ac.; Staphisagria; Aurum, 135; Bryonia, 107.

Motion, agg. by: Bryonia, 106; Colchicum, 281; Arnica, 99; Belladonna, 14; Ledum; Stannum, 157; Natrum mur., 70; Ranunculus, 297; Chamomilla; Cocculus, 277; Zincum, 160; Phosphorus, 255.

Motion, amel. by: Rhus tox., 101; Pulsatilla, 179; Rhododendron, 296; Sambucus; Capsicum, 12; Arsenicum, 198; Aurum, 135; Zinc. val.; Sabina; Kali iod., 48.

Motion, agg. after: Arsenicum, 197; Sepia, 185; Rhus tox., 104; Stannum, 157; Cannabis ind., 335; Agaricus, 347; Pulsatilla, 179.

Motion, agg. at beginning of: Rhus tox., 101; Capsicum, 12; Conium, 221; Euphorbium; Ferrum, 142; Lycopodium, 89; Phosphorus, 255.

Motion, car or boat, agg. by: Cocculus, 277; Colchicum, 281; Petroleum, 291; Sepia, 185; Tabacum; Lachesis, 218.

Music, agg. by: Sepia, 185; Phosphoric ac.; Natrum carb., 69; Graphites.

Music, amel. by: Tarantula.

Noise, agg. by: Belladonna, 14; Aconite, 1; Coffea, 276; Nux vom., 115; Causticum, 56; Chamomilla, 189; China, 211; Sepia, 185; Silica, 153; Spigelia, 227; Bryonia; Arnica.

Odors, agg. by: Colchicum, 281; Nux vom., 115; Coffea, 276; Belladonna, 14; Aurum, 135; Phosphorus, 255.

Lying down, agg. by: Rhus tox., 101; Aurum, 135; Arsenicum, 197; Capsicum, 13; Chamomilla, 189; Conium, 221; Drosera; **Platinum**, 145; Pulsatilla, 179; Sambucus; Sanguinaria, 26; Lycopodium, 89; **Mercurius**, 121.

Lying, amel. by: Bryonia, 106; Nux vom., 115; Calcarea carb., 60; Natrum mur.; Colocynth., 305; Magnesia phos., 83; Pulsatilla, 179.

Rising up, agg. from: Bryonia, 106; Rhus tox., 101; Aconite, 1; Nux vom., 115; Veratrum alb., 326 Capsicum, 13; Spigelia.

Rising up, amel.: Arsenicum, 199; Sambucus.

Sitting, agg. from: Platinum, 145; Capsicum, 13; Conium, 221; Cyclamen; Dulcamara; Verbascum; Viola tri.; Sepia, 185.

Sitting, amel.: Bryonia, 106; Sepia, 185; Colchicum, 281.

Standing, agg.: Sepia, 185; Sulphur, 5; Conium, 221; Pulsatilla, 179.

Pressure, agg.: Iodium, 169; Hepar, 110; Apis, 316; Lycopodium, 89; Cina, 244; Agaricus, 347; Baryta carb.

Pressure, amel.: Colchicum, 281; Bryonia, 106; Argentum nit., 130; Gelsemium, 207; Conium, 221; Actea, 175; Lilium tig.; **Natrum carb.**; Magnesia mur.; Pulsatilla, 179; Lachesis, 218.

Scratching, agg.: Rhus tox., 102; Capsicum; Anacardium; **Pulsatilla**, 181; Lachesis, 218.

Sleep, agg. just before: Pulsatilla, 184; Phosphorus; Sepia, 185; Arsenicum, 199.

Sleep, agg. during: Lachesis, 218; Cina, 244; Opium; Stramonium, 24; Bryonia, 106 Belladonna, 17; Hepar.

Sleep, agg. after: Lachesis, 218; Sepia; Causticum; **Calcarea carb.**; **Lycopodium**, 90; Staphisagria; Stramonium, 24.

Sleep, agg. from loss of: Cocculus, 278; Phosphorus, 25; Cuprum; Zinc.

Swallowing, agg.: Belladonna, 19; Bryonia; Phytolacca, 294; **Mercurius**, 125; Stramonium, 25; Lachesis, 218; Hepar, 112; Ignatia, 27; Hyoscyamus, 23.

Sweat, agg. or no relief from: Mercurius, 121; China, 213; Chininum ars., 216; Rhus tox.; Opium; Stramonium; Sepia, 188.

Sweat, amel. from: Bryonia, 110; Chamomilla, 17; Rhus tox.; Graphites, 94; Gelsemium, 21.

Touch, agg.: Lachesis, 218; Hepar, 110; Nux vom., 115; Ledum; China, 213; Cocculus; Arnica, 99.

Vaccination, agg.: Thuja, 340; Variolinum, 312.

Vertigo, agg.: Gelsemium, 207; Nux vom., 117.

Washing, agg.: Sulphur, 5; Rhus tox., 101; Clematis, 334; Ammonium carb., 267; Calcarea carb., 60; Sepia, 185; Psorinum.

Washing, amel.: Fluoric ac.; Ledum; Pulsatilla, 179; Argentum nit., 131.

SENSATIONS.

Aching: Bryonia; Gelsemium; Eupatorium; Arnica; Phytolacca; Ignatia; Nux vom.; Lycopodium; Baptisia; Stannum; Aconite.

Asleep, feeling as if: Lachesis; Nux vom.; Cocculus; Rhus tox.; Sepia.

Beaten, bruised, sore: Arnica; China; Bryonia; Nux vom.; Carbo veg.; Hepar; Cocculus; Ignatia; Rhus tox.; Ruta; Rhododendron.

Boring: Plumbum; Spigelia; Sepia; Asafœtida.

Broken, as if: Eupatorium perf.; Baptisia; Ruta; Ignatia.

Burning: Arsenicum; Phosphorus; Sulphur; Aconite; Belladonna; Bryonia; Sanguinaria; Nitric ac.; Secale; Cantharis; Mercurius cor.; Causticum.

Bursting, splitting: Bryonia; Gelsemium; Argentum nit.; Belladonna; Glonoine; Ignatia; Nux vom.

Cramping, colic, etc.: Cuprum; Nux vom.; Colocynth.; Plumbum; Veratrum alb.; Cocculus; Silica; Magnesia phos.; Magnesia mur.; Cina; Platinum.

Cutting: Colocynth.; Cantharis; Zinc.; Belladonna; Nux vom.

Dryness: Aconite.

Empty: Sepia; Sulphur; Phosphorus; Stannum; Ignatia; Cocculus.

Enlarged and full: Gelsemium; Argentum nit.; Pulsatilla; Hydrastis; Glonoine.

Fainting and Unconscious: Aconite; Cocculus; Ignatia; Nux m.; Opium; Sepia; Digitalis; Natrum mur.; Gelsemium; Glonoine.

Fullness: Aconite; Belladonna; Gelsemium.

Gnawing: Agnus cast.; Staphisagria; Ranunculus bulb.; Mezereum; Causticum.

Gurgling: Gambogia; Aloe; Rheum; Croton tig.

Heavy: Nux vom.; Aloe; Lycopodium; Pulsatilla; Rhus tox.; Calcarea carb.; Gelsemium; Sepia; Mercurius.

Increasing and decreasing slowly: Stannum; Natrum mur.; Spigelia; Cactus; Platinum.

Irritable; sensitiveness: Nux vom.; Bryonia; Phosphorus; Hepar; Chamomilla; Coffea; China; Ignatia; Lachesis; Nitric ac.; Zinc.; Arsenicum; Asafœtida; Cantharis; Antimonium crud.

Itching: Sulphur; Graphites; Calcarea carb.; Cyclamen; Arsenicum iod.

Jerking: Belladonna; Nux vom.; Ignatia; Spigelia; Stannum; Cicuta; Causticum; Colchicum; Sepia.

Knot or lump: Nux vom.; Pulsatilla; Ignatia; Zinc.; Sepia; Nux m.; Moschus.

Labor-like pains: Actea rac.; Secale; Sepia; Chamomilla; Sabina; Plumbum; Platinum.

Numbness: Platinum; Opium; Verbascum; Aconite; Plumbum; Pulsatilla; Rhus tox.; Phosphorus; Conium; Gnaphalium; Kalmia.

Plug, nail: Aloe; Ignatia; Thuja; Anacardium; Hepar; Platinum.

Pressure, squeezed: Verbascum; Platinum; Zinc.; Colocynth; Magnesia phos.; Plumbum.

Pulsating: Belladonna; Silica; Sulphur; Glonoine; Lachesis; Aconite; Gelsemium; Ferrum; Natrum mur.

Rending, torn: Rhus; Coffea; Nux vom.

Restlessness: Arsenicum; Aconite; Tarantula; Mercurius; Staphisagria; Actea rac.; Hyoscyamus; Stramonium.

Rough, raw: Phosphorus; Alumina; Nux vom.; Phytolacca; Æsculus; Mercurius; Sulphur.

Shaking: Nux vom.; Veratrum alb.; Ignatia; Platinum; China; Camphor; Capsicum, 14.

Shooting: Aconite.

Splinter-like: Hepar; Mercurius; Nitric ac.; Muriatic ac.; Kali bich.; Lachesis.

Sprained: Arnica; Bryonia; Rhus; Natrum carb.; Ruta.

Stiffness: Rhus tox.; Colocynth.; Cina; Causticum; Sepia; Bryonia; Ignatia.

Stitching: Bryonia; Argentum nit.; Kali carb.; Spigelia; Aconite; Sepia; Asafœtida; Nitric ac.; Cantharis; Aconite.

Tearing: Bryonia; Rhododendron; Arnica; Belladonna; Zinc.; Mercurius; Pulsatilla; Kali carb.; China; Carbo veg.; Hepar.

Tension, stretched: Bryonia; Causticum; Colocynth.; Rhus tox.; Sulphur; Nux vom.; Baryta carb.

Throbbing: Belladonna; Bryonia; Aconite; Glonoine; Gelsemium; Sepia; Kali carb.; Cocculus; Ignatia; Natrum mur.

Tingling, Crawling: Aconite; Platinum; Secale; Arnica; Rhus tox.; Zinc. phos.

Trembling: Gelsemium; Argentum nit.; Arsenicum; Actea rac.; Hyoscyamus; Ignatia; Syzygium; Zinc.; Arsenicum; Kali ars.

Urging: Nux vom.; Argentum nit.; Sepia; Lycopodium; Sulphur; Pareira; Lilium tig.

Wavelike: Arsenicum; China; Carbo veg.; Phosphorus; Veratrum alb.; Baptisia; Muriatic ac.; Stannum iod.; Gelsemium; Antimonium tart.; Ammonium carb.

COUGH.

Abdominal: Drosera; Conium; Sepia; Phosphorus; Rumex; Bryonia; Veratrum alb.

Constant: Sticta; Causticum; Ignatia; Rumex.

Dry at night, loose by day: Pulsatilla; Calcarea carb.; Phosphoric ac.; Sambucus.

Loose, rattling cough: Antimonium tart.; Ammonium carb.; Antimonium ars.; Hepar; Chelidonium; Silica; Grindelia rob.; Veratrum alb.; Kali bich.

Nervous cough: Coffea; Ignatia; Platinum; Sticta; Agaricus; Actea; Lachesis; Corallium.

Cough with hemorrhages: Ipecac; Bryonia; Arnica; Phosphorus; Crotalus; Drosera; Belladonna.

Urinating with cough: Pulsatilla; Phosphorus; Causticum; Veratrum alb.